Neuroplasticity: Advances in Brain Science and Neurology

Neuroplasticity: Advances in Brain Science and Neurology

Edited by Hudson Webb

STATES
ACADEMIC PRESS
www.statesacademicpress.com

States Academic Press,
109 South 5th Street,
Brooklyn, NY 11249, USA

Visit us on the World Wide Web at:
www.statesacademicpress.com

ISBN: 978-1-63989-373-7

Cataloging-in-Publication Data

Neuroplasticity : advances in brain science and neurology / edited by Hudson Webb.
p. cm.
Includes bibliographical references and index.
ISBN 978-1-63989-373-7
1. Neuroplasticity. 2. Cognitive neuroscience. 3. Neurosciences. 4. Neurology. I. Webb, Hudson.
QP363.3 .N48 2022
612.82--dc23

Table of Contents

Preface

The capacity of the brain to adapt and change through experience is known as brain plasticity or neuroplasticity. It can be broadly categorized into two types, functional plasticity and structural plasticity. The ability of the brain through which it can transfer functions to an uninjured area from an injured area is known as functional plasticity. Structural plasticity is used to define the capacity of the brain to change its structure through the process of learning. Neuroplasticity allows the human brain to recover from traumatic injuries to the brain, improves the health and well-being of the brain, and enhances the present cognitive abilities of the brain. This book provides significant information of this discipline to help develop a good understanding of brain science and neurology. It unfolds the innovative aspects of neuroplasticity which will be crucial for the progress of this field in the future. The book is appropriate for students seeking detailed information in this area as well as for experts.

All of the data presented henceforth, was collaborated in the wake of recent advancements in the field. The aim of this book is to present the diversified developments from across the globe in a comprehensible manner. The opinions expressed in each chapter belong solely to the contributing authors. Their interpretations of the topics are the integral part of this book, which I have carefully compiled for a better understanding of the readers.

At the end, I would like to thank all those who dedicated their time and efforts for the successful completion of this book. I also wish to convey my gratitude towards my friends and family who supported me at every step.

Editor

1

Brain Dynamics and Plastic Deformation of Self Circuitries in the Dementia Patient

Denis Larrivee

Abstract

Despite improved medical care that has resulted in greatly extended life expectancies, significant increases in numbers of individuals suffering age related cognitive defects is expected, making the improved understanding of normal and pathological aging an important priority. Current studies indicating that brain activity requires a dynamical architecture to preserve functional order in the face of persistent and extraneous activity suggests that cognitive impairments are likely to be closely linked to dysfunctional dynamical activity of brain systems. Cognitive impairments such as those introduced by Alzheimer's dementia (AD), that affect fundamental operational constructs like the self, are thus likely to implicate global dynamics that oversee whole brain operation. This paper explores plastic events associated with dynamical elements used in the normal construction of the self percept and the etiology of their deconstruction in the course of AD. It is proposed that the evolution of the disease involves the increasing impairment of a global dynamical operation that is normally engaged in forming a stable and coherent self image needed to flexibly engage task related, motor plans and effectors.

Keywords: brain dynamics, Alzheimer's dementia, dynamic neural fields, attractors, self circuits, oscillations

1. Introduction: the dynamical self and Alzheimer's dementia

United Nations' estimates project that by 2050 20% of the world's population will be nearly 60 or more years of age, with considerably higher percentages in developed nations [1]. Despite improved medical care resulting in greatly extended life expectancies, significant increases in numbers of those suffering age related cognitive defects, including various dementias, is expected. This reality makes the improved understanding of normal and pathological aging an important priority. Among the most promising avenues to such understanding today are studies related to brain dynamical systems and globally operant phenomena, including self awareness and consciousness. Significantly, and unlike the activity of peripheral sensory and motoric neural processes, brain activity is ongoing and not intermittent, dynamically sustaining a wide variety of metastable and plastic states, including such perceptual phenomena as the self that are progressively impaired in dementias. Changes in brain dynamics, therefore, are clearly evoked during the evolution of these pathologies.

Although promising, brain dynamical studies have yet to find a role in studies of self representation and its loss with pathological progression. This is especially pertinent since there is the increasing realization that self circuitries underlie global phenomena that are key to individual performance. Accordingly, this chapter will consider three themes that are intended to illustrate how the loss of self representation is related to plastic changes in brain system dynamics. The first theme will build upon the traditional linkage that has been forged between brain activity and its modulation by neuroplastic events underlying its physiological expression, Donald Hebb's oft-quoted rule, what fires together wires together [2]. Expanding on this foundation it will explore how connectivity changes modulate the stability of energetically favored resonances, for example, attractors, that are naturally exploited as operational motifs of larger scale networks [3] and how these are used to build a three-dimensional self image. The second will evidence how the regulation of motif stability assists the generation of self representations, particularly during development as sensorial, somatotopic input progressively shapes the brain, creating the self percept for mature interactivity with the world. The third will contextualize pathological distortions as loss of function etiologies that can be modeled by a change of system dynamics, evidenced in the loss of function of global dynamical systems underlying construction of the self image.

The outcome of this exploration will be the creation of a portrait of brain dynamics that both reciprocally and iteratively relates brain dynamics to the evolution of self representation in dementias. It will assist in clarifying the relationships between neuroplastic mechanisms of connectivity, their modulation of brain dynamical elements that create spatial representations of the embodied self, and distortions in regulating this representation as dementias increasingly impact global operation.

2. The self and its method of representation

Conceptions of the self adopt understandings that may be colloquial or intuited, philosophical or definitional, subjective or objective, functionalist or ontological, self contained or overlapping [4]. Cumulatively, these varied understandings provide a sense of what is generally meant by the self, yet the distributed nature of the definitions that contribute to its understanding mean that the conceptions that are intended to define the self can only approximately service the notion. Nevertheless, the self is a real construct, universally appealed to by professional and public alike. John Locke provided a definition more than 300 years ago that is still widely adhered to, and often regarded as definitional for personal identity

> *'the awareness of being the same person in different places and different times'.*

This self percept is usually taken in its subjective sense, yet the elements that contribute to the percept are objective features closely related to the neural architecture that underlies its subjective expression.

The present chapter will adopt a perspective of the self that is dynamical and interactivist, that is, an operational perspective of how the individual autonomously engages the exterior world [5, 6]. It will consider the self's role in initiating and structuring the actions that the individual carries out as it negociates a variable environment, that is, its interactive dimension, that will be termed here the performative self. There are several reasons for adopting this conception, that, while not covering the rich depth of understanding that is associated with the concept of the self [4, 6], are yet likely to be both valid and useful in the context of its contribution to understanding the etiology and evolution of dementias. First, it offers a tractable construct that possesses conceptual clarity vis-à-vis its behavioral and neural expression. The self is here understood to be that individual representation that acts to secure the vital dimensions needed for viability. Second, the neural and biological foundation of this conception of the self is increasingly well understood and likely to shed light on events that are abnormal, such as cognitive diseases like Alzheimer's dementia (AD). Current evidence, for example, indicates that the self is associated with the whole of the individual, that is, it is a totality whose origin and association is linked to the entire corpus, and not restricted to an isolated domain of representation lying within the brain [7], one that is the product of the progressive integration of regionally distributed, somatotopic afferent input. Significantly, this perceptual image appears to be invested with protagonist features and to assist in the construction of an intentional image used for counterfactual affordances [8]; in other words, this 3-D body image of the self enables the individual to 'situate and to conceive of himself' in different goal-directed planning trajectories.

There is good evidence to suggest, moreover, that the body image is the neural product of dynamical systems mechanisms that serve as its operational basis. Among other findings, for example, limb positions for navigation are topologically mapped [9] as are the external trajectories navigated, where they are linked to environmental cues later recalled to guide movement in association with exploration. The neurophysiological basis of such memories appears to involve dynamical systems processes that encapsulate the memories in energetically stable activity zones, such as Hopfield attractors [10]. Taken together, the performative self appears to be a construct that represents the whole individual bodily, engages dynamical neural processes, and is needed for unitary, goal-directed activity.

This performative model thus affords a physically defined and physiologically relevant neural terrain encompassing global brain and body operation that can be explored in terms of an ongoing etiological progression. In the next sections, I will consider underlying mechanisms of normal plastic changes involving dynamical system operation related to the self and then subsequently consider how these are likely to be affected by the progression of the disease.

2.1. Neuroplastic mechanisms in dynamical systems representations

The operational perspective of the self adopted here is situated by the need to sustain a continuous stream of neural activity. Constituted as a goal directed and autonomous entity the individual must possess a neural architecture whose operation, necessarily, remains persistently active in order to enable self directed action and maintain homeostatic autonomy. This requirement for independent and autonomous existence has clear implications for the form adopted by the neural architecture both anatomically and physiologically, a form that needs to be robustly maintained in the face of variable input activity while yet enabling behaviorally relevant responses.

Studies of brain operation are beginning to reveal how these requirements are met. Physically, they begin with the anatomical structure of the nervous system that in the brain exhibits an exceptionally high degree of recurrency. For example, nearly 95% of all brain neurons receive some level of feedback via nerve collaterals [11]. This organization creates neural topologies in which information flow cycles through preferred, low resistance pathways creating zones of stabilized activity, that is, basins of attraction to which the flow converges. What is significant about this observation is that it reveals that the brain's configuration is necessarily oriented to creating a dynamical setting where activity is used to create a functional order that resists the ravages of entropic deconstruction and is operationally reliable, that is, it can be described by mathematically ordered relations.

Constitutively, stability is the critical feature of dynamical system operation [12]. Stabilized activity is needed due to the susceptibility of information flow to external, that is, sensorial and internal, perturbing influences that are an ongoing and intrinsic aspect of brain operation. Such perturbing influences can only be circumvented by the creation of stabilized activity zones that foreclose interference to extraneous information flow that can and usually does originate in such sources. Because organisms are embodied their sensory, motor, and cognitive operations are continuously engaged in monitoring, interpreting, and responding to varied informational sources.

Stability is conferred in multiple ways that in addition to recurrency of information flow include appropriately adjusted connectivity strengths, leakage currents, glial barriers, and the like. The cumulative effect is the creation of energetically stabilized zones within an overall energy landscape that entrains and structures information flow, that have been termed attractors because of the convergence of flow to particular paths lying, appropriately, within basins of attraction. Thus, its characteristic feature is a zonal resistance to change that acts as a buffer to spurious sources of variable neural activity.

Dynamical system operation is characterized, additionally, not only by robustness and stability, but also by flexibility and the capacity for directed control. Thus, three features are incorporated into brain operation in the context of and need for accommodating ongoing brain activity that is required for sustaining interactive autonomy. Because brain activity determines motoric output energetic levels of information flow within stable zones must also remain sufficiently close to zonal instabilities in order to permit its exit from particular attractors and subsequent entry into alternative ones. This capacity for egress constitutes a principal means for achieving variable motor responsivity, a functional feature that also means that the particular form of behavioral output selected is directly related to the set of activity zones chosen. Physically, instabilities are forces of convergence that are relatively weaker in particular regions of the attractor. It becomes possible at such locations, accordingly, to induce transitions out of the stabilized zone, which therefore constitute bifurcations leading to new energy profiles [13]. Such transitions are characteristically abrupt, for example, like those observed in the hippocampus [14], and so represent a wholly new and nonlinear trajectory to a different energy locus. This sort of dynamical patterning suggests that functionally significant, motor output is characterized by its dependence on the assembly of discrete energy sets, rather than the deconstruction and reconstruction of parts of the dynamical elements themselves.

It is in the context of such selection that the role of the self is pertinent. A capacity for flexible responsivity means that there must also exists a reproducible and reliable manner of selecting particular sets of stabilized zones in order to yield a certain type or class of motor response. This capacity, further, must operate within the context of the demands of the whole individual, that is, it must benefit the individual as a whole, hence, the requirement for a performative self, that is, a representation that can guide goal-directed actions. Increasingly, neuroscientific evidence is revealing that this dynamic construct is systemically ordered, that is, it is globally distributed and operative [15], though more focally concentrated in regions, such as the Default Mode Network (DMN) [16], a feature that may be analogized by the DNA of eukaryotic cells. This global system, moreover, very likely operates by engaging select dynamical elements, which appears to be the basis of motor responsivity [17].

Importantly, since the neural substrate for the self is itself subject to the same operational constraint for persistent activity its operational configuration must also employ dynamical system operation. Overall, a critical operational dimension of the self that flows from this structure is that dynamical activity is constructed by a layered ordering of properties that while fundamentally dependent on underlying structural elements are nevertheless operationally independent from them. For example, while the brain uses spiking mechanisms to create information flow, that is, mechanisms described by Hodgkin Huxley action potential formulations, as do peripheral nerves, these constitute lower level operative features, whereas higher level dynamical systems like attractors and their assemblies constitute, in reality, the fundamental functional elements through which the brain conducts its operations [18].

2.2. Organizational mechanisms of the dynamical self percept

The use of dynamical stability to negociate biologically relevant outcomes, via the percept of the performative self, thus introduces the question of how the percept is structured and persists over time while yet remaining sensitive to ongoing input that may either facilitate its maintenance or induce an evolution in core features. A portion of the answer to this question can be gleaned from the distinctions between mechanisms used to create information flow, like the spiking mechanisms just mentioned, and those that employ these mechanisms to create distinctively new functional elements, like attractors. This is to say that the dynamical construction of this percept is a consequence of the nervous system's ability to construct a layered and dynamical order, with the progressive appearance of functionally significant new features at progressively higher levels. Thus, a fuller answer to this question is situated by the multiple layering of dynamical elements, and so relates to the question of the plasticity of the changes that transpire at various levels. Existing evidence indicates that these changes are likely to be multiple and to include specifically effects on connectivity modulation [11], dynamical motifs [19], higher order clustering [20], and/or symbolical representations [21].

Modulation of connectivity that transpires in recurrent networks constitutes a ground level for plastic changes that affect dynamical systems like attractors. Connectivity changes can influence signal transmission by controlling overall resistance to transmission among multiple synaptic contacts, for example. Underlying mechanisms mediating such changes via Hebbian or other processes, that is, synaptic activity dependent strengthening [2], can include molecular effects involving protein kinase modulation related to synaptic vesicle release, enhanced pre- or post-synaptic membrane conductances, increased synaptic size, and the like which modify information flow [22]. Significantly, connectivity weight changes can undergo dynamical variation with learning, habituation, or development, that is, weight changes that are mathematically described differentially by rates of change that assume different and variable time scales and which thus modulate the temporal evolution of higher order properties. For example, the time evolution of activation in a linear feed forward network described by $\Delta a_i = \lambda(net_i - a_j)$, where $net_i = \Sigma_i w_s a_s$ and w_{is} is the weight of a connection from neuron i to neuron s, creates a cascading effect of system dynamics over time [3]. Controlling connectivity changes over time, in fact, is a basic mechanism for introducing experiential effects into dynamical systems.

Such effects on higher properties are significant, moreover, for also revealing the existence of dependencies of dynamical processes on underlying network mechanics that sustain them, but which, nonetheless remain operationally and functionally independent of the connectivity arrangements themselves. This is seen, for example, in the Usher-McClelland model [3] for classification responses that are constructed from a single set of hidden neuron units receiving equal input with feedback excitation only to the units themselves while inhibitory to all other units. The significant feature of this relatively simple connectivity model is that the output of the network asymptotically approaches a steady state level as input levels to the hidden layer continue to rise over time. That is, while the output of this network depends on the existence of incoming spiking activity, it is only slightly and indirectly related to the magnitude of the activity entering the network at the onset and becomes altogether independent of its magnitude over time. Importantly, connectivity patterns are widely variable and of great complexity, not only between species, but in the structure of the human brain [23]. Thus they offer an extraordinary repertoire for introducing dynamical variation. Changes in ground state connectivity can lead, for example, to changes in the performance of given dynamical elements, or lead to the formation of new dynamical elements altogether.

The layering of properties, seen in the transition from the level of spiking activity to that of dynamical elements like attractors, is manifest at yet higher levels where dynamical units may combine to yield qualitatively and quantitatively differing sets of such elements. Shoner shows, for example, how an attractor and a divergent element like a repellor can combine to yield an entirely new attractor state [12]. Like the contributing elements, the assembled combinations are themselves robust to interference, as, for example, in the case of heteroclinic channels that are constructed from a series of attractors joined in sequence that effect unique trajectories through the dynamical state space [24]. Such combinations are potentially used for phoneme construction, a behavioral output that can be accommodated by effecting sequences within sequences through the creation of supraordinate heteroclinic activity at higher levels, that is, a hierarchically layered operational order that is functionally pertinent.

The significance of this layering, further, goes beyond the generation of robust patterns to their manner of combination and how their assembly is regulated since the former dictates what cognitive or motor effector is actuated and the latter how this actuation is subject to control. Because dynamical systems are persistent structures, due to their basins of attraction, the individual energetic profiles they assume cannot be randomly disassembled and then recombined but instead must be joined together in combinations of units which retain their individual profiles, that is, operative motifs, within the larger assembly. What this implies is that there are preferred ways in which these motifs can be joined to achieve functionally significant groupings. Evidence for functionally significant examples of this higher order association has been demonstrated in neural networks that control mouth motion 'chewing' in the roundworm *Caenorhabditis elegans*. Network clustering analyses show that the behavioral networks used for chewing are organized operationally into higher order clustering patterns that are made from combinations of lower level network motifs [20] which appear to be coordinated by primitive synchronizing mechanisms [25].

Such combinatorial products also enable the possibility for multiscaling, that is, combinatorial groupings that repeat at higher levels, and by so doing avail the possibility for accessing an extended operational repetoire of the sort suitable to symbolic representations. Cooperative behaviors like those of clustered networks can thus be exploited to greatly extend the range of representations that can be discriminated. Building on the work of Rodriguez [26], for example, that showed that simple recurrent networks could generalize from syntactical constructs with relatively few combinations of dynamical elements—in most cases an attractor and repellor sufficed—Tabor proposed that dynamical system elements could mediate between connectionist network structures and symbolical representations [21] by evolving combinatorial possibilities that could be scaled upwards by repeating lower level organizational combinations. Such scaling, significantly, means that these possibilities mathematically adopt fractal type organized patterns, which is to say that the self organized processes also found in physical structures like snowflakes, or protein molecules, retain their functional significance at increasingly hierarchical scales.

2.3. Constructing the self percept from dynamical elements

In keeping with much evidence the body is intrinsically involved together with the brain in establishing the performative self [7]. The layering of dynamical elements described above, accordingly, is framed by the dynamic between the two that involves the reciprocal and mutually dependent flow of information effected between brain regions such as the hippocampus and the distributed sensory and motor neural network that lies beyond the brain. This relationship is necessarily constrained by the dynamical nature of brain activity, which is continuous, and the need for stability, which remains the cornerstone of dynamical operation.

While it is clear that stability is needed for basic dynamical elements like attractors, it is not immediately clear why this should be required for global brain operation such as the self whose physiological basis seems to be underpinned by constraints beyond that of the buffering of spurious noise signals. Yet existing evidence indicates that stability and coherence are fundamental at this level as well. Hence, built into the dynamical layering is a predisposition to create coherent structures that can carry out the grander tasks of the neural architecture. Interestingly, this evidence has come from studies that explore the lack of certain cognitive capacities rather than their presence, such as the demonstration of perseveration in infants [27]. In the case of infant perseveration, that is, infant behavior when presented with an 'A not B' task, cognitive processing of the body's disposition in space is needed to relate the individual to the events of the world. This is to say that the whole body is needed to create a stable and coherent image that can be interactively and cognitively positioned in motor planning to create affordances enabling motor planning. Indeed, identity and self awareness are both linked to this embodied dimension [6, 7, 28]. For example, intentional acts in developing infants to either stand upright or to crawl, effect a differential brain mapping depending on the performative act intended, such as the acquisition of bimanual skills with the correspondent coupling of sensori-motor areas [28]. This observation reveals that task performance is related to the linkage made between the goal and the individual for whom the goal is intended, which is to say that intentional performance requires a stable representation of the individual that can be cognitively or physically mobilized as a whole.

Corbetta's [28] experiment is revealing in siting this representation to the performative dimension; that is, the representation of the self is set within the context of motor plans and is effected by sensorial, largely somatotopic, input. There appears, therefore, to be a constitutive requirement for a holistic and bodily contextualized, self representation for performance that can be employed in a wide variety of interactive and dynamic circumstances. This implies that mapping between levels must cohere, and can only do so to the extent that the dynamical elements themselves cohere and cooperatively engage to yield its global outcome. Due to the wide variety of interactive circumstances it also means that it must relate to the dynamical elements involved in effecting various acts at multiple levels that can then be reorganized according to the exigencies of interactive demands. Finally, it invokes the need for regulatory processes that are evoked by the self to accommodate the variability encountered in motor planning, that is, the regulation of the disassembly/reassembly processes that are mobilized to accommodate such possibilities.

The coherent self image is the basis on which the twin needs for stability and flexibility are satisfied and is used to dynamically frame individual motor acts in relation to the global self representation. In this way they can be understood as belonging to the self. It is in this context that Smith's [27] sensori-motor object can be understood, and also the way in which the infant perseveration studies are interpreted. In other words, the performative self arises from the need to frame the individual holistically for its interactive role, a framework that arises from somatotopic afferent input of the body schema and constituted by the three-dimensional body image [7].

Significantly, the body position undergoes its own temporal evolution that then becomes critical to the successful negociation of motor plans. This situates the juxtaposition of the whole against the elements of the body in a continually mobile frame where successive movements are always referenced to an immediately preceding spatiotemporal location, that is, at each dynamic moment there is a contrast between the spatiotemporal configuration of that which just was and the correspondingly new position of the here and now [27]. Thus, the sensorium is always placed in the role of needing to monitor the whole body, and so also of continually contextualizing the motor planning that may transpire. Decisional acts, additionally, that are associated with motor planning, must also participate in structuring motor plans in order to generate goal-directed activity.

This is also to imply that the sense of self in a minimal sense is a *persistent* process that provides the stable ground for decisional performance. That is, we consciously select among a range of potential acts suited to achieving a particular interactive goal [8] that must be understood to be the consequence of self made motions, in order to distinguish them from a sea of surrounding and non-cohering imagery. Here the infant perseveration results are again useful for understanding the need for a coherent image that can be directed to perform various motions. Consistent with this, Frith first proposed that the sense of agency was related to a comparison mediated correspondence between self made motions and selected motor plans [29], a genre of predictive processing models [6], thereby introducing the motor planning stage as the needed dimension for generating the sense of agency. In his Comparator Model a motor command termed corollary discharge is sent to the sensory cortex in advance of the execution of motor movement so that the sensorial observation of the expected movements can enable the distinction between movements of the individual and those of the surround. However, for the motor movements to be situated as an operation that is part of a whole means that the sensorial imagery of the body must also identify the motions as flexible ones against the stability and coherency of the self image. This makes it likely, and as the perseveration experiments seem to show, that there must be a sustained awareness of the self, with its corresponding need for persistent sensory input, from which such actions begin, depart, and end. Together, the performative self, motor planning, and decisional acts appear to share intimate relations that are mediated by the dynamical processes of the neural architecture, as Varela, Thompson, and Rosch earlier intuited [30].

2.4. Self mechanisms that effect operational order

How these dimensions overlap is thus crucial to a biological understanding of how the self percept is mediated performatively over time. Evidence indicating how these events occur implicates the sensorial control of dynamical elements, which are selectively appropriated for motor planning. Matching of sensorial input with special classes of attractors termed dynamic neural fields (DNFs) appears to underpin the unique structuring of motor element planning and execution [31]. DNFs, notably, are bistable or multistable attractor neural networks, that is, they are dynamical elements capable of being shifted into an activation mode by transitioning from lower attractor states to higher ones. Incoming sensoria generate peaks of activation that leverage the instabilities in the base states of these fields to induce transitions to the upper level ones [32]. Since motor plans must ultimately be transformed into effector actions it is likely that the upper states are also responsible for engaging the effectors and that sensorial input provides modal specific stimuli to insure the plan's performance by activating the transition from lower to higher level attractor states. Against this backdrop, and so providing overall coherence for the performative self, lie the lower attractor states that appear to act as the landscape for the three D body image, which contextualizes the respective effector events.

Understood systemically, global supervision implies that the whole of brain dynamical activity is accessible for a distributed oversight, which by extension means also that a smaller suite of behavioral repertoires are evoked for motor planning and motor activation. This oversight appears to involve the regulation of localized assemblies that are continually monitored by the global/self percept [15, 17]. The subordination of dynamical elements comprised of multiple neuronal units, in fact, is not unique to humans. *C. elegans* also exhibits a globally evoked dynamical operation in the form of coordinated sleep behaviors. Underlying this ability in humans and a number of other mammalian species, is a capacity for synchronizing activation of smaller subsets of dynamical elements, apparently regulated by a globally distributed oscillatory activity [33].

Governing how these assemblies become responsive, and thus regulating how dynamical units assemble into larger functional aggregates, are the relative free energy differences between units that regulate their assembly into the larger wholes along a descending free energy gradient [34]. In other words, higher order brain activity is organized naturally through energetic constraints that govern pattern assembly, an organizational strategy that is commonly used in biological systems in numerous other contexts. Such organized assemblies characterize numerous macromolecular events such as those of enzymatic catalysis. The combination of lower order monomers into combined polymer patterns yield novel cooperative effects that enhance function beyond a strict linear relation to the monomer alone, that is one greater than the sum of the parts. For example, cooperativity effects exhibited in hemoglobin multimers enhance oxygen binding to hemoglobin over and above a strict linear dependence on hemoglobin concentration, a feature critical to physiological performance.

Indeed, it is within the context of free energy efficiency that the selection of assemblies can be framed, that is, as a general principle determining brain responsivity. To permit information flow to exit attractor motifs, basins of attraction in attractors must be sufficiently shallow to overcome energy barriers dividing stabilized zones. This means that a key feature in creating and modifying assemblies is that of the intrinsic instabilities within the attractor space that can be accessed for egress. As with patterned assemblies that can form higher organizational layering, instabilities can form constituent features of stabilized zones at multiple levels that include motifs only, or higher levels that may be made of multiply clustered motifs including, for example, the exit from single attractor motifs that may occur at an instability creating a bifurcation, or in complex fields that may be composed of multiple single attractor states, such as, for example, dynamic neural fields, where field instabilities can be leveraged to generate a uniquely different field feature with a new output [12].

3. Modulating dynamical element stabilities across time scales: constructing the self percept during development

Inferences about neuroplastic changes to the self percept during dementias concern a construct that has itself been structured according to a pattern of organizational processes that together generate its mature form. Developmental events leading to the construct's mature expression can therefore be expected to inform not only mechanisms underlying its orderly developmental assembly, but also how it is deconstructed in etiologies whose progression may be variable and irregular. Driving the developmental events and constitutive of their mature expression are again the twin needs of operational stability and flexibility that are the hallmarks of the dynamical systems used in complex neural operation. How are these needs met in development?

The phenomenologist Merleau Ponty [35] was among the first to suggest that repetitive interaction between the body and environment structured a habitual, posturally determined perception of the world. This observation is germane for suggesting several features of the performative self that are needed for its generation. First, it underscores the importance of the body as a stable reference point for interaction; thus, a fundamental goal of the developmental process is the achievement of this functional objective. Second, it is from the perspective of the body that the self engages the world; hence, it is necessary to also situate the body in spatiotemporal terms to understand how this engagement occurs. As suggested by Merleau Ponty this is a process likely to develop only through interactions requiring significant repetition, of the sort that has been identified in Hebbian-like mechanisms of synaptic activity induced strengthening.

Evidence for the creation of this 'stable' and coherent self image indicates that it is mediated by afferent input from various modalities of the body that is qualitatively greatest in development, but nevertheless also achieved experientially throughout the life of the individual. For example, neuroscientific studies of monocular deprivation in kittens show that ocular dominance columns fail to form when deprivation occurs during a critical phase of synaptic organization during development [36]. In effect the kittens become permanently blinded because of the absence of cortical network structures that would otherwise have been properly ordered by light stimulation during this critical phase. Similarly, experience also shapes neural order, as demonstrated in adult rats where navigational forays establish topographical map relating the spatial environment to bodily structure, a posturally determined aspect essential for planning future maneuvers [8, 9].

A significant aspect of such mapping is its reliance on dynamical systems mechanisms to create stable processes that persist and can be used over time. The Traves and Rolls memory model, for example, relies on the use of attractors to encapsulate mapped memories for such planning [10]. By means of such repeated, environmentally interactive events the neural architecture is developmentally shaped [37] into the global dynamical organization of the self.

3.1. Neuroplastic shaping of the self image through reciprocal brain body exchange

As Merleau-Ponty observed, interaction of the body with the environment is, in fact, the fundamental feature shaping the self percept during development, up to and within the boundaries of the genetic envelope [38], meaning that the synaptic architecture of the brain is not wholly prespecified in the genetic code but is, rather, a product of development, learning and experience, a premise invoked in the epigenetic model of development. Sensory reception, in particular, extends the point of perception to its bodily mooring and is the key determinant in shaping the dynamical operation of the brain. By modulating information content both quantitatively and qualitatively, the body shapes the brain's perception of the world. The choice of sensory modality and the degree to which it ultimately activates brain neural fields is thus immediately influenced by the positioning of the body as it moves through the world [39]. For example, somatotopic zones that experience frequent contact are abundantly innervated, which seems to indicate that the body regulates the information delivered to the brain according to the degree of interaction that the body experiences; in other words, the body shapes the brain's perception according to the demands imposed upon it.

It is, in fact, by building upon the body's molding of the brain's perception through the reciprocal and perceptual dynamics of body brain neural exchange, that the unitary and performative dynamic of the self is generated, and wherein the individual is both perceived and actively engaged with the world [30]. Varela, Thompson, and Rosch propose, accordingly, a fundamental unity between perception and action

> *"By using the term action we mean to emphasize once again that sensory and motor processes, perception, and action, are fundamentally inseparable in the lived condition"*

which emphasizes the body's initiation of the brain's subsequent and reciprocal response, that is, a perception action loop that relates the perception of the individual to his actions. Esther Thelen proposes that the circuits participating in this cycle emerge from the activities that the loop generates [40]. Supporting these conclusions, the perceptual influence of body on brain has been demonstrated in studies on the perceptual and dynamical interaction with the environment in developing infants [41], acquired habitual motor abilities [42], biodynamic studies showing that movement and proprioception are intrinsically related to perception [43] and appears to relate to the need to construct a unitary construal of the body that can be used for action planning [8, 27].

Critical to the creation of this construct is the ability to relate the whole of ourselves to its performative role; thus, our holistic bodily perception is fundamental to the understanding of ourselves in an interactive context with the world, a developmental transition for this acquired ability that appears to take place around age three to four [8]. Existing evidence strongly suggests that before this time the self percept has not been sufficiently ordered to enable its use to guide the individual. This absence and the behavioral consequences that ensue nonetheless reveal its fundamental necessity to performance.

The objective of such development involves, necessarily, the recognition that we occupy a unique spatiotemporal location, that is, our recognition that we are the same individual in different places and at different times, as John Locke expressed. This holistic perception is achieved through a progressively entangled and dynamic framework that represents, as it were, a prototype and platform of peripherally initiated and increasingly complex integration of inwardly and outwardly directed exchange. Each interactive experience is recorded as a dynamic incident mapped to its respective body locus that yields a temporally successive series of individually contextualized events [7]. Building on this prototypical perceptual platform the performative and neural self construction extends inward and outward to its various peripheral sightings to assimilate this common representation, that is, a physical entity of which the representation is indicative. The performative self thus constitutes an ontological feature needed to confer individual unity that is employed not only performatively, but also for social and homeostatic viability [44].

3.2. Modulating performance elements during development

Key to autonomous behavior, further, is the ability to initiate and respond to environmental variation, meaning that the neural and bodily architecture must be made subject to suitable control. Thus, while the stable self percept forms the ground from which this performative dimension can emerge, action initiation must itself be open to a wide range of responses that are recognized as one's own; hence, another objective of the developmental process is the conferal of the ability to flexibly and selectively engage dynamical elements that can be accessed for a variety of neural trajectories.

Functionally meaningful events thus require that the selection and coordination of dynamical motor processes be amenable to self recruitment and capable of being disengaged when the motor plan has been executed. Importantly, functional behaviors must be reproducible, meaning that the coordinating network be sufficiently determinate that it can reliably account for metastable, multistable, and multifunctional patterns. Current work indicates that global brain networks, such as those likely to belong to the performative self, engage and disengage dynamically [15], that is, they are fundamentally required to be dynamical solutions. This sort of relation implies an operational configuration in which a global brain state entrains a localized network through the leveraging of local instabilities of the sort that have been described in large scale models of global dynamic density control [45] that are robust with persistent levels of activation that can assure delocalized and regionally distributed engagement [15]. However, it leaves open the question of the manner of eliciting local networks that govern various motor activities and of identifying them.

Developmental studies that implicate the need to evoke a coherent self image [27] as an a priori dimension of motor planning suggest that this elicitation of localized attractor assemblies occurs in relation to a sustained global brain state, against which they are framed; that is, they are recognized as constitutive actions emanating from the self. Critically, the activation of localized units in their mature stage must process through a stable trajectory, that is, there must be stable information flow that effects the motor plan. The origin of such information flow, however, cannot be wholly predetermined, but instead, as Merleau Ponty has observed and as can be seen from developmental sensory deprivation studies, is shaped by experience through empirically assessed corrective input to the flow path. The developmental process, accordingly, assembles the envelope within which the basic dynamical elements are structured through an initial activity dependent ordering, which is then later experientially refined via sequential, parallel, and hierarchically clustered patterns of activity strengthening. Accordingly, this developmental ordering suggests that the principle mechanism for evoking motor elements is through their developmentally defined, experientially sharpened, and regionally distributed, dynamical fields [31].

4. Alzheimer's dementia: the progressive loss of dynamical, global self systems

Although the etiological basis for AD has been studied from many different perspectives no single theory yet encompasses its neurological origin nor, correspondingly, have the many therapeutic proposals resulting from these studies yet yielded tangible benefits. Studies of the impact of the disease on dynamical system elements, on the other hand, have yet to be included in the exploratory spectrum, a reflection of the field's emphasis on theoretical issues concerning the relation of its theoretical models to the physical structure that is the object of the disease. Increasingly, however, not only are dynamical elements considered to be fundamental features of brain operation but their role in global operation are specifically targeted by the disease. This is also to say that their exploration is likely to prove fruitful to the understanding of the cognitive dimension that is specifically impacted by the disease and that constitutes its hallmark. This chapter builds on these observations to propose that the global dynamical operation targeted by the disease is constituted by a construct subsumed within the percept of the self.

The evidence for the specific effect on the dynamical systems that underlie the self is three fold and is framed against the backdrop of the studies just mentioned that demonstrate the basic need to dynamically structure a coherent and stable self image that can make and execute motor plans for interacting with events in the world beyond the self: first, Alzheimer's specifically affects a major brain network closely implicated with the self, the Default Mode Network (DMN); second, there is a specific loss in the ability to maintain functional integration over distributed regional zones that are likely to be subordinated to self performance; and third, parametric indices of dynamical metastability, an index relating global dynamics to coordinative oversight, is significantly altered in AD patients.

We begin with the evidence linking the DMN to the self percept [46]. The DMN was first identified by nuclear imaging studies that showed that this region displayed consistently higher levels of activity during passive task conditions. This led to the hypothesis of its role in monitoring the external environment, body, and even emotion [47]. Additionally, the DMN activity is generally and persistently elevated relative to a number of other areas of the brain, a feature needed for guiding global activity. Task related increases in activity in other zones, moreover, coincide with a relative decrease in DMN activity suggesting a reciprocal relation between the two that is related to the performative context of the task [17]. It is likely therefore that the dynamical ground state of the DMN situates the self image in the context of effecting motor plans and tasks in order to contextualize them as ones own. Consistent with this interpretation its high metastability index reflects a sustained exploratory state where the self image can be accessed for task execution. In other words, the DMN appears to function as the center of a global and distributed network system [16] that assimilates the body image as a coherent and stable self reference that is persistently ready to engage the environment [27].

Secondly, and strikingly, fMRI observed activity patterns in the DMN substantially change during the progression of Alzheimer's. Posterior cingulate and right inferior temporal cortical activities, for example, decline whereas the activity of the bilateral inferior parietal cortex increases [48]. What is significant about these zones is that they form central connectivity hubs within the DMN that exhibit causally influential connections. Thus changes in connectivity strength between these zones appear to reflect a weakening of causally influential, functionally significant, relations between the principal nuclei of the DMN, with a corresponding and decreasing ability to sustain the self percept.

Physiologically, the impact of altered connectivity appears to relate to global dynamical activity that can be observed in altered oscillatory patterns of the electroencephalogram (EEG) [49] in the AD patient. Source based EEG maps, for example, exhibit Alzheimer specific modulation, with changes in cortical spectral power that are related to attenuated alpha and beta and increased theta and delta in the posterior cingulate cortex and intraparietal cortex. Global oscillatory profiles, notably, are invoked as mechanisms for conferring inter areal coupling between brain regions that enables synchronization of activity; that is, brain oscillations are a major means by which the brain coordinates activity across extended spatial distances. The use of globally distributed voltage waveforms as a synchronization mechanism affords the brain the capacity to regulate and control activation by the entrainment of dynamical systems such as dynamical neural fields that are, accordingly, made subordinate to the global self construct [15]. The reduction in connectivity observed in Alzheimer's and the corresponding loss of oscillatory control, seems to imply, therefore, that Alzheimer's incurs a loss of the ability to entrain localized dynamical elements that are subordinate to the action of the self percept. Consistent with this interpretation, regional coherence significantly declines for the posterior cingulate cortex (PCC) relative to the precuneus, with increasingly greater decoherence as the disease progresses [50].

Third, metastability parameters appear to exhibit performative time scales physiologically consistent with normal brain activity in the context of motor responsivity to environmental demands. Measurements of metastability are currently revealing that the disease progression significantly lowers this index [51]. Revealingly, access to the exploratory repertoire of the DMN is counterbalanced in normal cognition by the frontoparietal network which lowers metastability and synchronizes activity [17]. Together, these observations are likely to mean that AD etiological and symptomatic features relate to a loss of global dynamical mechanisms for self representation used to entrain localized, motor planning, dynamical fields.

5. Conclusion

Though later years of life are often portrayed as a time of self realization, it is also the period of life when health related disabilities are especially protracted. Among the most debilitating is the loss of self awareness and self control experienced in advanced Alzheimer's dementia. This realization has impelled numerous studies seeking to identify its etiological roots; its physiological basis, nonetheless, remains uncertain and an overarching framework has yet to be determined. Increasingly, the realization that brain activity is dynamically sustained offers a prospectus within which to frame Alzheimer's related behavioral manifestations. Dynamical systems constitute an operational ground not only as processional motifs but as functional units at progressively higher levels where their coherent assembly is used to guide global operation. This chapter proposes that the peculiarly debilitating and widely regarded hallmark aspects of AD are likely to relate to its ravaging of a global dynamical system that serves as the neural substrate for our sense of self.

Author details

Denis Larrivee

Address all correspondence to: sallar1@aol.com

Loyola University Chicago, USA

References

[1] Kahlaoui K, Wilson M, Ansaldo AI, Ska B, Joanette Y. Neurobiologial and neuroethical perspectives on the contribution of functional neuroimaging to the study of aging in the brain. In: Illes J, Sahakian B, editors. Oxford Handbook of Neuroethics. Oxford: Oxford Press; 2011

[2] Hebb D. The Organization of Behavior. New York: Wiley Press; 1949

[3] McClelland JL, Vallabha G. Connectionist models of development: Mechanistic dynamical models with emergent dynamical properties. In: Spencer JP, Thomas MSC, McClelland JL, editors. Toward a Unified Theory of Development: Connectionism and Dynamic Systems Theory Re-considered. Oxford: Oxford University Press; 2009

[4] Morin A. Toward a glossary of self-related terms. Frontiers in Psychology. 2017;**8**(280):1-9

[5] Hooker CA. Interaction and bio-cognitive order. Synthese. 2008;**166**:513-346

[6] Allen M, Friston K. From cognitivism to autopoiesis: Toward a computational framework for the embodied mind. Synthese. 2016:1-24. DOI: 10.1007/s11229-016-1288-5

[7] Damasio A. Self Comes to Mind. New York: Pantheon Books; 2012

[8] Brinker M. Navigating beyond "here & now" affordances on sensorimotor maturation and "false belief" performance. Frontiers in Psychology. 2014;**5**(1433):1-5

[9] Moser MB, Moser EI, Forrest E, Andersen, Morris RGM. Spatial learning with a minislab in the dorsal hippocampus. Proceedings of the National Academy of Sciences of the United States of America. 1995;**92**:9697-9701

[10] Rolls ET, Deco G. Networks for memory, perception, and decision-making, and beyond to how the syntax for language might be implemented in the brain. Brain Research. 2015;**1621**: 316-334

[11] Fornito A, Zalesky A, Bullmore E. Fundamentals of Brain Network Analysis. London: Elsevier Press; 2016

[12] Schoner G. Development as change of system dynamics: Stability, instability, and emergence. In: Spencer JP, Thomas MSC, McClelland JL, editors. Toward a Unified Theory of Development: Connectionism and Dynamic Systems Theory Re-considered. Oxford: Oxford University Press; 2009

[13] Liz E, Ruiz-Herrera A. Attractivity, multistability, and bifurcation in delayed Hopfield's model with non-monotonic feedback. Journal of Differential Equations. 2013;**255**(11): 4244-4266

[14] Wills TJ, Lever C, Cacucci F, Burgess N, O'Keefe J. Attractor dynamics in the hippocampal representation of the local environment. Science. 2005;**308**:873-877

[15] Deco G, Jirsa V, Friston K. The dynamical and structural basis of brain activity. In: Rabinovich MI, Friston KJ, Varona P, editors. Principles of Brain Dynamics. Boston: MIT Press; 2013

[16] Raichle M. Two views of brain functioning. In: Auletta G, Colage I, Jeannerod M, editors. Brains Top Down: Is Top-Down Causation Challenging Neuroscience? London: World Scientific; 2013

[17] Hellyer PJ, Shanahan M, Scott G, Wise RJS, Sharp DJ, Leech R. The control of global brain dynamics: Opposing actions of frontoparietal control and default mode networks on attention. The Journal of Neuroscience. 2014;**34**(2):451-461

[18] Larrivee D. Brain implantable devices: A step forward or a step away? EC Neurology. 2017;**ECO.01**:9-11

[19] Muldoon SF, Pasqualetti F, Gu S, Cieslak M, Grafton ST, Vettel JM, Bassett DS. Stimulation based control of dynamic brain networks. PLoS Computational Biology. 2016;**12**(9):e1005076

[20] Benson AR, Gleich DF, Leskovec J. Higher order organization of complex networks. Science. 2016;**353**(6295):163-166

[21] Tabor W. Dynamical insight into structure in connectionist models. In: Spencer JP, Thomas MSC, McClelland JL, editors. Toward a Unified Theory of Development: Connectionism and Dynamic Systems Theory Re-considered. Oxford: Oxford University Press; 2009

[22] Benfenati F. Synaptic plasticity and the neurobiology of learning and memory. Acta BioMedica. 2007;**78**(1):58-66

[23] Sporns O. The nonrandom brain: Efficiency, economy, and complex dynamics. Frontiers in Computational Neuroscience. 2011;**5**:5

[24] Kiebel SJ, Friston K. Recognition of sequences of sequences using nonlinear dynamical systems. In: Rabinovich MI, Friston KJ, Varona P, editors. Principles of Brain Dynamics. Boston: MIT Press; 2013

[25] Kato S, Kaplan HS, Schrodel T, et al. Global brain dynamics embed the motor command sequence of *Caenorhabditis elegans*. Cell. 2015;**163**:656-669

[26] Rodriguez P. Simple recurrent networks learn context-free and context-sensitive languages by counting. Neural Computation. 2001;**13**(9):2093-2118

[27] Smith L. Stability and flexibility in development. In: Spencer JP, Thomas MSC, McClelland JL, editors. Toward a Unified Theory of Development: Connectionism and Dynamic Systems Theory Re-considered. Oxford: Oxford University Press; 2009

[28] Corbetta D. Brain, body, and mind: Lessons from infant motor development. In: Spencer JP, Thomas MSC, McClelland JL, editors. Toward a Unified Theory of Development: Connectionism and Dynamic Systems Theory Re-considered. Oxford: Oxford University Press; 2009

[29] Frith C. Explaining delusions of control: The comparator model 20 years on. Consciousness and Cognition. 2012;**21**(1):52-54

[30] Varela F, Thompson E, Rosch E. The Embodied Mind: Cognitive Science and Human Experience. Cambridge, MA: MIT Press; 1991

[31] Sandamirskaya Y, Zibner SKU, Schneegan S, Schoner G. Using dynamic field theory to extend the embodiment stance toward higher cognition. New Ideas in Psychology. 2013;**31**:322-339

[32] Spencer JP, Perone S, Johnson JS. Dynamic field theory and embodied cognitive dynamics. In: Spencer JP, Thomas MSC, McClelland JL, editors. Toward a Unified Theory of Development: Connectionism and Dynamic Systems Theory Re-considered. Oxford: Oxford University Press; 2009

[33] Reinhart R, Robert MG, Zhu J, Park S, Woodman GF. Synchronizing theta oscillations with direct current stimulation strengthens adaptive control in the human brain. PNAS. 2015;**112**(30):9448-9453

[34] Friston K, Senegupta B, Auletta G. Cognitive dynamics: From attractors to active inference. Proceedings of the IEEE. 2014;**102**(4):427-445

[35] Moya P. Habit and embodiment in Merleau-Ponty. Frontiers in Human Neuroscience. 2014;**8**:542-546

[36] Wiesel TN, Hubel DH. Single cell responses in striate cortex of kittens deprived of vision in one eye. Journal of Neurophysiology. 1963;**26**:1003-1017

[37] Gallagher S. How the Body Shapes the Mind. Oxford: Oxford University Press; 2005

[38] Changeux JP, Courrege P, Danchin A. A theory of the epigenesis of neuronal networks by selective stabilization of synapses. Proceedings of the National Academy of Sciences of the United States of America. 1973;**70**(10):2974-2978

[39] Shapiro L. Embodied Cognition. New York: Routledge; 2011

[40] Thelen E, Smith L. Dynamic Systems Approach to the Development of Cognition and Action. Cambridge, MA: MIT Press; 1994

[41] Campos JJ, Bertenthal BI, Kermoian R. Early experience and emotional development: The emergence of wariness of heights. Psychological Science. 1992;**3**:61-64

[42] Bushnell EW, Boudreau JP. Motor development and the mind: The potential role of motor abilities as a determinant of aspects of perceptual development. Child Development. 1993;**64**(4):1005-1021

[43] Lockman JJ, Thelen E. Developmental biodynamics: Brain, body, behavior connections. Child Development. 1993;**64**:953-959

[44] Carroll J. The truth about fiction: Biological reality and imaginary lives. Style. 2012;**46**:129-160

[45] Golos M, Jirsa V, Dauce E. Multistability in large scale models of brain activity. PLoS Computational Biology. 2015;**11**(12):e1004644

[46] Davey CG, Pujol J, Harrison BJ. Mapping the self in the brain's default mode network. NeuroImage. 2016;**132**:390-397

[47] Schulman GL, Corbetta M, Bruckner RL, Fiez JA, Miezin FM, Raichle ME, Petersen SE. Journal of Cognitive Neuroscience. 1997;**9**:648-663

[48] Zhong Y, Huang L, Cai S, Zhang Y, von Deneen KM, Ren A, Ren J. Altered effective connectivity patterns of the default mode network in Alzheimer's disease: An fMRI study. Neuroscience Letters. 2014;**578**:171-175

[49] Hsiao FJ, Wang YJ, Yan SH, Wei-Ta C, Lin YY. Altered oscillation and synchronization of default-mode network activity in mild Alzheimer disease compared to mild cognitive impairment: An electrophysiological study. PLoS One. 2017;**8**(7):e68792

[50] He Y, Wang L, Zang Y, Tian L, Zhang X, Li K, Jiang T. Regional coherence changes in the early stages of Alzheimer's disease: A combined structural and resting-state functional MRI study. NeuroImage. 2007;**35**:488-500

[51] Palomera A, Kaufamann T, Persson K, et al. Disrupted global metastability and static and dynamic brain connectivity across individuals in the Alzheimer's disease continuum. Scientific Reports. 2017;**7**(40268):1-14. DOI 10.1038/srep40268

2

Neuronal Plasticity in the Juvenile and Adult Brain Regulated by the Extracellular Matrix

Max F.K. Happel and Renato Frischknecht

Abstract

In brains of higher vertebrates, the delicate balance of structural remodeling and stabilization of neuronal networks changes over the life-span. While the juvenile brain is characterized by high structural plasticity, it is more restricted in the adult. During brain maturation, the occurrence of the extracellular matrix (ECM) is a critical step to restrict the potential for neuronal remodeling and regeneration, but providing structural tenacity. How this putative limitation of adult neuronal plasticity might impact on learning-related plasticity, lifelong memory reformation, and higher cognitive functions is subject of current research. Here, we summarize recent evidence that recognizes the ECM and its activity-dependent modulation as a key regulator of learning-related plasticity in the adult brain. We will first outline molecular concepts of enzymatic ECM modulation and its impact on synaptic plasticity mechanisms. Thereafter, the ECM's role in converting juvenile to adult plasticity will be explained by several key studies in wild-type and genetic knockout animals. Finally, current research evidences the impact of ECM dynamics in different brain areas including neocortex on learning-related plasticity in the adult brain impacting on lifelong learning and memory. Experimental modulation of the ECM in local neuronal circuits further opens short-term windows of activity-dependent reorganization. Malfunctions of the ECM might contribute to a variety of neurological disorders. Therefore, experimental ECM modulation might not only promote complex forms of learning and cognitive flexible adaptation of valuable behavioral options, but has further implications for guided neuroplasticity with regenerative and therapeutic potential.

Keywords: Learning, Plasticity, Memory, Cortex, Protein turnover

1. Introduction

In the brains of higher vertebrates, both neurons and glial cells produce and secrete the molecules that accumulate and form the extracellular matrix (ECM). In the nineteenth century, pioneers of brain cell biology including Camillo Golgi and Santiago Ramon y Cajal have discovered a mesh-like structure surrounding the most neurons and synapses in the adult brain [1]. This extracellular scaffold has been seen initially as a key component for ensuring the structural stability of the respective tissue [2]. Later research evidenced that the ECM has multiple functions including regulation of cell adhesion, cell-to-cell communication, cell differentiation, cellular compartmentalization, and several forms of neuronal plasticity [3]. During brain maturation, the ECM undergoes profound changes. In late embryonic phases, the ECM is composed of particular proteoglycans and glycoproteins like neurocan and tenascin-C, which are downregulated during adulthood. Other components like the glycoprotein tenascin-R and chondroitin sulfate (CS) proteoglycans (CSPGs), such as brevican and aggrecan, are the main molecular components of the adult brain ECM. One of the most important structural components in the adult ECM is the unbranched polysaccharide hyaluronic acid (HA). HA forms the backbone that structurally orchestrates the enmeshment of all other ECM components. Interestingly, it has been shown that this developmental shift of the juvenile and adult forms of the ECM coincides with the closure of the so-called critical periods during brain maturation of respective brain regions. This led to the hypothesis that the brain's ECM is involved in regulating the switch from juvenile to adult plasticity by structural tenacity restricting the potential for neuronal reorganization [4]. Thereby, the brain has evolved mechanisms that guarantee structural stability of the neuronal networks established during experience-dependent learning. This brain function is fundamental for strengthening neuronal connections and their respective forms of processing impacting on long-term memory storage and recall. Nevertheless, current research has shown that dynamic adaptations of the ECM can alter several forms of synaptic plasticity and thereby regulate flexible learning and memory organization in the adult brain.

2. The structural foundation of the ECM in the vertebrate's brain

Components of the ECM in the mature brain are interlinked in a complex netlike architecture [5]. The linear HA backbone binds and coordinates proteoglycans especially of the lectican family that are cross-linked by glycoproteins such as the tenascins. Thus, this form of ECM is referred to as HA-based ECM. It is rich in the glycosaminoglycan CS attached to CSPGs of the lectican family, as for instance brevican and aggrecan [6]. The main carrier of CS within the ECM is aggrecan with its multiple attachment sites, while Brevican is a part-time proteoglycan existing glycoprotein and proteoglycan [7,8]. Brevican and aggrecan both bind to the ECM glycoprotein tenascin-R (**Figure 1A**). Other so-called cartilage link proteins form a complex with N-terminal domains of the lecticans and HA and thereby contribute to the ECM stability [6]. A large variety of other components including reelin, laminins, thrombospondins, heparin-sulfate proteoglycans, guidance molecules, and even transcription factors are incorporated in the complex ECM structure (**Figure 1A**). This form of the homogenous HA-based ECM loosely enwraps cell bodies, dendritic, and synaptic structures of most neurons. Further, the mature brain contains a specialized glycosaminoglycan-rich ECM structure around synapses and somata of a small proportion of neurons. This more rigid form is called the perineuronal nets (PNNs), which are especially rich in aggrecan and CS. Such PNNs are most abundant on

GABAergic interneurons expressing the calcium buffer protein parvalbumin (PV; **Figure 1B**). Recent evidence shows that PNNs are highly heterogeneous and can be found on various types of neurons throughout the CNS. For the formation of WFA-positive PNNs, the cartilage link protein Crtl1/Hapln1 has been identified as a key regulator [9].

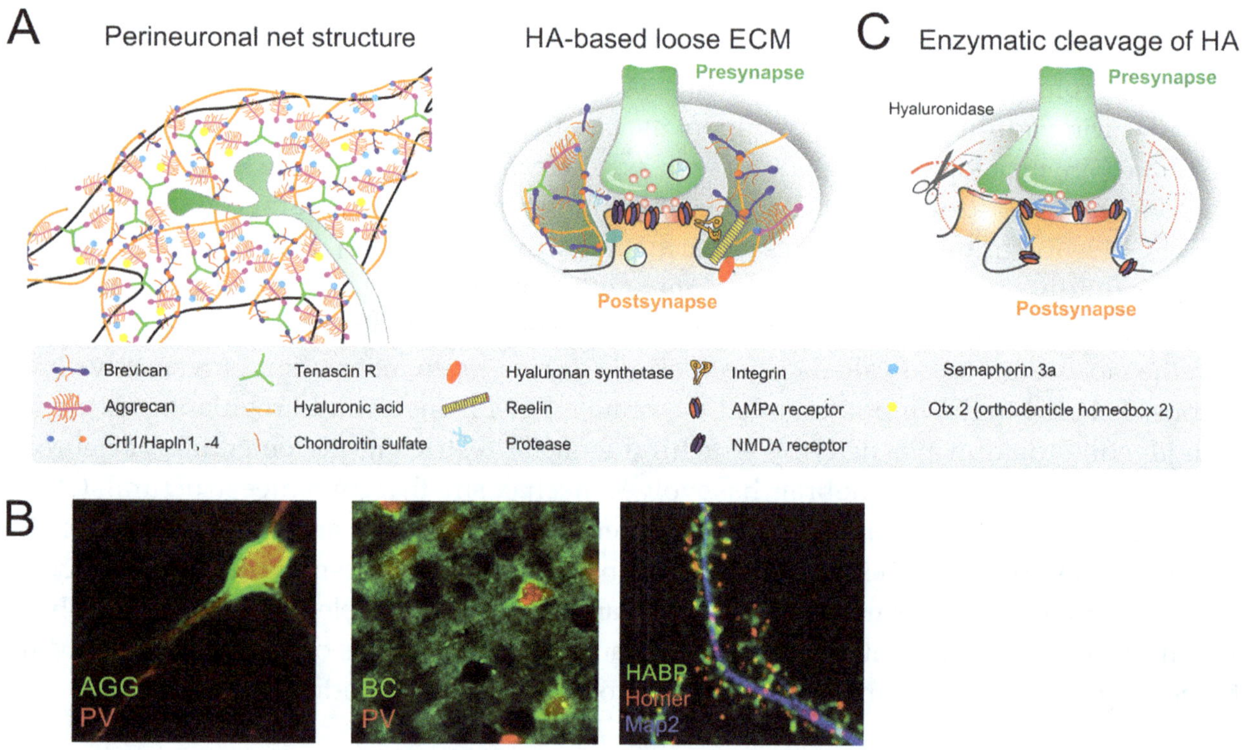

Figure 1. Cell types and their specific forms of the hyaluronan-based ECM. (**A**) The mature ECM is based on the backbone of hyaluronic acid (orange). Schematized are the specialized form of the PNN (*left*) and the loose ECM (*right*) around synaptic contacts. Densely packed PNNs are rich in CS and aggrecan. Small signaling molecules such as semaphorin 3a or Oxt2 are bound to CS within the PNN and mediate several functions or regulate gene expression. The loose ECM around excitatory, spiny synapses is rich in brevican and contains only little aggrecan and is thus less rich in CS. ECM proteins (e.g., reelin) signal through their receptors (e.g., integrins) and regulate several cellular processes including trafficking of glutamate receptors (see C). ECM function is modulated by proteases (scissors) that may free synapses by removing ECM or unmask signaling molecules. (**B**) *Left*, Parvalbumine positive interneuron (PV, red) with typical PNN stained for aggrecan (AGG, green). *Middle*, Dendritic spines and synapses of excitatory neurons (red) are also surrounded by brevican (BC, green), although it is less specific for PNN's. *Right*, Dissociated cortical neuron stained with the dendritic marker Map2 (blue) and Homer (red) to stain excitatory synapses and hyaluronic acid binding protein (HABP, green) to label extracellular matrix. Note the loose appearance around dendrites, spines, and synapses. (**C**) Enzymatic weakening of the ECM by glycosidases (e.g., hyaluronidase, see scissors) changes the micromillieu around synapses by for instance increased lateral diffusion and synaptic exchange of AMPA receptors (blue arrows). Further, removal of stabilizing cues facilitates structural plasticity such as *de-novo* formation of new synapses and synaptic scaling. Modified from Ref. [22].

The structural foundation of the mature ECM allows regulating several functions beyond mechanical stability of neuronal networks. In the juvenile brain, the ECM regulates neuro- and gliogenesis, cell migration, axonal pathfinding, and synaptogenesis. Adult forms of the HA-based ECM are in the service of multiple functions including regulation of synaptogenesis and synaptic plasticity, compartmentalization of the neuronal surface, neuroprotection, regulation of ion homeostasis, and neuron–glia interactions. The remainder of this review will consider several ECM-based mechanisms for regulating synaptic plasticity and its effects on brain development and adult learning behavior.

3. ECM-guided switch from juvenile to adult synaptic plasticity

Early in life, high structural plasticity allows profound shaping of brain circuits by experience. Such critical periods in the juvenile brain are limited by the occurrence of the ECM implementing adult brain plasticity modes. For instance, in wild-type animals, dark rearing delays not only the critical periods of developmental plasticity in visual cortex of rodents, but also the formation of PNNs. During the development, the cartilage link protein Crtl1/Hapln1 is organizing the formation of PNNs. Crtl1/Hapln1 k.o. mice do not develop normal PNN structures in the visual cortex. These mice show juvenile forms of ocular dominance (OD) plasticity and sensitivity of the visual system to deprivation throughout the life-span [9].

The seminal study by Pizzorusso et al. [10] has elucidated the ECM as the regulatory switch between juvenile and adult plasticity. The authors combined monocular deprivation with injection of the ECM-cleaving enzyme chondroitinase ABC (chABC) into visual cortex of adult rats (see also **Figure 1C**). The local weakening of the ECM "re-juvenated" the visual cortex and restored the critical period form of OD plasticity (**Figure 2**). By the same manipulation Pizzorusso and colleagues restored in a follow-up study, the visual acuity in adult animals grown up with long-term monocular deprivation [11]. Similarly, application of the serine protease tissue-type plasminogen activator (tPA) into the visual cortex can prolong or reactivate critical periods of OD plasticity in visual cortex [12] based on increased structural remodeling [13].

Later studies identified the regulatory role of the ECM in other forms of developmental plasticity during brain maturation of different vertebrate species. For instance, birdsong learning in the zebra finch occurs during a sensitive period similar to the language development in humans. It has been shown that with the end of this critical period PNNs around PV-positive neurons emerge in brain areas that are dedicated to singing [14]. In another set of experiments, Gogolla et al. [15] shown that the maturing ECM in the amygdala essentially makes fear memories erasure resistant in adult animals. In rats not older than 3–4 weeks, a conditioned fear memory trace can be erased permanently by extinction, that is, the presentation of the conditioned stimulus without the aversive stimulus. However, after this period extinction only attenuates the fear response, but it reinstates instantaneously if the aversive stimulus is presented again. Hence, a permanent loss of the fear memory is only found before the ECM in the amygdala is formed and is preserving established fear memories. Gogolla and colleagues now attenuated the ECM in the amygdala by chABC injections in adult rats. This led to a complete erasure of the fear response after an extinction phase even if the aversive stimulus is presented to these animals again. In addition, the early preweaning environment impacts on rodent ECM maturation in a functional manner. Improved performance in water maze learning in the adult age after early postnatal-enriched housing has been correlated with increased PNN formation in the striatum reflecting functional shaping of neuronal circuits involved in motor learning [16].

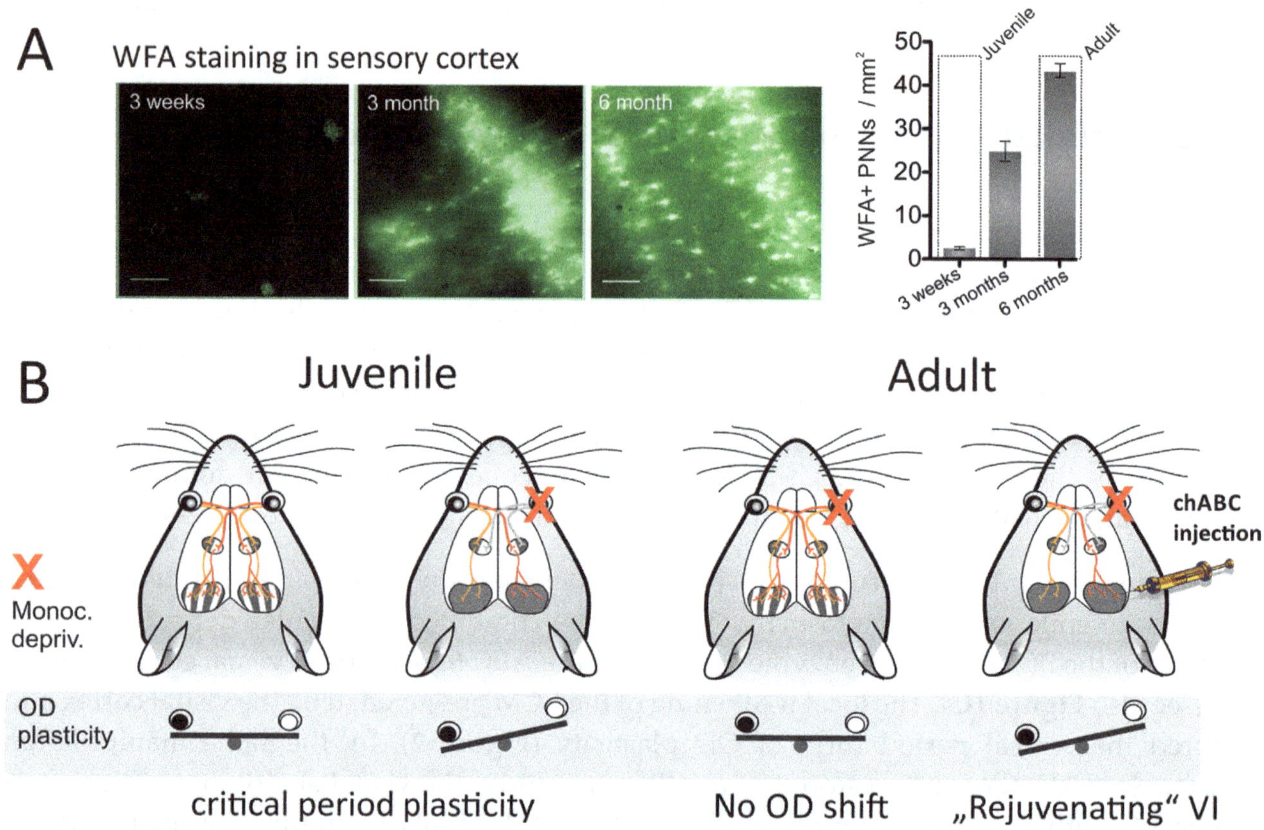

Figure 2. The emerging ECM during brain maturation and its regulatory role for juvenile brain plasticity (A) *Wisteria floribunda* (WFA) fluorescein staining against sugar chains of the CSPGs in rodent sensory cortex shows that the diffuse HA-based ECM and perineuronal nets around cells emerge with brain maturation (≥3 month), but were abundant in juvenile state (3 weeks). Modified from Ref. [42]. (**B**) Pizzorusso et al. [10] demonstrated the inhibitory role of the developmental maturation of the ECM in visual cortex of rats for early experience-dependent plasticity. In juvenile rats, monocular deprivation (MD) leads to an ocular dominance shift (left). After the critical period, MD alone did not cause such a shift in the adult. In this study, the authors found that weakening of the ECM by chABC treatment in visual cortex reactivated OD plasticity shifting toward the nondeprived eye.

The emerging ECM in the developing brain seems to be involved in a complex molecular machinery organizing the maturation of neuronal networks. For instance, in mouse visual cortex, it has been shown that critical periods are initiated, maintained, and closed by the action of the orthodenticle homeobox 2 homeoprotein (Otx2) on PV+-GABAergic interneurons [17]. Interestingly, Otx2 contains a glycosaminoglycan binding sequence that mediates its allocation to the PNNs by specific binding to CS D and E. Thereby, a constant level of Otx2 in PV+-neurons keeps a mature, consolidated, and persistent PNN-state in the adult brain. Hydrolysis of the PNNs by chABC reduces the amount of endogenous Otx2 in PV cells mediating the reopening of OD plasticity in adult mice [18].

The reviewed studies in this paragraph have shown how the change of the juvenile form of the ECM to a more rigid adult ECM mediates the different modes of neuronal plasticity during brain development. Why has this restriction of adult reorganizational and regenerative plasticity only evolved in higher vertebrates? The evolutionary benefit may be to preserve the costly acquired hardwired connections during early life experience, which are fundamental for rapid experience-based behavioral adaptations of higher vertebrates [4]. Nonetheless, the adult, healthy brain retains a remarkable capability of plastic reorganization that is essential for constantly adapting to our ever-changing environment.

4. The hyaluronic acid-based ECM regulates adult synaptic plasticity

The functional mechanisms by which the HA-based ECM implements adult forms of brain plasticity including classical (Hebbian) and homeostatic plasticity are still elusive (for an overview see [3]). Research investigating knockout models lacking particular components of the ECM have provided major insights into the impact of the ECM on adult synaptic plasticity. For instance, different mouse models deficient in specific matrix components, as tenascin-R, brevican, or neurocan, all showed impaired forms of hippocampal long-term potentiation (LTP). However, during the brain development of k.o.-models compensatory mechanisms might mimic the deficit of a particular matrix component and hence limit the significance of the findings. Therefore, another experimental strategy is to use acute enzymatic weakening of the ECM based on the local application of different matrix-degrading enzymes (**Figure 1C**). For instance, it has been shown that treatment with chABC impaired theta-burst-induced LTP in CA1–CA3 pyramidal synapses in hippocampal slices [19]. It has been suggested that this is due to an increased excitability of GABAergic perisomatic interneurons [3]. Similar findings have been found with Injection of the hyaluronidase (HYase) from *Streptomyces hyalurolyticus* [20]. In contrast to other hyaluronidases, this enzyme is highly specific to HA and does not digest CS. The phenotype in these experiments could be rescued by perfusion with HA. It has been suggested that this is due to the fact that HA directly regulates L-type voltage-gated calcium channels (L-VDCC; Cav1.2) of CA1 neurons and thus postsynaptic Ca^{2+} entry and hippocampal-dependent forms of learning [3,20]. In a recent study, we have described a molecular mechanism by which acute ECM removal was altering short-term-dependent forms of synaptic plasticity [21]. We measured paired pulse ratios in dissociated hippocampal cultures by cell-attached recordings. We found the typical robust paired pulse depression (PPD) under control conditions. Interestingly, digestion of the ECM by infusion of HYase prevented cells from expressing PPD. We further found increased lateral diffusion of extra-synaptic AMPA receptors after ECM digestion as key correlate of this effect [21]. This results in a higher exchange between synaptic desensitized receptors with extrasynaptic naïve ones, which quickly replenishes the pool of excitable receptors in the active zone of a synapse (**Figure 1C**). In such conditions, synapses are able to follow higher firing frequencies. Blockade of lateral diffusion of AMPA receptors by cross-linking with antibodies, on the other hand, led to stronger PPD caused by accumulated desensitized synaptic AMPA receptors [22]. Similarly, mobility of other receptor types can be modulated by specific proteolytic enzymes. For instance, MMP9 increases the mobility of NMDA-type, but not AMPA receptors. These results have shown that the perisynaptic ECM forms surface compartments that act as diffusion barrier for membrane proteins such as AMPA receptors. Modulation of lateral receptor diffusion provides a novel mechanism of short-term plasticity due to a changed extracellular micromillieu at individual synapses. Interestingly, lack of the major hyaluronan synthetase

HAS3 in the hippocampus did not lead to a striking morphological change in the ECM. However, the extracellular space was reduced, which resulted in a more dense packing of cells and lower diffusion of soluble molecules in the CA1 *stratum pyramidale* [23]. Further, these animals were prone to epileptic seizures which underlines the importance of the regulatory function of the HA-based ECM that is required for instance for volume transmission and ion homeostasis.

Weakening of the ECM and the corresponding synaptic networks might further promote architectural remodeling and even increased spine motility. In *in vitro* hippocampal cultures, microinjections of chABC treatment increased the motility of local spines and induced spine remodeling in a β1-integrin-dependent manner [24].

5. ECM proteolysis and the generation of synaptic signaling molecules

Endogenous ECM-modulating enzymes regulate synaptic function in the juvenile and adult brain [25,26]. Such enzymes can exert their function by either altering the extracellular milieu via digestion of the ECM or by generating proteolytic fragments that may act as signaling molecules. An important group of such enzymes are the metalloproteases of the ADAMTS-family (a disintegrin and metalloproteinase with thrombospondin motifs). Within this family, ADAMTS-4/-5 are particularly interesting, as they are known for their ability to digest aggrecan and brevican. Therefore, they have been termed previously aggrecanase-1/-2. The current terminology, however, better reflects the ability of these enzymes to digest all members of the lectican family. Interestingly, their activity is increased after epileptic seizures and regulates homeostatic plasticity [27]. However, their impact on synaptic plasticity remains elusive and is subject of current research. The best-studied extracellular protease is the matrix metalloprotease 9 (MMP9). The activity-dependent expression of MMP9 influences synaptic plasticity by regulating spine enlargement and synaptic potentiation [25]. Recently, a molecular signaling cascade regulating synaptic plasticity has been identified based on the MMP-9-dependent cleavage of neuroligin-1 [28]. This study has demonstrated that focal activation of a single spine by glutamate uncaging is sufficient to cleave neuroligin-1. Moreover, the activity of MMP9 has been shown to be NMDA-receptor dependent and hence implemented locally input-specific forms of synaptic plasticity. Thereby, extracellular MMP-9 triggers a specific retrograde regulation of presynaptic efficacy by targeting postsynaptic neuroligin-1 [26,28]. Similarly, the brain-specific serine protease neurotrypsin is regulated in an activity-dependent manner and requires concomitant activation of the postsynaptic neuron [29]. Proteolytic cleavage of agrin by neurotrypsin unmasks a signaling molecule harboring a single laminin G3 domain. This 22 kDa molecule can further regulate spine morphology and de-novo synapse generation. Together, this suggests that proteolysis of components of the ECM by exoenzymes not only modify the structural rigidity, but also activates instructive signal molecules that locally modulate synaptic functions [25]. This may temporally restore local divisions of "juvenile" environments as a major constituent of the balance between plasticity and tenacity in the mature brain.

We have shown that the ECM in the adult brain is a plastic structural scaffold shaped by network activity. Depending on the current activity level, the ECM can incorporate secreted components or release signaling messengers by proteolytic cleavage. Cleaved products can trigger signaling through diverse ECM receptors and modulate the activities of transmitter receptor, ion channels, or integrin signaling impacting on plastic shaping of individual synapses.

6. Role of the ECM in control of adult learning behavior and cognitive flexibility

Experimental weakening of the ECM by local injection of matrix-digesting enzymes can promote functional neurorehabilitation in the injured brain. This has been related mostly to injuries on the level of the peripheral nervous system and spinal cord [4,30,31]. Experience-driven plasticity does, however, not only lead sensory development or neuronal rehabilitation, but is also indispensable during learning, memory formation, and re-consolidation throughout life. The question now arises how forms of ECM-dependent plasticity in the adult brain might govern learning-related plasticity, lifelong memory reformation, and the organization of cognitively flexible behavior. In this respect, several studies have investigated the involvement of ECM functions in memory storage in adult animals. This has been characterized the best for long-term plasticity in the hippocampus and fear memory in the amygdala. However, available evidence is controversial about how ECM functions may impact on learning and memory processes.

For instance, it has been reported that tenascin-R knockout mice show normal hippocampus-dependent spatial memory acquisition in a Water maze. In subsequent reversal learning though animals showed more vulnerable spatial long-term memory yielding enhanced relearning performance due to less conflicting past and actual learning contingencies [32]. Another study found an already impaired acquisition of hippocampus-dependent contextual memory in same knockout mice [33]. Injection of chABC in the bilateral striatum, however, has been related to an improvement of water maze acquisition learning, while the recall of the learned values was unaffected [34].

In addition to deficits in matrix components, studies also found effects of deficits in exoproteases modeling the ECM. Loss of MMP9 activity has been associated with impaired hippocampal-dependent learning and amygdala-dependent learning. This is in line with findings of wild-type mice trained in an inhibitory avoidance (IA) learning paradigm [35,36]. Hippocampal LTP has been related to increased levels of MMP3 and MMP9. Both proteases were upregulated for at least ~48 h promoting local plastic synaptic environments underlying the learning performance. Intra-hippocampal injections of MMP9 blockers completely abrogated memory for the IA response when tested days later. Comparably, hippocampal MMP3 and MMP9 were found to be increased during water maze acquisition learning in a NMDA-dependent manner. Hippocampal injection of the broad-spectrum MMP9 inhibitor FN-439 also prevented elevated MMP9 levels, altered hippocampal LTP, and prevented spatial acquisition learning [35].

Similarly, spatial training in a water maze in wild-type rats has been found to correlate with increased levels of hippocampal brevican and versican in the membrane fraction [37]. These findings indicate that hippocampal-dependent learning induced a period of intrinsic activity-induced focal MMP-mediated proteolysis driving long-lasting synaptic modifications underlying learning and memory consolidation. Effects of changes in the ECM on initial learning are, however, still unclear [25,33].

More recently, insights into the impact of the ECM onto behavior came from studies using experimental, enzymatic, and local weakening of the ECM. The study of Gogolla et al. manipulating adult fear extinction suggested that memory acquisition differs in juvenile and adult brains due to changes of the mature ECM functions. The authors further argued that intra-amygdala injections of chABC in adult rats had no effect on acquisition learning of fear, but only on extinction, reinstatement, and renewal of the fear memory [15]. A further study showed that intra-hippocampal and prefrontal injection of chABC and HYase in mice impair long-term trace contextual fear conditioning [38]. This finding has been related to the impairment in the L-VDCC-dependent component of hippocampal LTP by cleaved extracellular HA [20].

In addition to spatial memory, another set of studies examined the function of the ECM in memory consolidation of drug seeking. A recent study showed that intracerebral injection of FN-439 impaired the acquisition of a cocaine-induced conditioned place preference (CPP) of rats. FN-439 injection 30 min prior to cocaine memory re-activation further attenuated the reinstatement of CPP in extinguished animals. The study further showed that intra-amygdala injections of chABC during active extinction of cocaine-induced CPP prevented its subsequent priming-induced reinstatement. ChABC injections alone had no effect on the retention, retrieval, or relearning of CPP [39]. Similarly, enzymatic weakening of PNNs in the prelimbic cortex or in the amygdala of adult rats impaired the acquisition and reconsolidation of drug-induced memories [40,41].

With respect to cognitively flexible adaptation of behavior, we have recently shown that weakening of the ECM in auditory cortex promotes complex forms of cortex-dependent relearning in the Mongolian gerbil [42]. In our experiments, we trained animals on frequency-modulated tone discrimination based on the rising or falling modulation direction in a go-/nogo-task. Such auditory learning is known to depend on learning-induced plastic reorganization of neuronal circuits in the auditory cortex. After acquiring robust discrimination of the stimulus contingencies, the animals were trained to reverse their choice. We found that ECM weakening by local HYase injection in bilateral auditory cortex accelerated the demanding relearning performance (**Figure 3**). Specifically, animals had to inhibit the obsolete initial behavioral strategy and then establish its successful reversal. Importantly, attenuation of the ECM did neither affect the acquisition learning nor erased already established, learned memory traces (**Figure 3B**). That means attenuation of the ECM in sensory cortex of these animals promoted the flexible adaptation of the effectively appropriate strategy during cortex-dependent learning behavior that bases on "reprogramming" previously acquired auditory memories. The ECM reconstitutes after several days to weeks limiting again the promoting effects onto cognitive flexibility (**Figure 3A**). A comparable finding investigated log-term object recognition memory in knockout mice of the link protein Crtl1/Hapln1—a key molecule for stabilization of PNNs. The Ctrl1/Hapln1 knockout mice have attenuated PNNs in the perirhinal cortex. Long-term object recognition memory, a task depending on perirhinal cortex, was enhanced in these mice. Local injection of chABC in wild-type mice had the same memory-prolonging effect in the object recognition task, but also attenuated over time [43]. In this study, the attenuation of the PNNs was accompanied by enhanced perirhinal LTD, which is thought to be the major synaptic mechanism underlying object recognition memory.

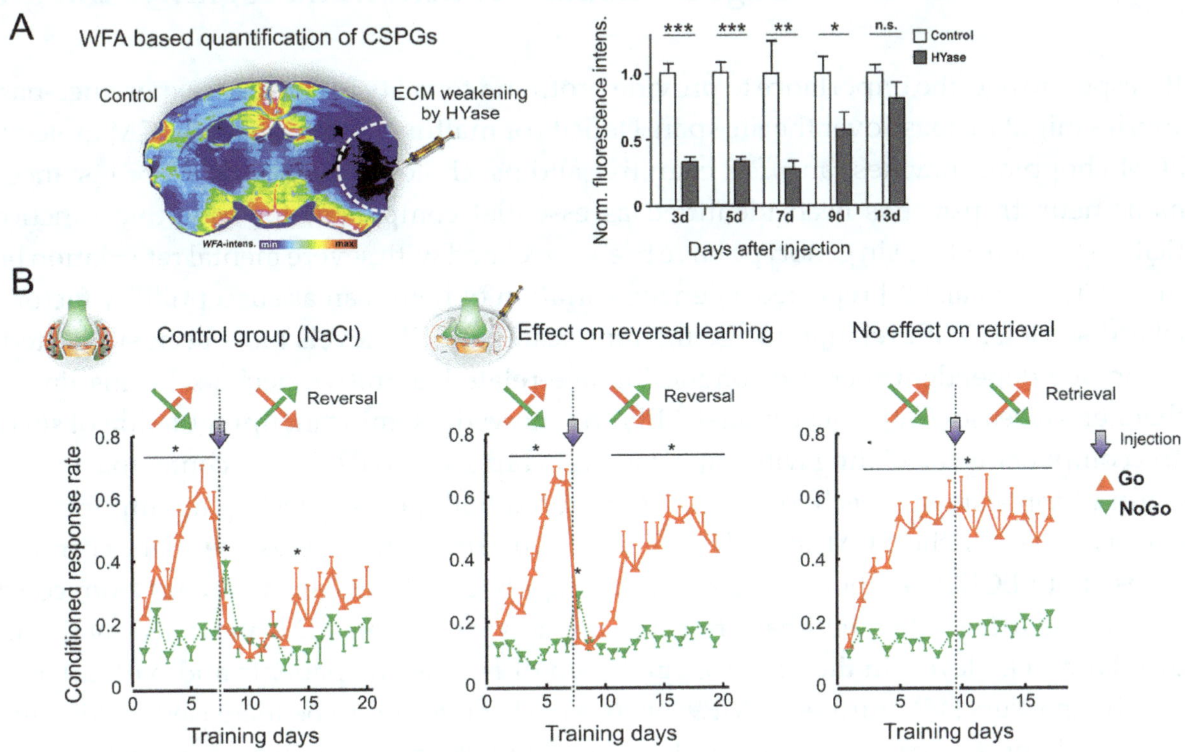

Figure 3. Local enzymatic weakening of the ECM in auditory cortex of Mongolian gerbils enhanced the cognitive flexibility in a relearning paradigm. (**A**) *Right*, Quantification of ECM weakening after local injection of HYase in unilateral auditory cortex of Mongolian gerbils (right) compared to control (left) based on WFA staining. *Left*, HYase injection significantly weakened the ECM for about 1 week and reconstituted fully after 2 weeks. (**B**) Mongolian gerbils were trained in a two-compartmental go/no-go Shuttle-box in order to discriminate two frequency-modulated sounds (modulation direction indicated by rising and falling arrows). Gerbils showed successful acquisition depending on the contingency of the stimuli as a go-stimulus (red) or Nogo-stimulus (green). In two groups, the contingency was reversed after seven training days (*left and middle*). Conditioned response rates were strongly reduced in both experimental groups indicating the active inhibition of the previously established discrimination strategy. HYase-treated animals were significantly better in correcting the behavioral strategy and successfully relearn the task (middle). Interestingly, HYase treatment did not interfere with the recall of already established cortex-dependent auditory memories (*right*). Modified from Ref. [42].

The both last-mentioned studies therefore promote the view that the perineuronal ECM in the adult brain actively organizes the balance between memory stability and flexibility. Cortical attenuation of the ECM in the mature brain might hence promote the cognitive flexibility that can build on learned behaviors and allows for an enhanced activity-dependent memory reorganization (see also Ref. [44]). And regeneration of the ECM gradually restores normal, restrictive adult plasticity levels. Generally, all studies summarized in this review emphasized that the increased experience-based plasticity by acute, enzymatic PNN diminution is activity-dependent and the rather inconspicuous effect of mere ECM attenuation in general. Mechanistically, enzymatic ECM degradation might facilitate the rearrangement of functional network connectivity by a shift in the balance between excitation and inhibition leading to destabilized existing patterns of neuronal network interactions [45].

7. Impact of the ECM in old age on memory function and cognitive integrity

With respect to age, the importance to provide profound tenacity to conserve experience-based memories might increase over the life span. Deficits or malfunctions of several ECM molecules or ECM-chopping enzymes can affect cognitive and psychological conditions. For instance, in humans neurotrypsin has been identified as essential component for cognitive functions. Deficits in the neurotrypsin genotype have been correlated with severe mental retardation [46]. Further, Cichon et al. [47] reported a genetic variation of neurocan as susceptibility factor for bipolar disorders. With relation to ageing, hippocampal ECM levels have been suggested to show an age-dependent increase conquering age-related cognitive decline. In this line, the Alzheimer's disease (AD) mouse model APP/PS1 showed a significant upregulation of several matrix components correlating with impairments in hippocampal LTP and contextual memory [48]. Intra-hippocampal injections of chABC restored both [48] suggesting an important, but yet elusive role for the ECM in early memory impairment in AD, as the mere correlative findings about ECM alterations in dementia are highly controversial and are far from conclusive [33]. That these data might have relevant impacts for human AD is indicated by findings of correlating HA levels in the cerebrospinal fluid of female AD patients and particular AD-related biomarkers [49]. Further, MMP9 levels have been found to be increased in Alzheimer patients [50] and to cleave the amyloid beta peptide leading to AD-typical neuritic plaques [51]. Its role in Aβ-induced cognitive decline is however elusive [52].

8. Outlook

We have summarized recent evidence showing that experimental modulation of the ECM promotes "windows of opportunities" with an increase in learning-related plasticity yielding cognitively flexible adaptation of learned behaviors and the underlying memories. How the ECM, in addition, impacts onto several mental disorders that generally develop after the closure of major critical periods for higher brain functions, as for instance affective disorders or schizophrenia, are exciting new research directions. We are envisaging future challenges in developing new tools for guided neuroplasticity with therapeutic potential for memory disorders, stroke, or neuroprosthetic applications based on ECM manipulations.

Author details

Max F.K. Happel[1,2*] and Renato Frischknecht[3*]

*Address all correspondence to: mhappel@lin-magdeburg.de and rfrischk@lin-magdeburg.de

1 Department Systems Physiology of Learning, Leibniz-Institute for Neurobiology, Magdeburg, Germany

2 Institute for Biology, Otto-von-Guericke University Magdeburg, Magdeburg, Germany

3 AG Perisynaptic Extrazellular Matrix, Department Neurochemistry and Molecular Biology, Leibniz-Institute for Neurobiology, Magdeburg, Germany

References

[1] Celio MR, Spreafico R, De Biasi S, Vitellaro-Zuccarello L: Perineuronal nets: past and present. *Trends Neurosci* 1998, 21:510–5.

[2] Berardi N, Pizzorusso T, Maffei L: Extracellular matrix and visual cortical plasticity: freeing the synapse. *Neuron* 2004, 44:905–8.

[3] Dityatev A, Schachner M, Sonderegger P: The dual role of the extracellular matrix in synaptic plasticity and homeostasis. *Nat Rev Neurosci* 2010, 11:735–46.

[4] Gundelfinger ED, Frischknecht R, Choquet D, Heine M: Converting juvenile into adult plasticity: a role for the brain's extracellular matrix. *Eur J Neurosci* 2010, 31:2156–65.

[5] Berardi N, Pizzorusso T, Ratto GM, Maffei L: Molecular basis of plasticity in the visual cortex. *Trends Neurosci* 2003, 26:369–78.

[6] Yamaguchi Y: Lecticans: organizers of the brain extracellular matrix. *Cell Mol Life Sci* 2000, 57:276–89.

[7] Giamanco KA, Morawski M, Matthews RT: Perineuronal net formation and structure in aggrecan knockout mice. *Neuroscience* 2010, 170:1314–27.

[8] Frischknecht R, Seidenbecher CI: Brevican: a key proteoglycan in the perisynaptic extracellular matrix of the brain. *Int J Biochem Cell Biol* 2012, 44:1051–54.

[9] Carulli D, Pizzorusso T, Kwok JCF, Putignano E, Poli A, Forostyak S, Andrews MR, Deepa SS, Glant TT, Fawcett JW: Animals lacking link protein have attenuated perineuronal nets and persistent plasticity. *Brain* 2010, 133:2331–47.

[10] Pizzorusso T, Medini P, Berardi N, Chierzi S, Fawcett JW, Maffei L: Reactivation of ocular dominance plasticity in the adult visual cortex. *Science* 2002, 298:1248–51.

[11] Pizzorusso T, Medini P, Landi S, Baldini S, Berardi N, Maffei L: Structural and functional recovery from early monocular deprivation in adult rats. *Proc Natl Acad Sci USA* 2006, 103:8517–22.

[12] Oray S, Majewska A, Sur M: Dendritic spine dynamics are regulated by monocular deprivation and extracellular matrix degradation. *Neuron* 2004, 44:1021–30.

[13] Hensch TK: Critical period plasticity in local cortical circuits. *Nat Rev Neurosci* 2005, 6:877–88.

[14] Balmer TS, Carels VM, Frisch JL, Nick TA: Modulation of perineuronal nets and parvalbumin with developmental song learning. *J Neurosci* 2009, 29:12878–85.

[15] Gogolla N, Caroni P, Lüthi A, Herry C: Perineuronal nets protect fear memories from erasure. *Science* 2009, 325:1258–61.

[16] Simonetti T, Lee H, Bourke M, Leamey CA, Sawatari A: Enrichment from birth accelerates the functional and cellular development of a motor control area in the mouse. *PLoS One* 2009, 4:e6780.

[17] Sugiyama S, Di Nardo AA, Aizawa S, Matsuo I, Volovitch M, Prochiantz A, Hensch TK: Experience-dependent transfer of Otx2 homeoprotein into the visual cortex activates postnatal plasticity. *Cell* 2008, 134:508–20.

[18] Beurdeley M, Spatazza J, Lee HHC, Sugiyama S, Bernard C, Di Nardo AA, Hensch TK, Prochiantz A: Otx2 binding to perineuronal nets persistently regulates plasticity in the mature visual cortex. *J Neurosci* 2012, 32:9429–37.

[19] Bukalo O, Schachner M, Dityatev A: Modification of extracellular matrix by enzymatic removal of chondroitin sulfate and by lack of tenascin-R differentially affects several forms of synaptic plasticity in the hippocampus. *Neuroscience* 2001, 104:359–69.

[20] Kochlamazashvili G, Henneberger C, Bukalo O, Dvoretskova E, Senkov O, Lievens PM-J, Westenbroek R, Engel AK, Catterall WA, Rusakov DA, Schachner M, Dityatev A: The extracellular matrix molecule hyaluronic acid regulates hippocampal synaptic plasticity by modulating postsynaptic L-type Ca(2+) channels. *Neuron* 2010, 67:116–28.

[21] Frischknecht R, Heine M, Perrais D, Seidenbecher CI, Choquet D, Gundelfinger ED: Brain extracellular matrix affects AMPA receptor lateral mobility and short-term synaptic plasticity. *Nat Neurosci* 2009, 12:897–904.

[22] Heine M, Groc L, Frischknecht R, Béïque J-C, Lounis B, Rumbaugh G, Huganir RL, Cognet L, Choquet D: Surface mobility of postsynaptic AMPARs tunes synaptic transmission. *Science* 2008, 320:201–5.

[23] Arranz AM, Perkins KL, Irie F, Lewis DP, Hrabe J, Xiao F, Itano N, Kimata K, Hrabetova S, Yamaguchi Y: Hyaluronan deficiency due to Has3 knock-out causes altered neuronal

activity and seizures via reduction in brain extracellular space. *J Neurosci* 2014, 34:6164–76.

[24] Orlando C, Ster J, Gerber U, Fawcett JW, Raineteau O: Perisynaptic chondroitin sulfate proteoglycans restrict structural plasticity in an integrin-dependent manner. *J Neurosci* 2012, 32:18009–17, 18017a.

[25] Huntley GW: Synaptic circuit remodelling by matrix metalloproteinases in health and disease. Nat Rev Neurosci. 2012, 13(11):743–57

[26] Shinoe T, Goda Y: Tuning synapses by proteolytic remodeling of the adhesive surface. *Curr Opin Neurobiol* 2015, 35:148–55.

[27] Juan RV, Christopher H, Gilbert F, Jeet S, Barbara S, Constanze S, Frischknecht R: Hyaluronan-based extracellular matrix under conditions of homeostatic plasticity. *Philos Trans R Soc B Biol Sci* 2014. 19;369(1654):20130606

[28] Peixoto RT, Kunz PA, Kwon H, Mabb AM, Sabatini BL, Philpot BD, Ehlers MD: Transsynaptic signaling by activity-dependent cleavage of neuroligin-1. *Neuron* 2012, 76:396–409.

[29] Frischknecht R, Fejtova A, Viesti M, Stephan A, Sonderegger P: Activity-induced synaptic capture and exocytosis of the neuronal serine protease neurotrypsin. *J Neurosci* 2008, 28:1568–79.

[30] Bowes C, Massey JM, Burish M, Cerkevich CM, Kaas JH: Chondroitinase ABC promotes selective reactivation of somatosensory cortex in squirrel monkeys after a cervical dorsal column lesion. *Proc Natl Acad Sci USA* 2012, 109:2595–600.

[31] Fawcett JW: The extracellular matrix in plasticity and regeneration after CNS injury and neurodegenerative disease. *Prog Brain Res* 2015, 218:213–26.

[32] Morellini F, Sivukhina E, Stoenica L, Oulianova E, Bukalo O, Jakovcevski I, Dityatev A, Irintchev A, Schachner M: Improved reversal learning and working memory and enhanced reactivity to novelty in mice with enhanced GABAergic innervation in the dentate gyrus. *Cereb Cortex* 2010, 20:2712–27.

[33] Dityatev A, Wehrle-Haller B, Pitkänen A: *Brain extracellular matrix in health and disease.* Progress in Brain Research Vol. 214; 2014 - Elsevier.

[34] Lee H, Leamey CA, Sawatari A: Perineuronal nets play a role in regulating striatal function in the mouse. *PLoS One* 2012, 7:e32747.

[35] Meighan SE, Meighan PC, Choudhury P, Davis CJ, Olson ML, Zornes PA, Wright JW, Harding JW: Effects of extracellular matrix-degrading proteases matrix metalloproteinases 3 and 9 on spatial learning and synaptic plasticity. *J Neurochem* 2006, 96:1227–41.

[36] Nagy V, Bozdagi O, Huntley GW: The extracellular protease matrix metalloproteinase-9 is activated by inhibitory avoidance learning and required for long-term memory. *Learn Mem* 2007, 14:655–64.

[37] Saroja SR, Sase A, Kircher SG, Wan J, Berger J, Höger H, Pollak A, Lubec G: Hippocampal proteoglycans brevican and versican are linked to spatial memory of Sprague–Dawley rats in the morris water maze. *J Neurochem* 2014, 130:797–804.

[38] Hylin MJ, Orsi SA, Moore AN, Dash PK: Disruption of the perineuronal net in the hippocampus or medial prefrontal cortex impairs fear conditioning. *Learn Mem* 2013, 20:267–73.

[39] Brown TE, Forquer MR, Cocking DL, Jansen HT, Harding JW, Sorg BA: Role of matrix metalloproteinases in the acquisition and reconsolidation of cocaine-induced conditioned place preference. *Learn Mem* 2007, 14:214–23.

[40] Xue Y-X, Xue L-F, Liu J-F, He J, Deng J-H, Sun S-C, Han H-B, Luo Y-X, Xu L-Z, Wu P, Lu L: Depletion of perineuronal nets in the amygdala to enhance the erasure of drug memories. *J Neurosci* 2014, 34:6647–58.

[41] Slaker M, Churchill L, Todd RP, Blacktop JM, Zuloaga DG, Raber J, Darling RA, Brown TE, Sorg BA: Removal of perineuronal nets in the medial prefrontal cortex impairs the acquisition and reconsolidation of a cocaine-induced conditioned place preference memory. *J Neurosci Off J Soc Neurosci* 2015, 35:4190–202.

[42] Happel MFK, Niekisch H, Castiblanco Rivera LL, Ohl FW, Deliano M, Frischknecht R: Enhanced cognitive flexibility in reversal learning induced by removal of the extracellular matrix in auditory cortex. *Proc Natl Acad Sci USA* 2014, 111:2800–5.

[43] Romberg C, Yang S, Melani R, Andrews MR, Horner AE, Spillantini MG, Bussey TJ, Fawcett JW, Pizzorusso T, Saksida LM: Depletion of perineuronal nets enhances recognition memory and long-term depression in the perirhinal cortex. *J Neurosci* 2013, 33:7057–65.

[44] Tsien RY: Very long-term memories may be stored in the pattern of holes in the perineuronal net. *Proc Natl Acad Sci USA* 2013, 110:12456–61.

[45] Bikbaev A, Frischknecht R, Heine M: Brain extracellular matrix retains connectivity in neuronal networks. *Sci Rep* 2015, 5:14527.

[46] Senkov O, Andjus P, Radenovic L, Soriano E, Dityatev A: Neural ECM molecules in synaptic plasticity, learning, and memory. *Prog Brain Res* 2014, 214(January 2016):53–80.

[47] Cichon S, Mühleisen TW, Degenhardt FA, Mattheisen M, Miró X, Strohmaier J, Steffens M, Meesters C, Herms S, Weingarten M, Priebe L, Haenisch B, Alexander M, Vollmer J, Breuer R, Schmäl C, Tessmann P, Moebus S, Wichmann HE, Schreiber S, Müller-Myhsok B, Lucae S, Jamain S, Leboyer M, Bellivier F, Etain B, Henry C, Kahn JP, Heath S, Hamshere M, et al.: Genome-wide association study identifies genetic variation in neurocan as a susceptibility factor for bipolar disorder. *Am J Hum Genet* 2011, 88:372–81.

[48] Végh MJ, Heldring CM, Kamphuis W, Hijazi S, Timmerman AJ, Li K, van Nierop P, Mansvelder HD, Hol EM, Smit AB, van Kesteren RE: Reducing hippocampal extracel-

lular matrix reverses early memory deficits in a mouse model of Alzheimer's disease. *Acta Neuropathol Commun* 2014, 2:76.

[49] Nielsen HM, Palmqvist S, Minthon L, Londos E, Wennstrom M: Gender-dependent levels of hyaluronic acid in cerebrospinal fluid of patients with neurodegenerative dementia. *Curr Alzheimer Res* 2012, 9:257–66.

[50] Asahina M, Yoshiyama Y, Hattori T: Expression of matrix metalloproteinase-9 and urinary-type plasminogen activator in Alzheimer's disease brain. *Clin Neuropathol* 2001, 20:60–3.

[51] Backstrom JR, Lim GP, Cullen MJ, Tökés ZA: Matrix metalloproteinase-9 (MMP-9) is synthesized in neurons of the human hippocampus and is capable of degrading the amyloid-beta peptide (1–40). *J Neurosci* 1996, 16:7910–9.

[52] Mizoguchi H, Yamada K, Nabeshima T: Matrix metalloproteinases contribute to neuronal dysfunction in animal models of drug dependence, Alzheimer's disease, and epilepsy. *Biochem Res Int* 2011, 2011:681385.

3

Development of Human Pancreatic Innervation

Alexandra E. Proshchina, Yuliya S. Krivova, Olga G. Leonova, Valeriy M. Barabanov and Sergey V. Saveliev

Abstract

Human pancreatic innervation is of particular interest due to its possible role in the pathogenesis of such diseases as diabetes mellitus, pancreatitis and pancreatic cancer. Despite the clinical importance, data concerning pancreatic innervation during human ontogeny and in various disorders are very limited. In this chapter, we present a review on human pancreatic autonomic innervation on the basis of the literature data and our previous results. Special attention is paid to the innervation of the endocrine pancreas. Gradual branching of neural network was seen during human pancreatic development. Innervation of the foetal pancreas is more abundant than in adults. In agreement with previous observations, we have revealed a close integration and similarity between endocrine cells and nervous elements in the developing human pancreas. Moreover, simultaneous interactions between the nervous system components, epithelial cells and endocrine cells were detected in the pancreas during prenatal human development. It has been suggested that pancreatic innervation plays an important role not only in regulation of endocrine and exocrine activity but also in normal islet morphogenesis.

Keywords: pancreatic innervation, islets of Langerhans, human development, sympathetic system, parasympathetic system

1. Introduction

The pancreas of most vertebrates is an organ that combines both endocrine and exocrine functions. Functions of the exocrine pancreas are the synthesis, accumulation and secretion of digestive enzymes (protease, amylase, lipase and nucleases) and preferment (elastase, procarboxypeptidase, trypsinogen, pepsinogen, deoxyribonuclease and ribonuclease). The main function of the endocrine pancreas is regulation of carbohydrate metabolism. Specialised endocrine cells are grouped in units called pancreatic islets or islets of Langerhans. Islets of mammals (including humans) contain four major types of endocrine cells: beta cells secreting insulin, alpha cells secreting glucagon, delta cells secreting somatostatin and PP cells that synthesise pancreatic polypeptide [1]. Recently, another type of pancreatic endocrine cells was described—ghrelin-containing cells (epsilon cells) [2]. Pancreatic innervation is of interest due to its role in the pathogenesis of some diseases including chronic pancreatitis, pancreatic cancer and type 1 diabetes. Pain is the dominant clinical symptom in the majority of cases (73–93%) in patients with pancreatic cancer and pancreatitis. At the same time, the aetiology and pathogenesis of pain in chronic pancreatitis and pancreatic cancer are still unclear and are the subject of numerous studies [3].

In experiments on rodents (mice and rats) and cell cultures, it was indicated that nerve fibres and glial cells located in pancreatic islets may be the first target of autoimmune attack in type 1 diabetes [4–7]. Recently, there were reports of involvement of the peripheral nervous system in the pathogenesis of types 1 and 2 diabetes in humans [8, 9]. Moreover, the participation of the nervous system in the regulation of maturation, level of proliferation and number of insulin-producing beta cells, both in prenatal pancreatic development and in the postnatal period, was indicated in a number of experimental studies. Therefore, detailed information about the innervation of the endocrine pancreas is needed for understanding the mechanisms of beta cell pool renewal.

The pancreas is well innervated by the autonomic nervous system in various mammalian species [3, 10–15]. Rich innervation of the blood vessels and the exocrine part of the pancreas as well a more abundant innervation of the islets compared with the surrounding acinar part was detected already in the early studies [16, 17].

Connections between neurons are usually studied using anterograde and retrograde labelling of pathways. Pancreatic innervation was studied in various animal species using different tracing methods involving viruses, cholera toxin B, horseradish peroxidase, True Blue or DiI. It is believed that nerve fibres enter (and exit) in the pancreas as a part of neurovascular trunks. Within the pancreas, they also pass along the blood vessels and terminate (or, conversely, begin) near to the capillary wall and endocrine cells [18]. At the same time, they do not form classical synapses with target cells, but release neurotransmitters into the intercellular space, thus affecting more than one target simultaneously (i.e. they are enpassant synapses) [14]. Using retrograde labelling, the connection of pancreatic innervation with the central parasympathetic and sympathetic neurons in the brain stem, midbrain, hypothalamus and forebrain was shown [19–21]. Some of these brain centres are involved in monitoring of food intake or circadian rhythms, and it would be logical to assume that they send signals to the pancreas to adapt the digestive ferments and pancreatic hormone secretion to behavioural status. However, the central regulation of these processes has not yet been sufficiently studied [14].

In the pancreas, nerve endings were shown around blood vessels, as well as pancreatic acinar, ductal and endocrine cells, using immunohistochemistry and electron microscopy [17, 18]. Four types of plexuses (perivascular, periductal, periacinar and peri-insular) have been identified in the mouse pancreas [18]. Similar data were obtained in studies on the pancreas of the rat and nutria [22, 23]. One of the most interesting features of the mammalian pancreas is that endocrine cells may form highly organised complexes with structures of the nervous system, so-called neuro-insular complexes (NICs). The structure of NIC in the human pancreas has not been studied in detail since their first description by van Campenhout [24] and Simard [25]. Fujita described two types of NIC, which he observed in the foetal and adult pancreas of the dog, cat and rabbit [26]. Some of the pancreatic ganglia contained endocrine cells forming NIC type I (NIC I). In NIC type II (NIC II), endocrine cells lie on the surface of, or even in the midst of, the nerve bundle. However, the distinction between these two types of complexes is conditional because there is an intermediate type of complex in which islets associate with nerve cells and nerve fibres simultaneously. Thus, in the pancreas, endocrine islets are closely associated with a dispersed neural network, which consists of autonomic nerves including sympathetic, parasympathetic and sensory nerves. Unfortunately, because of depth limitations in microscopy, this network cannot be easily portrayed by standard microtome-based two-dimensional (2D) histology. The systematic development of three-dimensional (3D) islet neurohistology has provided insight into neural-islet regulatory mechanisms and the role of neural tissue remodelling in the development of diabetes [27–29].

In addition, endocrine cells of pancreatic islets are similar to nervous cells in some biochemical and physiological characteristics. Some proteins expressed in endocrine cells of pancreatic islets are also specific to the nervous system: S100, GFAP (glial fibrillary acidic protein), GAD (glutamic acid decarboxylase), TH (tyrosine hydroxylase), NPY (neuropeptide Y), NSE (neuron-specific enolase) and others [6, 7, 30–32]. Moreover, a number of transcription factors that are characteristic of the nervous system, such as Ngn3 (neurogenin3), BETA2/NEUROD, etc., are expressed during the differentiation of pancreatic endocrine cells [33–35]. The cells of the endocrine pancreas are classified as cells of a dispersed (diffuse) endocrine epithelial system. The cells of the dispersed endocrine system are a part of the so-called APUD (amine precursor uptake and decarboxylation) system [36]. These cells have the combined ability to the capture and deposit amine precursors and synthesise biogenic amines. The obvious similarity between the pancreatic endocrine cells and nerve tissue leaves the issue of its causes open to discuss.

The precise innervation patterns of islets are unknown, particularly in humans [37]. Every year reviews are published, in which morphology and function of pancreatic innervation are discussed (see for review [10, 11, 14, 15, 38–40]). However, the nature and distribution of the nervous system structures in the pancreas were studied mainly in rodents. Interspecies differences in the structure and innervation of the pancreas between humans and experimental animals (mice and rats) are quite large. In humans, the pancreas is a compact organ, while in rodents it is treelike, distributed over the mesentery of the small intestine. Therefore, it is impossible to automatically transfer the data obtained on experimental animals to humans.

In addition, knowledge about the dynamics of innervation during ontogenesis and in various diseases of the pancreas is very limited. Single studies are devoted to the formation of innervation in prenatal human development (mainly in the last century, without the use of modern methods). Therefore, the fine details of pancreatic innervation (such as the distribution of sympathetic and parasympathetic fibres and the formation of neuro-insular complexes) in human ontogenesis are insufficiently studied. This is mainly due to the inaccessibility of the material and to a number of technical difficulties, including the quality of pancreatic autopsy samples due to the activity of enzymes of the exocrine part [40].

However, over the past 10 years, different groups of researchers have made significant progress in the study of the peculiarities of innervation in rodents. The most attention was paid to the influence of the nervous system on the endocrine pancreas. It has been shown that both sympathetic and parasympathetic nervous systems affect postnatal development of the endocrine pancreas and its plasticity in adult animals [9, 41]. For example, after vagotomy there was a decrease in insulin-containing cell proliferation in mice and rats [42]. The important role of the sympathetic innervation for the formation of islet cytoarchitecture and their functional maturation during development was also shown [43].

Thanks to recent progresses in the field of islet research (including the study of isolated islets, in thick slices and in vivo), a number of issues concerning the structure and functions of pancreatic innervation have been clarified (see, e.g. [44–47]). In this chapter, we summarise the literature data and our previous results concerning the morphological organisation of autonomic innervation in the human foetal and adult pancreas. We also discuss the possible role of the close integration between the nervous system and epithelial and endocrine cells in the development of the endocrine pancreas.

2. Sources of pancreatic innervation

The pancreas is innervated by sympathetic and parasympathetic nerve fibres [11, 13]. The literature data indicate poor innervation of adult human pancreatic islets in comparison with rodents [44, 48–50]. At the end of the twentieth century, pancreatic innervation by postganglionic adrenergic and cholinergic fibres was intensively studied (for references, see [51]). Single nerve cells and nerve ganglia, both myelinated and unmyelinated nerve fibres of various diameters, have been detected in the human pancreas [23, 37, 48, 49]. In a simplified form, it can be considered that pancreatic sympathetic innervation is effected by the fibres of the ventral trunk and the parasympathetic innervation by the vagus nerve.

2.1. Efferent sympathetic fibres

Bodies of neurons, which form the efferent preganglionic sympathetic nerve fibres, are localised in the thoracic and upper lumbar segments of the spinal cord (T5–L1) [37, 52] or, according to some literature, in C8–L3 [21, 53]. Myelinated axons of these cells leave the ventral roots of the spinal cord and terminate on the bodies of neurons that lie in the ganglia of the paravertebral sympathetic chain, or pass through this chain via the n. splanchnicus to the celiac (*celiac*) and superior mesenteric (*mesenteric*) ganglia, and then terminate on neurons localised in these ganglia [54, 55]. The preganglionic fibres of the sympathetic system secrete acetylcholine (Ach). Postganglionic nerve fibres go to the pancreas, where they secrete norepinephrine, which binds to α and β adrenergic receptors and the neuropeptides galanin and NPY (neuropeptide Y) [10, 11, 53, 56].

In humans, the body and tail of the pancreas are innervated by nerve fibres originating from the ventral plexus and accompanying two arteries: the splenic artery and the transverse artery of the pancreas. The pancreatic head receives the largest number of nerve fibres [57, 58].

In the exocrine pancreas, sympathetic axons contact mostly with intrapancreatic ganglia, blood vessels and ducts. In mice, the innervation of the exocrine part is less pronounced than in humans. The major nerves run along the interlobular arteries and form the peri-insular plexus [18]. At the same time, in mice axons of sympathetic nerves contact alpha cells, while contact with beta cells is not found [44]. The axons of sympathetic nerves also innervate smooth muscle cells and pericytes of blood vessels and perivascular space, forming the so-called sympathetic neurovascular complex. In humans, sympathetic fibres innervate smooth muscle cells and pericytes and rarely contact directly with the endocrine cells. Apparently, the effects of the sympathetic innervation are likely mediated through indirect effects on local blood flow within the islet microcirculation [44, 59].

2.2. Efferent parasympathetic fibres

The bodies of the neurons forming the parasympathetic preganglionic nerve fibres lie in the dorsal motor nucleus of the n. vagus (X) [60–62] and, possibly, in the *nucleus ambiguus* [11–13]. Both of these nuclei are under the control of the hypothalamus. Preganglionic parasympathetic fibres are directed to the pancreas as a part of the vagus nerve branches. In the pancreas, parasympathetic fibres terminate on the bodies of parasympathetic neurons lying in intrapancreatic ganglia [38, 63]. These ganglia contain from 3 to 30 neurons and are usually located in intralobular connective tissue, within lobules or in close proximity to islets [13, 27, 29]. It is also important that these ganglia receive input not only from the parasympathetic nervous system but also from the sympathetic nervous system, as well as fibres from other intrapancreatic ganglia and also from the *myenteric plexus* [13]. Parasympathetic fibres are also involved in the formation of nerve plexuses around the arteries and mingle with sympathetic fibres.

Preganglionic parasympathetic fibres secrete acetylcholine (Ach), which binds to nicotine receptors on the membranes of neurons [53]. Short, unmyelinated postganglionic fibres terminate on the epithelial cells of acini and ducts, smooth muscle cells and islet cells. Postganglionic parasympathetic fibres release several neurotransmitters (Ach (acetylcholine) and NO (nitric oxide)) and neuropeptides (VIP (vasoactive intestinal peptide), GRP (gastrin-releasing peptide) and PACAP (pituitary-activating adenyl cyclase polypeptide)) [10, 11, 13, 56]. Postganglionic nerve fibres perform their functions mainly via Ach by binding to muscarinic receptors found, in particular, in the endocrine cells of the islets [12, 53]. In mice, postganglionic parasympathetic nerve fibres innervate all types of islets cells [10, 11, 44]. Recently, it was found that parasympathetic islet innervation in humans differs from that in mice: first, it was shown that only a small number of fibres penetrate inside the islets (most of the axons terminate in the exocrine part of the pancreas) [44], and, secondly, it was recently shown that stimulation with Ach mostly stimulates beta and delta cells, whereas alpha cells react to a lesser extent [64]. Interestingly, alpha cells themselves may be the primary source of Ach in human islets [45]. Apparently, in human islets, this classical neurotransmitter regulates the activity of other cell types in a paracrine manner. However, now, this concept is again under revision thanks recently to the work of Tang et al. [29].

2.3. The afferent fibres

In the pancreas, there are afferent (sensory) nerve fibres in addition to efferent sympathetic and parasympathetic innervation [10–12, 53, 54]. Bundles of sensory nerve fibres leave the pancreas and follow the sympathetic (*n. splanchnicus*) and vagus nerves. The bodies of sensory sympathetic neurons are localised in the ganglia of the dorsal roots in the spinal cord, mainly at the level of the lower thoracic segments (the so-called spinal afferents) projected on interneuron plates I and IV [52, 65]. For the parasympathetic system, the bodies of afferent neurons are localised in the ganglion nodosum, sending information to the nucleus of tractus solitarii [12, 54]. The neurotransmitters of the sensory nerve fibres are CGRP (calcitonin gene-related peptide) and SP (substance P). Most sympathetic and parasympathetic afferent nerves are sensitive to capsaicin [14]. Capsaicin (vanillin) receptors mainly transmit pain information [66]. In addition, Pacinian corpuscles were described in the pancreas of various mammalian species. The suggested function of this receptor is to transmit information about pressure and vibration stimuli. In the human pancreas, they were discovered in the early twentieth century [67]. Despite this fact being presented in many histology textbooks, in the modern literature, only three cases of these findings (all in pancreatic cancer) were described [67, 68]. In our research, we have studied pancreatic autopsies of 42 foetuses and neonates aged from the 10th to 40th week of gestation and of 65 adults, 18 of whom suffered from diabetes mellitus type 2. In total, more than 1000 sections were investigated. However, Pacinian corpuscles are a rare finding in the human pancreas: we were able to detect Pacinian corpuscles only in one pancreatic section of a newborn with diagnosed diabetic fetopathy. Thus, Pacinian corpuscles do not appear to play a significant role in the sensory innervation of the human pancreas.

2.4. Enteric nervous system

In some studies on pancreatic innervation, it is assumed that the pancreas is innervated not only by extrinsic efferent and afferent nerves but also by intrinsic enteric neurons of the so-called enteric nervous system (ENS) [12, 69]. The ENS controls the motor, secretion and other functions of the gastrointestinal tract and is closely related with the diffuse endocrine system [70]. Enteric ganglia have some morphological and functional differences from sympathetic and parasympathetic ganglia:

1. The ENS performs complex integrative functions independently of higher nerve centres.
2. In the ENS, a large number of various neurotransmitters, many of which are characteristic of the central nervous system, are produce.
3. Unlike other autonomous ganglia, enteric ganglia do not contain connective tissue and blood vessels. Enteric ganglia are demarcated from the surrounding tissue of the so-called blood-ganglionic barrier, similar to the blood–brain barrier. It is insufficiently studied, and not all researchers agree with its existence.
4. Glial cells of enteric ganglia are similar in morphology, cell markers and functions with astrocytes of the CNS.

The complex structure of the enteric nervous system, containing a variety of morphological and functional types of neurons and their neurotransmitters, allows the ENS to perform complex reflex acts, some of which are implemented autonomously and some in interaction with the central nervous system and other parts of the autonomous nervous system. Intrapancreatic ganglia are connected with autonomous ganglia in the intestinal nerve plexus [71–73]. Neurotransmitters for neurons of these ganglia are, among others, serotonin and nitric oxide (NO) [73]. However, according the dominant viewpoint, intramural pancreatic neurons belong to the parasympathetic system.

3. Functional role of pancreatic innervation

As was mentioned earlier, the pancreas combines exo- and endocrine functions, secreting digestive enzymes and hormones, which regulate glucose homeostasis. The nervous system regulates the activity of both the endocrine and exocrine pancreas. However, it is problematic to separate the innervation of the pancreatic endocrine part from the innervation of the exocrine, since the tracing method used for this purpose belongs to the pancreas as a whole. In addition, the activity of both endocrine and exocrine parts of the pancreas depends on food intake. Therefore, it is not surprising that the cephalic phase has been described for both pancreatic parts. Although the stimulation of the ventromedial hypothalamus and efferent sympathetic and parasympathetic neurons affects the secretion of islet hormones (see below), it is unknown whether this stimulation is direct through axons innervating the islet or indirect by activating other organs, which affect insulin and glucagon secretion [14]. Moreover, it is very difficult to separate the nervous system effects from other (e.g. humoral) influences.

So, in the laboratory of I.P. Pavlov, in 1895, I.L. Dolinsky conducted an experiment in which he established that acid injection into the duodenum causes a release of pancreatic juice [74]. In 1901, British physiologists William Baileys and Ernest Starling concluded that there is some substance released by the duodenum that stimulates secretion by the pancreas. In the following year, 1902, this substance was discovered and named secretin. Secretin was the first such "chemical messenger" identified. This type of substance is now called a hormone.

At the same time, in the classic studies of I. P. Pavlov with M. A. Afanasiev, the nervous mechanism of pancreatic secretion was found. In the work "On secretory nerves of the pancreas" (1877), they showed that vagus nerve stimulation causes pancreatic secretion. Moreover, I. P. Pavlov with his colleagues detected that imaginary feeding in animals with chronic pancreatic fistula causes an abundant release of pancreatic juice. Later, this was confirmed by the studies of K. M. Bykov and G. M. Davydov in patients with pancreatic fistula. An abundant pancreatic juice released by this patient occurred while talking about delicious food [74]. However, pancreatic juice obtained after vagus nerve stimulation is released in a small quantity and is rich in proteins and enzymes, whereas after the secretin injection, it contains little proteins and enzymes and is released in large quantities [74]. It should be noted that both these factors (nervous and humoral) act simultaneously and synergistically.

Currently, it is considered that efferent sympathetic nerve fibres indirectly inhibit the release of enzymes of the exocrine pancreas by suppressing the stimulating effects of ganglia and constriction of vessels (vasoconstriction), thereby reducing blood flow [13, 59]. The stimulation of short, unmyelinated postganglionic parasympathetic fibres increases release from secretory cells of the exocrine pancreas and ducts causing vasodilation [13, 57].

The autonomous nervous system also regulates hormone release in the endocrine pancreas, thereby affecting glucose metabolism [10, 11, 14, 53]. Many various chemical factors affect insulin and glucagon expression. Auto-, juxta-, para- and endocrine ways potentially regulate secretion of islet hormones. Since the classical studies of Claude Bernard, which showed that injection into the floor of the fourth ventricle causes hyperglycemia, the involvement of the nervous system in the regulation of pancreatic endocrine function and metabolic control has been shown in many studies. It is, therefore, rather difficult to separate one effect from the other [14, 53].

The cellular architecture of islets affects paracrine regulation and synchronises the release of insulin [75]. All pancreatic islets secrete hormones consistently, with an approximately 5-min interval [76]. In order to create this secretion pattern, the activity of insulin-containing beta cells must be consistent both within the individual islet and between the islets [14]. At the same time, the secretory activity of other islets endocrine cells, such as glucagon-secreting alpha cells that have opposite effects on glucose homeostasis, should be consistent with the activity of beta cells. Thanks to this interaction, endocrine cells can simultaneously send signals regulating the effective delivery of islet hormones into the circulatory system and, ultimately, to the liver, regulating the maintenance of glucose homeostasis [76].

However, the islets of Langerhans are a part of a complex coherent system. They are also exposed to humoral factors such as circulating plasma hormones (e.g. epinephrine). The brain also regulates the secretion of islet hormones via the autonomic nervous system [14]. Thus, in works by Akmaev et al. [19], it was shown that the hypothalamus is able to stimulate insulin secretion from beta cells of pancreatic islets along the nerve pathway, which was named "paraventricular-vagal." This pathway starts from small neurons of the paraventricular nucleus (PVN) of the hypothalamus, synaptically switches in the medulla oblongata to neurons of the dorsal nucleus of the vagus nerve and reaches the pancreatic islets in the composition of the vagus nerve. In this pathway, beta cells receive stimulating signals. Inhibitory signals come from neurons by a humoral way: PVN neurons secrete corticotropin-releasing hormone, which stimulates the secretion of adrenocorticotropic hormone in the pituitary gland that induces the secretion of glucocorticoids in the adrenal cortex. Glucocorticoids inhibit insulin release from beta cells. This kind of double control, according to the authors, is typical for the regulation of endocrine functions. Recently, there has been data that significantly complements this concept: various areas of the hypothalamus have different effects on the secretion of insulin and/or glucagon [77]. So, a detailed study of this system is needed to further identify both neurons and functionally related projections of the central nervous system regulating islet functions.

For most species studied, it is characteristic that nerve fibres are localised mainly at the periphery of the pancreatic islets, forming a peri-insular nervous network [17]. Only single nerve fibres are detected within islets. The bodies of ganglion neurons are also rarely localised in the pancreatic islets and may be in direct contact with endocrine cells [17, 27, 29, 78, 79].

It is believed that autonomic innervations indirectly affect the release of insulin in the cephalic phase during food intake and also take part in the increase of glucagon and decrease of insulin release by sympathetic stimulation [10, 80]. Stimulation of the splanchnic nerve increases the release of glucagon and reduces the release of insulin and somatostatin from endocrine cells of the pancreas [12, 14, 15]. Sympathetic nerves are also believed to be involved in islet response for hypoglycemia, which includes increased glucagon secretion and inhibition of insulin secretion. The general sympathetic effect is expressed by reducing the insulin concentration in plasma (by increasing the concentration of catecholamines that inhibit insulin secretion) [10, 11].

Parasympathetic nerves are responsible for the early phase of insulin secretion, including the cephalic phase (i.e. insulin secretion, which occurs during anticipation of eating). In general, parasympathetic stimulation is believed to increase the release of insulin, glucagon, somatostatin and pancreatic polypeptide in many different species (for review, see [10, 11, 14, 15]).

Sensory nerves are also involved in the regulation of hormone secretion by endocrine cells [11]. Following chemical destruction of sensory nerves (capsaicin treatment) in mice, there is an increase in insulin secretion in response to glucose compared to control [81].

In conclusion, it should be added that pancreatic innervation is insufficiently studied, especially in humans [40, 44]. Interestingly, the innervation of the islets is very plastic: it has been shown that islets transplanted into the portal vein of diabetic rats were reinnervated by the nerves of the liver [82]. This makes it necessary to further study the role of innervation in the regulation of glucose homeostasis and plasticity of the endocrine part of the pancreas.

4. Pancreatic innervation during prenatal development

Despite the clinical importance, data concerning pancreatic innervation during human ontogeny and in diseases are very limited [37]. Such studies have been performed on rodents and mostly concern the sympathetic innervation [43, 55, 83]. The embryonic sources of neural elements are fibres of the vagus (*n. vagus*) and splanchnic nerves (*n. splanchnicus*) growing into the developing pancreas and neurons that differentiate from the neural crest cells migrating to the pancreas. Sympathetic fibres innervate the developing mouse pancreas starting from the 15th day of embryonic development (E14.5) [43]. Consequently, the degree of sympathetic innervation increases until 20 days of postnatal development (P20) [55]. The development of the pancreatic sympathetic innervation depends on nerve growth factor (NGF) [43].

The human pancreas receives extensive innervation, showing peculiar growth dynamics during gestation [37]. Ingrowths of nerves in the human pancreas start at 6 weeks of development. Further morphogenesis of pancreatic innervation is characterised by the increase of sources of innervation and degree of nervous element differentiation [84, 85]. Large bundles of nerve fibres and groups of poorly differentiated neurons are found in the human pancreas starting from the 8th week of development. At the end of the 9th week, the pancreas is innervated from almost all sources, characteristic of adults (celiac plexus, superior mesenteric plexus and posterior vagal trunk) [85]. In 1940, it was shown that pancreatic nerve cells migrate from the solar plexus and from ganglia located in the wall of the duodenum and along the branches of the vagus nerve (mainly right). At the same time, neuroblasts were detected in the pancreas of 20-week-old foetuses. Moreover, even in newborns pancreatic nerve cells were neuroblastic [86].

The gradual branching of the vascular and neural networks is observed in the human pancreatic development. Primitive free nerve endings are detected starting from the 12th week of development. In an immunohistochemical study of pancreatic innervation development in human foetuses, two peaks of increase in the number of structures of the nervous system in the head of the gland were revealed at the 14th and 22th weeks. In the pancreatic body and tail, the number of nerve structures increases from the 20th week [37]. By 30–32 weeks of development, the density of nerve endings is reduced compared to previous periods [85]. The innervation of pancreatic islets in humans is formed from the 14 to 15th weeks of the development. It differs from experimental mammals (rodents): the development of pancreatic islet innervation in rodents (mouse, Mongolian gerbil and golden hamster) is observed in the first weeks after birth [83, 87, 88].

Our study was performed on a collection of pancreatic autopsies, which allows us to explore the features of intrapancreatic innervation directly in humans using a variety of methods: classical histology; immunohistochemistry; light, fluorescent and confocal microscopy; morpho- and stereometry; statistical analysis; 3D histology; and computer reconstruction. The study was performed on 50 pancreatic autopsies of foetuses from the 10th to 40th gestational week (g.w.). Foetal pancreatic autopsies were divided into four groups according to the classification of the foetal period: pre-foetal period (10–12 g.w.), early foetal period (13–20 g.w.), middle foetal period (21–28 g.w.) and late foetal period (29–40 g.w.). A panel of antibodies for nervous system proteins (chromogranin A, neuron-specific enolase (NSE), neural cell adhesion molecule (NCAM), synaptosomal-associated protein of 25 kDa (SNAP-25, peripherin, S100 protein and neuron-specific class III β-tubulin), endocrine cell hormones (insulin, glucagon and somatostatin) and epithelial cells (cytokeratin 19 (CK19)) were used in this work [89, 90]. We generated new data concerning the spatio-temporal distribution of the innervation in the human pancreas during prenatal development.

In the pre-foetal period (10–12 g.w.), large weakly branched bundles of nerve fibres and nerve ganglia were detected already at the 10th week of gestational development using antibodies to NSE, NCAM and neuron-specific β-III tubulin (**Table 1**). The largest bundles of nerve fibres were detected in the dense peri-pancreatic mesenchyme, and the group of neurons and bundles of nerve fibres of smaller diameter were located in the loose mesenchyme between pancreatic ducts (**Figure 1a**). A network of fine nerve fibres was not developed. In some cases, bundles of nerve fibres were found near large vessels. Nerve ganglia in the pancreas of 10–12 week foetuses were small groups of cells.

Starting from 12 weeks, cells immunopositive for antibodies to S100 protein were found in nervous system structures. Localisation of neuromarkers was different. In the nerves, NSE-positive

Markers	NSE	NCAM	Neuron-specific β-III tubulin	S100 protein	Chromogranin A	SNAP-25	Peripherin
Nerve fibres and ganglions	10 weeks	10 weeks	10 weeks	12 weeks	14 weeks (weak staining)	14 weeks	14 weeks
Endocrine cells	12 weeks	14 weeks	14 weeks	15–16 weeks (some islets cells)	12 weeks	16 weeks	—

Table 1. Appearance of immunopositive reactions to neural proteins in the developing human pancreas.

fibres formed the core, while small S100-positive cells surrounded them. The ganglionic cells were NSE-positive, and the small cells surrounding them S100-positive. The bodies of ganglion neurons were immunonegative to S100, that is, the positive reaction to S100 protein was observed in satellite cells of intrapancreatic ganglia and in Schwann cells of nerve fibre bundles, while NSE was detected in neuronal bodies and processes. In addition, NSE- and chromogranin A-positive endocrine cells were first found in 12-week foetuses (**Table 1**).

The formation of the human pancreatic islets starts only at 12 weeks of development. In the pre-foetal period, only contacts between single endocrine cells or small groups and fine nerve fibres were detected, and classical NIC I and NIC II were not found. At gestational week 10 (postconception week 8), thickening of the ductal epithelial layer was found, in which endocrine cells were concentrated forming "buds" on pancreatic ducts. As development proceeds, buds containing different types of endocrine cells separate from the ducts forming small clusters or mantle-type islets. In our studies, contacts between the structures of the nervous system and epithelial cells of primitive ducts were detected in the foetal pancreas at early stages of development (10–13 weeks) before the formation of islets.

The formation of the pancreatic lobules begins in the early foetal period, from 13 weeks. At the same time, active formation of the islets of Langerhans and innervation of the endocrine part starts (**Figure 1b**). Nervous system of the pancreas of 14–15 week foetuses becomes more branched in comparison with 10–12 weeks of development. Large bundles of nerve fibres are localised in the connective tissue of gland's capsule. Smaller nerves pass into the interlobular connective tissue separately or along the blood vessels. Nerve fibres and ganglia are first found within the lobules. At the 16th week of development, the nervous apparatus of the pancreas is presented by bundles of nerve fibres of different diameters and nerve ganglia, which are located in the interlobular connective tissue and within the lobules. The nerve fibres connecting two nerve ganglia were found in 14–15 week foetuses, i.e. the first clearly detected integration of the nervous system structures was shown.

Localisation of antigens in the structures of the nervous system was also similar with the pre-foetal period. In addition, the immunopositive cells for chromogranin A, SNAP-25 and peripherin were detected in the nerve fibres and ganglia starting from 14 to 15 weeks of the development (**Table 1**). SNAP-25, NCAM, NSE, peripherin and neuron-specific β-III tubulin

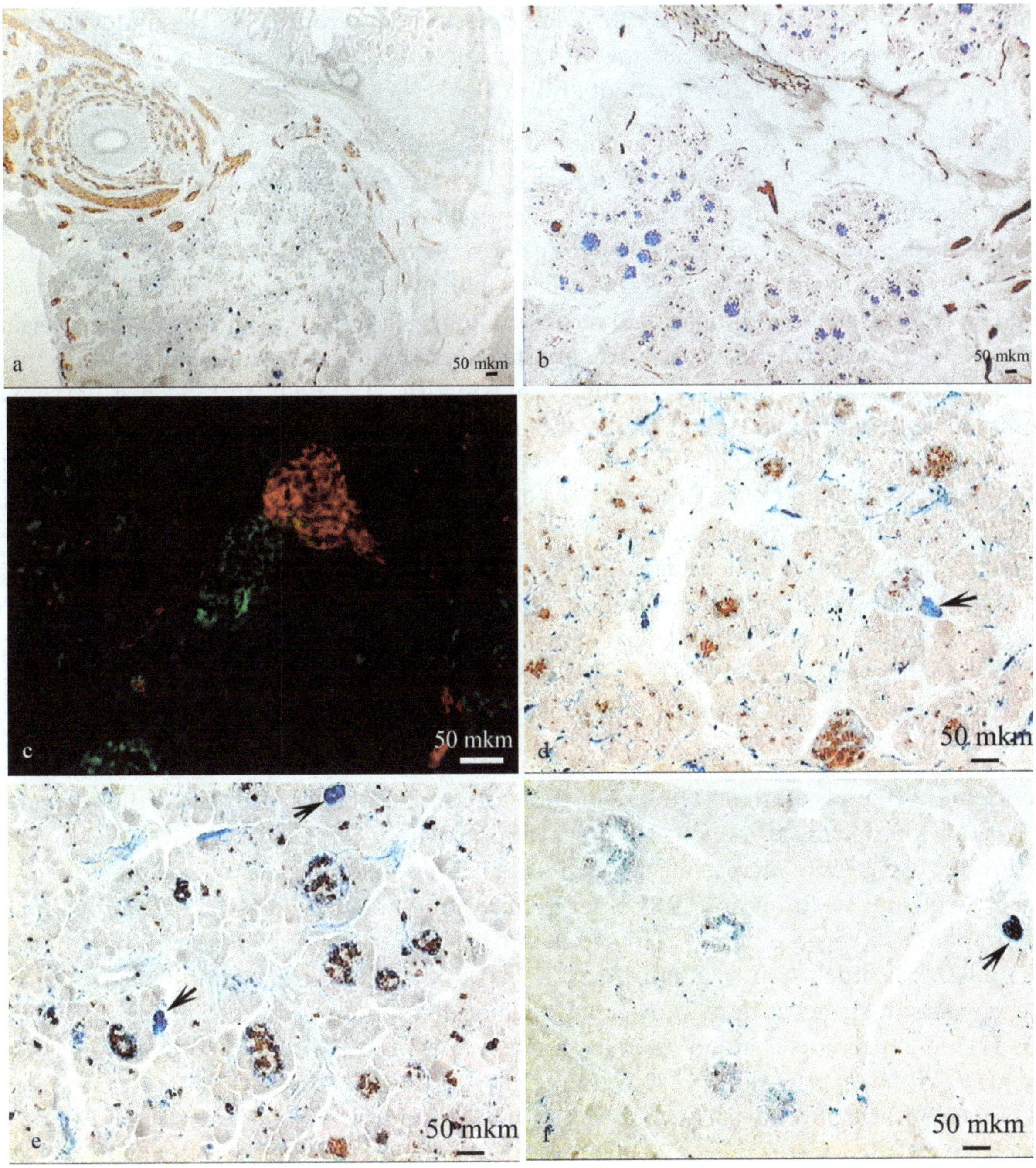

Figure 1. Spatio-temporal distribution of the nervous system structures in the human pancreas during ontogenesis. (a, b, d–f) double immunohistochemistry on the pancreatic slices of foetuses ((a) 12 g.w., (b) 16 g.w., (d) 28 g.w.), child ((e) 3 months) and adult ((f) 88 years): (a, b) insulin (blue) + S100 (red), (d, e) insulin (red)+ NSE (blue) and (f) glucagon (red) + NSE (blue). Arrows indicate some ganglia. (c) Stack of serial immunofluorescence images of NIC in the foetal pancreas (20 g.w.) (sum thickness of slices 90 mkm): Glucagon (green) + S100 (red).

were detected in bundles of nerve fibres of different diameters and the bodies of neurons in human foetuses. However, there were fine nerve fibres located in the acinar parenchyma that were immunonegative for peripherin but reacted with other markers in all investigated cases. This suggests that nerve fibres of the human pancreas differ according to the set of expressed proteins. In addition, positive immunostaining for NCAM and neuron-specific β-III tubulin was observed in endocrine cells starting from 14 weeks of development, while SNAP-25-positive endocrine cells were detected only from 16 weeks of development. Immunopositivity to antibodies against S100 protein was found only in some islet cells starting from 15 to 16 weeks of development (**Table 1**).

The contacts of nerves fibres with endocrine cells were detected starting from 12 weeks of development. Already in the early foetal period, it was possible to identify NIC I (single insulin- or glucagon-containing cells in ganglia (Supplementary Video 1) or ganglia associated with the islets) and NIC II (single endocrine cells in the nerve (Supplementary Video 2), nerve endings associated with single endocrine cells or with the islets) and make their 3D reconstruction. The analysis of three-dimensional reconstructions allowed us to show ganglia associated with two islets at once, islets associated simultaneously with two ganglia, and NIC of mixed (intermediate) type [91]. Moreover, in the foetal pancreas, starting from 13 weeks, we showed simultaneously neuro-insular complexes and contacts between the structures of nervous system and epithelial cells located in ducts as well as in cell clusters that were often connected with the ducts. Based on these findings, we suggested that the development of neuro-insular complexes may be due to integration between the structures of the nervous system and epithelial progenitors at the initial stages of islet formation. Furthermore, endocrine cells are supposed to migrate along nerve fibres from the ducts, small clusters of endocrine cells and islets to the other islets, which are located a distance from pancreatic ducts, due to exocrine pancreatic growth, thus increasing their pool of endocrine cells. We suppose that the mechanism of pancreatic islet formation is similar to the formation of some peripheral analysers.

The pattern of immunoreactivity of neural markers during the middle (21–28 g.w.) and late foetal periods is similar to those in the early foetal period. In the middle of the foetal period, the density of pancreatic innervation is higher than in the early foetal period (**Figure 1c**, **d**). Despite increasing the size of pancreatic lobules and more sparse distribution of large and medium bundles of nerve fibres, the network of fine nerve fibres gradually branch and become denser. However, during late foetal and neonatal development, this network is much sparser (**Figure 1e**). This is due to the increase in the size of lobules. However, at all stages of human prenatal development, density of distribution of the nervous system structures is higher than in adults (**Figure 1f**). The density of NIC distribution also gradually decreases at birth. Our quantitative data indicate that the largest number of NIC I was observed in the early and middle foetal periods, during the active morphogenesis of pancreatic islets, whereas at birth (in the late foetal period) and in the adult, NIC II became more prevalent [91]. During the middle and late foetal periods, the nervous system components also contact epithelial cells located in ducts or in clusters outside the ductal epithelium and form complexes with separate epithelial cells. We observed CK19-positive cells inside the ganglia and nerve bundles, which were located separately or integrated within the islets [90].

In this study, our previous data were confirmed and refined [89] that the formation of the nervous system in the development of human pancreas can be divided into three stages. In the pre-foetal period, the nervous apparatus of the pancreas is represented by slightly branched bundles of nerve fibres and nerve ganglia. However, the structures of the nervous system differ from the late foetuses and adults by antigenic composition. Expression of various neural proteins does not begin simultaneously in the foetal pancreas.

The second stage of development of the nervous apparatus of the pancreas (during the early and middle foetal periods) is characterised by gradual branching of the neural network and formation of connections between the structures of the nervous system and exocrine and endocrine parts. In the early foetal period, nerve fibres gradually branch, nerve fibres and nerve ganglia appear localised between the acini, and a network of fine nerve fibres starts to form. In the later stages of development, the distribution of neural structures (nerve fibres, nerve ganglia and parenchymal network of fine nerve fibres) become sparser with increase in the size of the pancreas. Thus, innervation of the pancreas at this stage of development gradually becomes similar to the distribution structures of the nervous system in the adult pancreas.

In our studies, we demonstrated close integration between the structures of the nervous system and endocrine cells in the human pancreas, which were more frequently observed during prenatal development. Thus, a dense network is formed in the developing human pancreas, in which the structures of the nervous system are associated with the islets of Langerhans. The close relationship between developing islets and structures of the nervous system suggests that neuroendocrine interactions can influence not only the secretion of hormones but also to participate in the morphogenesis of the islets, presumably due to the participation in migration of endocrine cells from ducts to islets. Understanding the role of NICs in islet formation can lead to new approaches to understanding the mechanisms and treatment of diabetes.

5. Conclusions

Thus, our knowledge about the peripheral nervous system in the human pancreas is limited. Importantly, human islet development has not been examined for the presence of classical markers of the parasympathetic and sympathetic nervous systems. Furthermore, the exact location where neuronal axons terminate within the human islets in adults was not shown until recently.

However, the human pancreas is abundantly innervated during the gestational period. The value of such an abundant innervation of the pancreas and pancreatic islets, in particular, in human development is not clear. The observed differences between the nervous apparatus of foetuses and adults may have functional significance for pancreatic morphogenesis. Interestingly, some authors have described similar dynamics of innervation development in other internal human organs. The close relationship between the nervous and endocrine systems makes it necessary to further study the role of innervation in the plasticity of the endocrine pancreas both during formation of endocrine function and disorders of carbohydrate metabolism.

Acknowledgements

This work was supported by the Russian Foundation for Basic Research, project no. 18-015-00146.

Conflict of interest

The authors declare no competing interests.

Author details

Alexandra E. Proshchina[1]*, Yuliya S. Krivova[1], Olga G. Leonova[2], Valeriy M. Barabanov[1] and Sergey V. Saveliev[1]

*Address all correspondence to: proshchina@yandex.ru

1 Research Institute of Human Morphology, Moscow, Russia

2 Engelhardt Institute of Molecular Biology, Russian Academy of Sciences, Moscow, Russia

References

[1] Veld In't P, Marichal M. Microscopic anatomy of the human islet of Langerhans. In: Islam MS, editor. The Islets of Langerhans. Netherlands: Springer; 2010. pp. 1-19

[2] Wierup N, Sundler F, Heller RS. The islet ghrelin cell. Journal of Molecular Endocrinology. 2013;**52**(1):R35-R49. DOI: 10.1530/JME-13-0122

[3] Lindsay TH, Halvorson KG, Peters CM, Ghilardi JR, Kuskowsk MA, Wong GY, et al. A quantitative analysis of the sensory and sympathetic innervation of the mouse pancreas. Neuroscience. 2006;**137**(4):1417-1426. DOI: 10.1016/j.neuroscience.2005.10.055

[4] Mei Q, Mundinger TO, Lernmark A, Taborsky GJ Jr. Early, selective, and marked loss of sympathetic nerves from the islets of BioBreeder diabetic rats. Diabetes. 2002;**51**(10):2997-3002. DOI: 10.2337/diabetes.51.10.2997

[5] Razavi R, Chan Y, Afifiyan FN, Liu XJ, Wan X, Yantha J, Tsui H, Tang L, Tsai S, Santamaria P, Driver JP, Serreze D, Salter MW, Dosch HM. TRPV1+ sensory neurons control beta cell stress and islet inflammation in autoimmune diabetes. Cell. 2006;**127**(6):1123-1135. DOI: 10.1016/j.cell.2006.10.038

[6] Tsui H, Winer S, Chan Y, Truong D, Tang L, Yantha J, et al. Islet glia, neurons, and beta cells. Annals of the New York Academy of Sciences. 2008;**1150**(1):32-42. DOI: 10.1196/annals.1447.0330

[7] Winer S, Tsui H, Lau A, Song A, Li X, Cheung RK, et al. Autoimmune islet destruction in spontaneous type 1 diabetes is not beta-cell exclusive. Nature Medicine. 2003;**9**(2):198-205. DOI: 10.1038/nm818

[8] Mundinger TO, Mei Q, Foulis AK, Fligner CL, Hull RL, Taborsky GJ. Human type 1 diabetes is characterized by an early, marked, sustained and islet-selective loss of sympathetic nerves. Diabetes. 2016;**65**(8):2322-2330. DOI: 10.2337/db16-0284

[9] Thorens B. Neural regulation of pancreatic islet cell mass and function. Diabetes, Obesity & Metabolism. 2014;**16**(S1):87-95. DOI: 10.1111/dom.12346

[10] Ahren B. Autonomic regulation of islet hormone secretion–Implications for health and disease. Diabetologia. 2000;**43**(4):393-410. DOI: 10.1007/s001250051322

[11] Ahrén B. Islet nerves in focus—Defining their neurobiological and clinical role. Diabetologia. 2012;**55**(12):3152-3154. DOI: 10.1007/s00125-012-2727-6

[12] Gilon P, Henquin JC. Mechanism and physiological significance of the cholinergic control of pancreatic b-cell function. Endocrine Reviews. 2001;**22**(5):565-604. DOI: 10.1210/er.22.5.565

[13] Love JA, Yi E, Smith TG. Autonomic pathways regulating pancreatic exocrine secretion. Autonomic Neuroscience. 2007;**133**(1):19-34. DOI: 10.1016/j.autneu.2006.10.001

[14] Rodriguez-Diaz R, Caicedo A. Novel approaches to studying the role of innervation in the biology of pancreatic islets. Endocrinology and Metabolism Clinics of North America. 2013;**42**(1):39-56. DOI: 10.1016/j.ecl.2012.11.001

[15] Dolenšek J, Rupnik MS, Stožer A. Structural similarities and differences between the human and the mouse pancreas. Islets. 2015;**7**(1):e1024405. DOI: 10.1080/19382014.2015.1024405

[16] Coupland RE. The innervation of pancreas of the rat, cat and rabbit as revealed by the cholinesterase technique. Journal of Anatomy. 1958;**92**(1):143-149

[17] Sunami E, Kanazawa H, Hashizume H, Takeda M, Hatakeyama K, Ushiki T. Morphological characteristics of Schwann cells in the islets of Langerhans of the murine pancreas. Archives of Histology and Cytology. 2001;**64**(2):191-201. DOI: 10.1679/aohc.64.191

[18] Ushiki T, Watanabe S. Distribution and ultrastructure of the autonomic nerves in the mouse pancreas. Microscopy Research and Technique. 1997;**37**(5-6):399-406. DOI: 10.1002/(SICI)1097-0029(19970601)37:5/6<399::AID-JEMT4>3.0.CO;2-9

[19] Akmaev IG. Neuroimmunoendocrine aspects of the pathogenesis of diabetes mellitus [article in Russian]. Diabetes Mellitus. 2005;**3**:8-12

[20] Beall C, Ashford ML, McCrimmon RJ. The physiology and pathophysiology of the neural control of the counterregulatory response. American Journal of Physiology. Regulatory, Integrative and Comparative Physiology. 2012;**302**(2):R215-R223. DOI: 10.1152/ajpregu.00531.2011

[21] Osundiji MA, Evans ML. Brain control of insulin and glucagon secretion. Endocrinology and Metabolism Clinics of North America. 2013;**42**(1):1-14. DOI: 10.1016/j.ecl.2012.11.006

[22] Chumasov EI, Petrova ES, Korzhevskii DE. Distribution and structural organization of the autonomic nervous apparatus in the rat pancreas (an immunohistochemical

study). Neuroscience and Behavioral Physiology. 2012;**42**(8):781-788. DOI: 10.1007/s11055-012-9635-6

[23] Krivova IS, Barabanov VM, Savel'eva ES, Savel'ev SV. Neuroendocrine complexes in the pancreas of nutria (*Myocastor coypus*) (an immunohistochemical study) [article in Russian]. Morfologiia. 2009;**135**(3):59-62

[24] Van Campenhout E. Contributions a l'etude de l'histogenese du pancreas, chez quelques mammiferes. Les complexes sympathico-insulaires. [Contributions to the study of the histogenesis of the pancreas in some mammals. The sympathico-insular complex]. Archives de Biologie. 1927;**37**:121-171

[25] Simard LC. Les complecses neuro-insulaires. [The neuro-insular complex]. Archives d'anatomie microscopique. 1937;**33**:49-64

[26] Fujita T. Histological studies on the neuro-insular complex in the pancreas of some mammals. Zeitschrift fur Zellforschung und Mikroskopische Anatomie. 1959;**50**(1):94-109. DOI: 10.1007/bf00342656

[27] Tang SC, Shen CN, Lin PY, Peng SJ, Chien HJ, Chou YH, Chamberlain CE, Pasricha PJ. Pancreatic neuro-insular network in young mice revealed by 3D panoramic histology. Diabetologia. 2018;**61**(1):158-167. DOI: 10.1007/s00125-017-4408-y

[28] Chien HJ, Peng SJ, Hua TE, Kuo CH, Juang JH, Tang SC. 3-D imaging of islets in obesity: Formation of the islet-duct complex and neurovascular remodeling in young hyperphagic mice. International Journal of Obesity. 2015;**40**(4):685-697. DOI: 10.1038/ijo.2015.224

[29] Tang SC, Baeyens L, Shen CN, Peng SJ, Chien HJ, Scheel DW, Chamberlain CE, German MS. Human pancreatic neuro-insular network in health and fatty infiltration. Diabetolo gia. 2018;**61**(1):168-181. DOI: 10.1007/s00125-017-4409-x

[30] Von Dorsche HH, Falt K, Hahn HJ, Reiher H. Neuron-specific enolase (NSE) as a neuroendocrine cell marker in the human fetal pancreas. Acta Histochemica. 1989;**85**(2):227-228. DOI: 10.1016/s0065-1281(89)80073-x

[31] Kim J, Richter W, Aanstoot HJ, Shi Y, Fu Q, Rajotte R, et al. Differential expression of GAD65 and GAD67 in human, rat, and mouse pancreatic islets. Diabetes. 1993;**42**(12):1799-1808. DOI: 10.2337/diabetes.42.12.1799

[32] Teitelman G, Alpert S, Polak JM, Martinez A, Hanahan D. Precursor cells of mouse endocrine pancreas coexpress insulin, glucagon and the neuronal proteins tyrosine hydroxylase and neuropeptide Y, but not pancreatic polypeptide. Development. 1993;**118**(4):1031-1039

[33] Schwitzgebel VM, Scheel DW, Conners JR, Kalamaras J, Lee JE, Anderson DJ, Sussel L, Johnson JD, German MS. Expression of neurogenin3 reveals an islet cell precursor population in the pancreas. Development. 2000 Aug;**127**(16):3533-3542

[34] Bonal C, Herrera PL. Genes controlling pancreas ontogeny. The International Journal of Developmental Biology. 2008;**52**(7):823-835. DOI: 10.1387/ijdb.072444cb

[35] Naya FJ, Huang HP, Qiu Y, Mutoh H, DeMayo FJ, Leiter AB, Tsai MJ. Diabetes, defective pancreatic morphogenesis, and abnormal enteroendocrine differentiation in BETA2/

neuroD-deficient mice. Genes & Development. 1997 Sep 15;**11**(18):2323-2334. DOI: 10.1101/gad.11.18.2323

[36] Pearse AG, Polak JM. Neural crest origin of the endocrine polypeptide (APUD) cells of the gastrointestinal tract and pancreas. Gut. 1971;**12**(10):783-788. DOI: 10.1136/gut.12.10.783

[37] Amella C, Cappello F, Kahl P, Fritsch H, Lozanoff S, Sergi C. Spatial and temporal dynamics of innervation during the development of fetal human pancreas. Neuroscience. 2008;**154**(4):1477-1487. DOI: 10.1016/j.neuroscience.2008.04.050

[38] Cerf ME. Islet organogenesis, angiogenesis and innervation. Cell Biology International. 2011;**35**(11):1065-1078. DOI: 10.1042/CBI20100780

[39] Pan FC, Brissova M. Pancreas development in humans. Current Opinion in Endocrinology, Diabetes, and Obesity. 2014;**21**(2):77-82. DOI: 10.1097/MED.0000000000000047

[40] Abdulreda MH, Rodriguez-Diaz R, Cabrera O, Caicedo A, Berggren PO. The different faces of the pancreatic islet. Advances in Experimental Medicine and Biology. 2016;**938**:11-24. DOI: 10.1007/978-3-319-39824-2_2

[41] Kiba T. Relationships between the autonomic nervous system and the pancreas including regulation of regeneration and apoptosis: Recent developments. Pancreas. 2004;**29**(2):e51-e58. DOI: 10.1097/00006676-200408000-00019

[42] Lausier J, Diaz WC, Roskens V, Larock K, Herzer K, Fong CG, et al. Vagal control of pancreatic beta-cell proliferation. American Journal of Physiology. Endocrinology and Metabolism. 2010;**299**(5):E786-E793. DOI: 10.1152/ajpendo.00202.2010

[43] Borden P, Houtz J, Leach SD, Kuruvilla R. Sympathetic innervation during development is necessary for pancreatic islet architecture and functional maturation. Cell Reports. 2013;**4**(2):287-301. DOI: 10.1016/j.celrep.2013.06.019

[44] Rodriguez-Diaz R, Abdulreda MH, Formoso AL, Gans I, Ricordi C, Berggren PO, et al. Innervation patterns of autonomic axons in the human endocrine pancreas. Cell Metabolism. 2011;**14**(1):45-54. DOI: 10.1016/j.cmet.2011.05.008

[45] Rodriguez-Diaz R, Dando R, Jacques-Silva MC, Fachado A, Molina J, Abdulreda MH, Ricordi C, Roper SD, Berggren PO, Caicedo A. Alpha cells secrete acetylcholine as a non-neuronal paracrine signal priming beta cell function in humans. Nature Medicine. 2011;**17**(7):888-892. DOI: 10.1038/nm.2371

[46] Chiu YC, Hua TE, Fu YY, Pasricha PJ, Tang SC. 3-D imaging and illustration of the perfusive mouse islet sympathetic innervation and its remodelling in injury. Diabetologia. 2012;**55**(12):3252-3261. DOI: 10.1007/s00125-012-2699-6

[47] Stožer A, Dolenšek J, Rupnik MS. Glucose-stimulated calcium dynamics in islets of Langerhans in acute mouse pancreas tissue slices. PLoS One. 2013;**8**(1):e54638. DOI: 10.1371/journal.pone.0054638

[48] Fink T, Di Sebastiano P, Bochlerj M, Beger HG, Weihe E. Growth-associated protein-43 and protein gene-product 9,5 innervation in human pancreas: Changes in chronic pancreatitis. Neuroscience. 1994;**63**(1):249-266. DOI: 10.1016/0306-4522(94)90020-5

[49] Castorina S, Romeo R, Marcello MF. Immunohistochemical study of intrinsic innervation in the human pancreas. Bollettino della Società Italiana di Biologia Sperimentale. 1996;**72**(1-2):1-7

[50] Pour PM, Saruc M. The pattern of neural elements in the islets of normal and diseased pancreas and in isolated islets. Journal of the Pancreas: JOP. 2011;**12**(4):395-403

[51] Böck P. Fine structure of the neuro-insular complex type II in the cat. Archivum Histologicum Japonicum. 1986;**49**(2):189-197. DOI: 10.1679/aohc.49.189

[52] Furuzawa Y, Ohmori Y, Watanabe T. Anatomical localization of sympathetic postganglionic and sensory neurons innervating the pancreas of the cat. The Journal of Veterinary Medical Science. 1996 Mar;**58**(3):243-248

[53] Brunicardi FC, Shavelle DM, Andersen DK. Neural regulation of the endocrine pancreas. International Journal of Pancreatology. 1995;**18**(3):177-195. DOI: 10.1007/BF02784941

[54] Salvioli B, Bovara M, Barbara G, De Ponti F, Stanghellini V, Tonini M, et al. Neurology and neuropathology of the pancreatic innervation. Journal of the Pancreas: JOP. 2002;**3**(2):26-33

[55] Cabrera-Vasquez S, Navarro-Tableros V, Sanchez-Soto C, Gutierrez-Ospina G, Hiriart M. Remodelling sympathetic innervation in rat pancreatic islets ontogeny. BMC Developmental Biology. 2009;**9**(1):34. DOI: 10.1186/1471-213x-9-34

[56] Myojin T, Kitamura N, Hondo E, Baltazar ET, Pearson GT, Yamada J. Immunohistochemical localization of neuropeptides in bovine pancreas. Anatomia, Histologia, Embryologia. 2000 Jun;**29**(3):167-172. DOI: 10.1046/j.1439-0264.2000.00257.x

[57] Tiscornia OM. The neural control of exocrine and endocrine pancreas. The American Journal of Gastroenterology. 1977 Jun;**67**(6):541-560

[58] Yi SQ, Miwa K, Ohta T, Kayahara M, Kitagawa H, Tanaka A, Shimokawa T, Akita K, Tanaka S. Innervation of the pancreas from the perspective of perineural invasion of pancreatic cancer. Pancreas. 2003;**27**(3):225-229

[59] Almaça J, Weitz J, Rodriguez-Diaz R, Pereira E, Caicedo A. The pericyte of the pancreatic islet regulates capillary diameter and local blood flow. Cell Metabolism. 2018;**27**(3):630-644.e4. DOI: 10.1016/j.cmet.2018.02.016

[60] Rinaman L, Miselis RR. The organization of vagal innervation of rat pancreas using cholera toxin-horseradish peroxidase conjugate. Journal of the Autonomic Nervous System. 1987;**21**(2-3):109-125

[61] Chen XH, Itoh M, Sun W, Miki T, Takeuchi Y. Localization of sympathetic and parasympathetic neurons innervating pancreas and spleen in the cat. Journal of the Autonomic Nervous System. 1996;**59**(1-2):12-16

[62] Browning KN, Coleman FH, Travagli RA. Characterization of pancreas-projecting rat dorsal motor nucleus of vagus neurons. American Journal of Physiology. Gastrointestinal and Liver Physiology. 2005 May;**288**(5):G950-G955. DOI: 10.1152/ajpgi.00549.2004

[63] Berthoud HR, Powley TL. Morphology and distribution of efferent vagal innervation of rat pancreas as revealed with anterograde transport of Dil. Brain Research. 1991;**553**(2):336-341

[64] Molina J, Rodriguez-Diaz R, Fachado A, Jacques-Silva MC, Berggren PO, Caicedo A. Control of insulin secretion by cholinergic signaling in the human pancreatic islet. Diabetes. 2014;**63**(8):2714-2726. DOI: 10.2337/db13-1371

[65] Won MH, Park HS, Jeong YG, Park HJ. Afferent innervation of the rat pancreas: Retrograde tracing and immunohistochemistry in the dorsal root ganglia. Pancreas. 1998;**16**(1):80-87

[66] Szallasi A, Blumberg PM. Vanilloid (capsaicin) receptors and mechanisms. Pharmacological Reviews. 1999;**51**(2):159-212

[67] Standop J, Ulrich A, Schneider MB, Andrén-Sandberg A, Pour PM. Pacinian corpuscle in the human pancreas. Pancreas. 2001;**23**(1):36-39

[68] García-Suárez O, Calavia MG, Pérez-Moltó FJ, Alvarez-Abad C, Pérez-Piñera P, Cobo JM, Vega JA. Immunohistochemical profile of human pancreatic pacinian corpuscles. Pancreas. 2010;**39**(3):403-410. DOI: 10.1097/MPA.0b013e3181bc0372

[69] Watari N. Fine structure of nervous elements in the pancreas of some vertebrates. Zeitschrift für Zellforschung und Mikroskopische Anatomie. 1968;**85**(3):291-314

[70] Khochanskij DN, Makarova OV. Current views on the structure and function of enteric nervous system [article in Russian]. Morphological Newsletter. 2015;**1**:106-117

[71] Kirchgessner AL, Gershon MD. Innervation of the pancreas by neurons in the gut. The Journal of Neuroscience. 1990;**10**(5):1626-1642

[72] Kirchgessner AL, Pintar JE. Guinea pig pancreatic ganglia: Projections, transmitter content, and the type-specific localization of monoamine oxidase. The Journal of Comparative Neurology. 1991;**305**(4):613-631

[73] Love JA, Szebeni K. Morphology and histochemistry of the rabbit pancreatic innervation. Pancreas. 1999;**18**(1):53-64

[74] Shelagurov AA. Pancreatitis [in Russian]. Moscow: Medicine; 1967. 360 p

[75] Halban PA, Wollheim CB, Blondel B, Meda P, Niesor EN, Mintz DH. The possible importance of contact between pancreatic islet cells for the control of insulin release. Endocrinology 1982;**111**(1):86-94

[76] Tengholm A, Gylfe E. Oscillatory control of insulin secretion. Molecular and Cellular Endocrinology. 2009;**297**(1-2):58-72. DOI: 10.1016/j.mce.2008.07.009

[77] Rosario W, Singh I, Wautlet A, Patterson C, Flak J, Becker TC, et al. The brain to pancreatic islet neuronal map reveals differential glucose regulation from distinct hypothalamic regions. Diabetes. 2016;**65**(9):2711-2723. DOI: 10.2337/db15-0629

[78] Kobayashi S, Fujita T. Fine structure of mammalian and avian pancreatic islets with a special reference to D-cells and nervous elements. Zeitschrift für Zellforschung und Mikroskopische Anatomie. 1969;**100**(3):340-363. DOI: 10.1007/bf00571491

[79] Donev S. Ultrastructural evidence for presence of a glial sheath investing the islets of Langerhans in the pancreas of mammals. Cell and Tissue Research. 1984;**237**(2):343-348. DOI: 10.1007/bf00217154

[80] Gilliam LK, Palmer JP, Taborsky GJ Jr. Tyramine-mediated activation of sympathetic nerves inhibits insulin secretion in humans. The Journal of Clinical Endocrinology and Metabolism 2007;**92**(10):4035-4038. DOI: 10.1210/jc.2007-0536.

[81] Karlsson S, Scheurink AJ, Steffens AB, Ahrén B. Involvement of capsaicin-sensitive nerves in regulation of insulin secretion and glucose tolerance in conscious mice. The American Journal of Physiology. 1994;**267**(4 Pt2):R1071-R1077

[82] Gardemann A, Jungermann K, Grosse V, Cossel L, Wohlrab F, Hahn HJ, Blech W, Hildebrandt W. Intraportal transplantation of pancreatic islets into livers of diabetic rats. Reinnervation of islets and regulation of insulin secretion by the hepatic sympathetic nerves. Diabetes. 1994;**43**(11):1345-1352

[83] Burris R, Hebrok M. Pancreatic innervation in mouse development and β-cell regeneration. Neuroscience. 2007;**150**(3):592-602. DOI: 10.1016/j.neuroscience.2007.09.079

[84] Pervushin VI, Stavrova NP. Comparison between the development of the nervous apparatus and parenchymatous units of the pancreas in human embryogenesis [article in Russian]. Arkhiv Anatomii, Gistologii i Émbriologii. 1973;**65**(8):68-74

[85] Bashkin AD. Development of the neural apparatus of the human pancreas in prenatal ontogeny [article in Russian]. Arkhiv Anatomii, Gistologii i Émbriologii. 1988;**94**(2):13-18

[86] Jabotinsky YM. Normal and pathological morphology of vegetative ganglia [in Russian]. Moscow: AMS USSR; 1953. 291 p

[87] Cegrell L. The postnatal occurrence of biogenic monoamines in pancreatic islets of golden hamsters. Acta Endocrinologica. 1975;**78**(2):289-293

[88] Thomas NW, Findlay JA. Innervation of the endocrine pancreas in the mongolian gerbil (*Meriones unguiculatus*). In: Coupland RE, Forssmann WG, editors. Peripheral Neuroendocrine Interactions. New York: Springer Verlag; 1978. pp. 134-143

[89] Krivova YS, Proshchina AE, Barabanov VM, Saveliev SV. Development of the islets of Langerhans in the human fetal pancreas. In: Satou A, Nakamura H, editors. Pancreas: Anatomy, Diseases and Health Implications. Nova Science Publishers: NY; 2012. pp. 53-88

[90] Krivova Y, Proshchina A, Barabanov V, Leonova O, Saveliev S. Structure of neuro-endocrine and neuro-epithelial interactions in human foetal pancreas. Tissue & Cell. 2016;**48**(6):567-576. DOI: 10.1016/j.tice.2016.10.005

[91] Krivova YS, Proshchina AE, Barabanov VM, Saveliev SV. Neuro-Insular Complexes in the Human Pancreas. In: Seicean A, editor. Challenges in Pancreatic Pathology. Rijeka, Croatia: InTech; 2017. pp. 3-17. DOI: 10.5772/65059

4

Plastic Adaptation: A Neuronal Imperative Capable of Confounding the Goals of Stem Cell Replacement Therapy for either Huntington's or Parkinson's Disease

Michael I. Sandstrom, Kevin A. Anderson, Naveen Jayaprakash, Parnit K. Bhupal and Gary L. Dunbar

Abstract

Although stem cell transplant therapy offers considerable promise for deteriorative diseases, the efficacy of its application may be mitigated by endogenous compensatory mechanisms in the host brain. Plastic compensation follows neurodegeneration, beginning at its very onset and minimizing early symptom expression. As researchers attempt to correlate symptom remission with the ability of transplanted cells to adopt specific cell phenotypes, they need to be vigilant of the possibility that competing, local compensatory effects may be altering the outcome. Clearly plastic compensatory mechanisms could confound desired transplant-derived improvements by supplanting the beneficial contributions of the transplants. As circuit-level adaptations occur, more explicit explorations of their relevance to neuronal transplantation success are needed. Conceptual models of undirected transplanted cells adopting preconceived appropriate roles require revision. The notion that newly transplanted neuronal precursors will incorporate themselves into host circuitry with mutual cooperation across both parties (i.e., transplant and host) without some symbiosis-promoting mechanism is naïve. Undirected local circuits could react to newly transplanted additions as intruders. We advocate that appropriate signaling from transplanted cells to the host environment is required to optimize the therapeutic relevance of transplantation. This review surveys critical signaling mechanisms that might promote symbiotic interdependence between the host and new transplants.

Keywords: stem cells, transplantation, Parkinson's disease, Huntington's disease, adaptive plasticity, development

1. Introduction

For several years now, efforts have been underway to examine and refine technology associated with promoting the incorporation of pluripotent stem cells from various origins following transplantation into the brains of patients suffering from various deteriorative diseases [1–3], or to test the viability of such treatments using experimental animal models [4–6]. The typical pattern of findings associated with clinical efforts is initial moderate symptom improvement, followed by either resumption of symptoms over time or highly variable therapeutic outcomes [7–9]. Common arguments raised for the mechanism underlying inconsistent effectiveness are that either the transplanted cells are not merging sufficiently with the host brain due to a timely competition-related synaptogenesis process, that transplanted cells are not surviving in the harsh environment of the host due to immune-system/inflammatory host responses, or both [8–11] (also see the extensive review by cell type [12]). While evidence for these arguments certainly exists, it remains unclear whether those arguments cover all the relevant possibilities that threaten the longevity of the transplanted stem cells' utility. One potential threat to the long-term efficacy of this treatment, or to stem cell transplant therapies in general, which is frequently overlooked, would be *plastic adaptation*. Briefly, plastic adaptation represents a multitude of cellular responses that occur with the apparent role of maintaining cellular homeostasis, yet within the nervous system also supports the maintenance of a sort of dynamic status quo in which compensatory changes adjust the actions or response capacities of local healthy neurons in support of a superseding circuit-associated need. Plastic adaptation also occurs within the physiologically healthy brain in order to adjust for novel needs, supporting changes such as long-term memory, habit formation, and other sorts of behavioral adaptation of organisms to new surroundings and demands (for examples see [13, 14]). A surge of inquiry into what are now known as epigenetic mechanisms supports the notion of a clear capacity of cells to respond to environmental stimuli by generating enduring changes in their genetic expression [15–18]. This, combined with numerous demonstrations of more transient receptor plasticity [19–22], defines neuronal cells as versatile in both short- and long-term periods in adjusting to their neurochemical and electrophysiological circumstances at their membranes and within their nuclei, respectively. Following transplantation, it is likely that plastic adaptation responses could occur in both populations of neuronal cells of concern, either the transplanted cells or the surrounding host cells that likely interact with the transplanted cells.

During nervous system development, the mechanisms that guide the distributions of cells and their connectivity offer a far more forgiving flexibility when compared to the harsher, more demanding adult environment we face when attempting to correct deterioration with transplants [23–26]. Growth distances for neurites are shorter given the smaller neuropil, and more overt chemical gradients support pathfinding [27–29]. A developmental neurogenesis surge supports self-repair in the event of cell destruction because phenotype commitment is guided by a progressive fulfillment of niches and feedback signals once niches are filled [30–34]. Differential neuronal responsibilities within developing circuits are coaxed into existence in the context of an enhanced adaptive plasticity on either side of synaptic clefts, where each contributes to phenotype adoption of the other while it is determined what they might contribute to the developing circuit [35, 36]. As needs are met, postsynaptic neurons decrease their encouragement of subsequent equivalent connections by adapting their signaling [37–40]. How new afferents drive or control action potentials contributes significantly to circuit behavior, depending on factors as subtle as the proximity of synapses to a target neuron's trigger zone, while on the postsynaptic side the development of the trigger zone may modify when and how action potentials arise [41–46]. Incorporation into circuits relates to both identity and survival as neurons develop. As the neuronal phenotype is established, developing cells become increasingly dependent upon both afferent and efferent connections to other neurons. Neuronal fate seems to result from aspects of stimulation in the context of neurotrophic factors such as brain-derived neurotrophic factor (BDNF). Excitatory postsynaptic potentials known to increase intracellular calcium seem to participate in driving developmental determinations. This was shown by a series of experiments performed on precursor cells *in vitro* where calcium chelation blocked the establishment of neuronal phenotypes normally induced by either electrical or NMDA-glutamate stimulation in conjunction with BDNF [47–49]. Thus, precursors that receive insufficient controlling input to engage their activity likely adopt non-neuronal, glial, or support cell status, modifying or diminishing their contribution to circuits. When growing neurons establish connections to other neuronal populations, this provides them with target-derived trophic support that staves off programmed cell death that is likely to occur in its absence [50–53]. Surviving long enough to establish contributions is of course also important for transplanted populations, but evidence indicates that this is easier in the more forgiving context of development. A very useful series of explorations documenting how transplantation faces diminished success as the host ages was thoroughly documented in a mini-review by Sally Temple [54]. In addition, often the younger and less "experienced" or "committed" precursor cells are shown to more easily adapt into their transplanted roles than similar, yet older, populations [55–57]. In other contexts, such as the ability to properly generate blood cells following bone marrow transplants, younger donors seem to yield more successful results than older donors, indicating this age-dependency is not limited to neuronal populations [58, 59]. The similar goals of establishing appropriate cell populations to fill various niches following transplantation suggest if the environment were less competitive or more accommodating, and cells were guided by the more overt signals available during development, the process of incorporation would be more straightforward. In the adult brain, the mechanisms of plasticity engage to maintain the continuity of established function with mechanisms to prevent deviation from working systems; otherwise all nervous systems would constantly deteriorate into chaos. Thus, while similar concerns are present with transplantation, (i.e., coaxing the new cells to make useful and appropriate contributions to established circuitry), we cannot expect that new additions will naturally get swept into correct and working interactions the way they do during development.

To tease out the contributions of plastic adaptation to the success or longevity of stem cell transplantation therapy, it seems there is a need to expand inquiry further than whether transplanted cells develop into neurons, survive, or form mutually integrative connections with endogenous neurons. It appears equally important to determine how the cell populations influence each other and how each population adapts to this influence over time. There may be important clues to the mysteries surrounding the impermanence of replacement therapy in how these populations adjust to the presence of the *other*. This chapter was written to consider current knowledge about plastic adaptation as it pertains to the act of incorporating transplanted neuronal cells or precursors into a damaged host brain. In addition, this review represents a general call for more direct inquiry into this subject in future efforts to explore and hone such a promising therapeutic technology. If plastic changes compromise the capacity to maintain symptom-suppressing benefits of these transplants, solutions to this will likely require more than tracking the quality and longevity of behavioral benefit or the anatomical persistence of the transplants over extended periods. Success may be enhanced by recognizing the ongoing patterns of plasticity with which transplanted neuronal cells must cooperate to earn the opportunity to contribute. Given that the age of both the cells transplanted and the host into which they have been transplanted are relevant to their incorporation and therapeutic efficacy, it appears that the capacity to adapt into the new environment depends on factors or signals from both elements that need to be understood to support moving forward intelligently with this therapeutic endeavor. The remainder of this review will address concerns regarding the host adaptive responses to the transplant as well as the transplant's adaptive response to the host that ought to be considered in this regard, focusing largely on efforts with Huntington's and Parkinson's disease.

2. Achievements of "successful" transplantations

Therapeutic support derived from neural transplantation likely necessitates circuit-level reconstruction so that certain missing neurobehavioral actions are restored. However, it is important to acknowledge that circuits can be supported by either the addition of new neuronal contributions that might restore disconnected components or by bolstering the inherent capacity of compromised circuits to adjust or compensate. The brain's inherent capacity to compensate for damage/disruption or "repair itself" is considerable and likely the reason why physical or occupational therapies support function restoration. Trophic support and other general support of persisting residual circuit components, receptor sensitivity adjustments, sprouting, and several other inherent mechanisms contribute to reparation (for an extensive review of these mechanisms see [60]). These trophic or supportive contributions can be accomplished by non-neural cells or glia that likely contribute mostly indirectly to neuronal circuit actions. In fact, Blurton-Jones and colleagues [61] demonstrated that transplant-derived BDNF was eventually responsible for supporting cognitive improvements in a rodent Alzheimer's model by promoting enhanced synaptic density in the hippocampus between preexisting neurons. Thus, it appears that either the transplanted cells become active contributors to the circuit or they support the existing circuit that itself seems to engage compensatory mechanisms supporting at least partial function. Therefore, it appears beneficial to respect that plastic adaptation persists as an ongoing process, regularly promoting positive improvements in functional circuits, and that a *successful* contribution of transplanted stem cells to existing neural circuitry necessitates a recognizable supportive contribution to this endeavor. It is our overarching concern that transplant efforts do not typically respect this context, usually holding a more direct circuit reconstruction as paramount with the presumption that the host brain will somehow also recognize our clinical perspective and modify ongoing adaptive mechanisms accordingly. When this does not happen, we appear surprised that transplantation efforts impede healthy behavior restoration over time, or show diminished effectiveness over time—but we should not be.

While beyond the scope of this chapter, we nonetheless feel it is important to also acknowledge the prominence of neuronal circuit dependence on both use and the ongoing local actions of the immune system. It is likely that a repetitive drive on the circuit due to the person or animal engaging in systemic practice to recapture the skill they once had also supports circuit-level adaptation. This is likely why Parkinson's patients who regularly move and push themselves to actively engage compromised limbs rather than remaining sedentary reap clinical benefits from those actions [62, 63]. It is intriguing to consider these effects in the context of their ultimate therapeutic mechanisms which promote restoration or strengthening of key circuits with positive contributions to adaptation efforts, as well as the fact that once a part of a circuit, transplant-derived neurons may require practice to become proficient in their established roles. Of course, immune rejection and the broader context of inflammation also enter into this equation, given the common desire to utilize transplants in the context of deteriorative diseases or trauma-related damage. While it is arguable that convincing the immune system not to overreact has been extensively studied as a factor in this context (e.g., [64]), the inflammatory response certainly has the capacity to tailor the very adaptation mechanisms we will discuss (e.g., [65]). For extensive reviews of the reciprocal interactions between neural systems and inflammatory systems relevant to plasticity see Di Filipo and colleagues [66], or Xanthos and Sandkuhler [67].

Do the new additions engage with the existing circuits in positive adaptation-enhancing ways? Along the way it appears that there are adaptations on both sides that might enhance or diminish this relationship. If the adaptations diminish this circuit-supporting relationship, then the ability of the new transplanted cells to continue their presence and effectively support positive behavioral improvements will likely be lost and the clinical efforts of transplantation will likely be considered insufficient or transient. Alternatively, if the adaptations that occur enhance the circuit-supporting relationship while avoiding interfering with ongoing adaptive efforts, the success may extend further than the initial witnessed improvements into continuous ongoing improvements, rather than plateauing at some yet incomplete recovery. In this chapter we will divide our appreciation of transplantation-related plasticity as new cells establish roles contributing to existing yet compromised circuits first into whether the endogenous circuit adopts the newcomers as team players, and second whether the transplanted cells adopt the roles required of them to contribute to the circuit or not.

3. Adaptation of endogenous host tissue to neural transplantation

Although adult neurogenesis was overlooked in the past and neuroscientists were convinced that new neurons were not produced beyond the early stages of development, it has now been demonstrated conclusively that there are select regions in the brain that regularly accept new neurons into established circuits that are derived from precursor neuroblasts that retain mitotic capacity throughout our lives, and divide asymmetrically to produce new neurons as daughter cells (for review see [68]). Two key areas that benefit from this neurogenesis would be the hippocampus and olfactory bulb, and the degree of this natural new neuron incorporation depends on the activity levels generated in these regions. Specific functions that rely upon neurogenesis include new learning for the hippocampus [69], and rich olfactory sensory experience for the olfactory bulb [70]. As this occurs regularly in an activity-dependent manner already, it stands to reason that neuronal precursors transplanted into these regions would be more likely to receive signals encouraging their incorporation into either the hippocampus or the olfactory bulb, and in fact, this seems to be the case [71, 72]. Yet in other regions such as the striatum (the main input structure of the basal ganglia), the capacity of endogenous neuronal progenitors to become neurons seems reduced compared to exogenous transplantations [73]. The answer to why this distinction exists has been a top priority among those of us who foresee more successful replacement therapies. While the whole picture is not available, what seems clear is that there is an interactive relationship between the endogenous host cells and transplanted cells at the center. The so-called "neurogenic" regions (hippocampus and olfactory bulb) where replacement happens regularly as part of the natural progression throughout our lives would likely not be a useful target region for clinical transplantation for any key neuronal disorders, given that their potential for reconstructive replacement remains high. Yet we might initially presume that the mechanisms encouraging incorporation, such as the guidance molecules used and trophic factors encouraging survival as connections are established, or the afferent connections grown into and onto the transplant cells as the afferent component, may follow rules similar to transplant events elsewhere.

When precision is required in the placement of axon terminals, it would seem that the parameters for what might be considered functional success would be correspondingly more restrictive or demanding. Here it is appropriate to briefly describe how establishing a wide range of general chronic dopamine can provide considerable benefit in Parkinson's disease, and the distinction between "open" diffusion-capable release mechanisms versus "closed" synaptic connections circumscribed by glial borders. Due to the chronic widespread levels of dopamine persisting in extracellular space, simple diffusion-based neurotransmitter delivery is often discussed without emphasizing the more nuanced details of precise release. To illustrate, in the case of dopamine loss in Parkinson's disease, the standard drug levodopa promotes endogenous release to higher global levels without significant dependence on direct synaptic integration of the remaining endogenous dopamine neurons, as a large majority of these are gone when this treatment is prescribed (presumably after at least 70% of the endogenous innervation deteriorates). Also, dopamine-lesioned experimental model animals have been improved by treatment with synthetic slow-release nanoparticles [74] or transplantation of genetically modified fibroblasts [75] that likely neither need, nor have the capacity to respond to, afferent control. In this context these treatments, as well as the dopamine systems considered, are seen as utilizing volume transmission or "open" synapses that tend to increase release levels over larger areas, based either on simple diffusion mechanisms or low-level chronic stimulation. By contrast, there are systems that rely on comparatively local transmission or "closed" synapses that are locally circumscribed by glial cells to certain synaptic junctions, and usually depend much more heavily on the timing of inputs for their function. Systems utilizing volume transmission would, by this definition, present an ambiguity to whether they necessitate as much acceptance into the network [76, 77]. So long as they provide the requisite compound this contribution may suffice, at least initially, in bolstering the circuit in question, though release would need to take place in key areas to be effective. Dopaminergic inputs seem to exhibit both of these characteristics ("open" and "closed"). This concept, commonly overlooked in the clinic, will be expanded upon later.

Another aspect of transplant-related plasticity is the extent to which neurons are transplanted into a typical or atypical host environment for the neuron type that is their intended end-point for the current therapy. It is clear that during early fetal periods, useful progenitor populations can naturally undergo sufficient prior developmental modification to become predisposed to becoming a certain common neural type and can be found in regionally distinct populations in the fetus. For example, cells from the lateral ganglionic eminence show a high propensity to become GABAergic striatal neurons [78], or cells from the fetal mesencephalic region show a high propensity to become dopaminergic type neurons (e.g., [79]). Specific developmental trajectory predispositions can also be coaxed from progenitor cell populations *in vitro*, where the approximate mitogens, epigenetic cues, and morphogenic signals are maintained and progressively modified to encourage specific phenotype development trajectories [6, 80, 81]. Once neural developmental predisposition is established, it is perhaps fair to suggest that there are some host regions in which predisposed neurons would thrive as they would be placed into a "familiar" environment (i.e., a *homotypic* host region; e.g., GABAergic medium spiny predisposed neurons transplanted into the striatum) and some host regions that would *not* represent environments that might foster familiarity (i.e., an *ectopic* host region; e.g., dopaminergic destined neurons transplanted into the striatum). Precedent for this homotypic versus ectopic distinction has been set [82, 83]. Keep in mind that this distinction is made to capture the regional relations of predisposed neurons for certain locations, and functional benefit concerns are secondary.

For years, neuroscientists have been studying the anatomy of neuronal populations of various types that produce different neurochemical compositions throughout the brain and the corresponding afferent connections that grow into and drive activity in these different regions. Establishing appropriate afferent drive onto the neurons that are transplanted would be a clear sign that the circuit into which the transplanted cells need to merge has accepted them as part of the equation. Clearly then, when placed into a homotypic host region this sort of acceptance would be more likely based on the proximity of the transplanted cells to appropriate afferent input that such cells need to be driven properly by the host brain architecture. The prime example of this sort of transplant that has shown considerable acceptance into the host circuit and was extensively characterized by Klas Wictorin in 1992 is the intrastriatal transplant of striatal-predisposed precursor cells obtained from the embryonic day 14–15 fetal lateral ganglionic eminence following an excitotoxic lesion of the host striatum [84]. The extensive host innervation of this transplant along with the extensive growth and integration of the transplant with the host in the context of circuit re-establishment was dramatic, long-lasting, and seemed to contribute considerable support to the lesioned circuit as seen by neurobehavioral improvement. Wictorin indicated that the initial destructive lesion to destroy local endogenous striatal neurons is crucial for enabling the sort of host integration seen, as the absence of such a lesion (i.e., transplantation into an intact striatum) yielded far less integration [85]. It stands to reason this would occur because afferent inputs would find greater ease in filling an open void or niche so long as it maintains a general presence after the lesion. A transplant without deteriorative or destructive loss would also be unnecessary because, as stated, the transplant is meant to restore the lost contribution. Wictorin describes a considerable ingrowth of afferent inputs from the host brain into the transplant with cortical, thalamic, nigral dopaminergic, and serotonergic inputs from the raphe that showed extensive yet differential degrees of penetration into the graft [84]. Also relevant was the point made about how regions that did not appear "striatum-like" seemed far less capable of inducing dopaminergic ingrowth and that specific transplants of cerebellar or cortical tissue into the excitotoxin-lesioned striatum of adult rats yielded no such dopaminergic innervation. Electrophysiological experiments demonstrated that these innervations of the graft were synaptically functional, supporting host-originating cortical drive [86, 87], and functional dopaminergic modification of GABA release from transplanted cells into the globus pallidus and the substantia nigra reticulata [88].

Although speculative, it is possible that even if the neurons transplanted into the striatum that became GABAergic did not grow extensively into the host tissue and participate more fully in the host basal ganglia circuitry, some circuit support might be established by enhancing only local GABA release from these neurons with limited incorporation as exclusively interneurons. It has become clear that in the context of the Huntington's disease condition, even prior to the major deterioration of striatal cells, there is considerable and abnormal spontaneous activity within the dorsal striatum [89, 90], and it appears that overactive glutamate release or diminished reuptake transport of glutamate is at least partially to blame for this [91, 92]. Under these circumstances, a considerable disruption of striatal function might arise due largely to this main input region being considerably noisier than normal (electrophysiologically speaking), and under such circumstances the proper selection of outputs would necessarily become challenged. If transplanted cells were simply driven by locally increased glutamatergic inputs or the ambient glutamate levels, after which they proceeded to feed back onto local medium spiny projection neurons in a manner that minimized this noise, some presumed information processing capacity might be restored, despite the lack of full integration.

To highlight the behavioral relevance of induced electrophysiology on transplanted cells, our laboratory initiated a project that involved preliminary transduction of transplant-destined neuronal precursor cells harvested from the subventricular zone of neonatal rats (P1 to P2) with Channelrhodopsin-2 (ChR2). This receptor construct allowed for rapid and exclusive optogenetic stimulation of these cells as they became functional neurons activated by blue light. The construct also contained a transgene with a synapsin promoter as well as code for enhanced yellow fluorescent protein (EYFP) for visualization post-euthanasia. It was our interest to explore the propensity of these transplanted cells to incorporate with the circuitry of the otherwise intact dorsal striatum in a manner that would allow a movable skull-mounted iontophoresis/single-unit electrophysiology electrode with fiber optic light incorporation to locate transplanted cells by slowly moving dorsoventrally across the striatum of a freely-moving rat and searching for units that would respond to various local stimulations. There were three stimulation types that could be generated: iontophoresis of glutamate, stimulation with 473 nm blue light, and behavioral stimulation. The advantage of this strategy was that only cells transduced with ChR2 (i.e., the cells to be transplanted) would show photosensitivity to blue light. Several interesting findings arose from this work. Previous work with a similar iontophoresis electrode (modified merely to allow the inclusion of a narrow fiber optic cable for light stimulation in the present study) had clearly shown that rats with intact striata exhibit largely low levels of spontaneous activity [93]. Thus this technique that uses pulled 4-barrel glass electrodes (recording via 3 M NaCl, and iontophoresis of 0.25 M glutamate with a 0.25 M NaCl balance barrel and a narrow fiber-optic cable delivering blue light through the final barrel, wiring and fiber-optic cable connected to a combined swivel apparatus above the chamber) took advantage of a movable electrode holder allowing multiple exploratory passes through the dorsomedial striatum while monitoring the extracellular field for potential signs of single unit activity. Iontophoresis of glutamate was our global stimulant capable of activating any striatal neuron in proximity whether it originated endogenously or from the transplant.

We went in expecting a low yield of photosensitive units given established findings that transplanted neurons tend not to incorporate well in an intact striatum (e.g., [84]). In our experiments, each animal received approximately 40,000 neuronal stem cells as 8–10 neurospheres per animal except "controls." The distribution of behaviorally responsive units was similar to previous work with similar electrodes employed without light [93] among controls. Among our main findings was that none of the units that responded to light or light/glutamate combinations also responded to the behavior of the animal. This suggests that although glutamatergic inputs from both cortex and thalamus synapsed functionally with grafts placed into the striatum following an ibotenic acid lesion [84], we saw little evidence of the corresponding freely-moving-animal incorporation that likely would have generated behavior-induced responses in our localized and verified transplanted cells. Of the 40,000 potential contributors placed directly into the pathway of our electrodes, we recorded from approximately 20 light-sensitive cells per animal at 2 weeks and then found a far smaller number (approximately 2-3) at 4 weeks. However it was not the case that the neurons derived from transplants were unable to form connections, as on multiple occasions with the subjects tested at 2 weeks post-transplantation we witnessed responses of what we predicted were spontaneously active endogenous units that were clearly inhibited during light stimulation (see **Figure 1**). None of these light-induced inhibitions were found at 4 weeks, in part because spontaneous activity was also harder to find at this later date. However, this finding and the fact that 2–3 out of the average 20 light stimulation events yielded this sort of response at 2 weeks but not at 4 weeks also suggests the possibility of temporary local synaptic connections being formed and then lost between the periods explored. While it is possible that a certain lack of drive (evidenced by the lack of behavioral drive on light-activated units) may have contributed to their demise as well as inflammatory or immune responses, another finding from this study was particularly intriguing. During the search for EYFP-expressing units at the final stages of these experiments, rats euthanized after explorations at 4 weeks contained far higher levels of fluorescent units merging into the olfactory-destined rostral migratory stream (see **Figure 2**). Newly produced neurons from the subventricular zone (where our neural stem cells were originally harvested) initially follow the edges of the lateral ventricles and then proceed ventrally into the stream headed for the olfactory bulb [94]. Fluorescent cells were consistently found to be incorporated into this system in a more rounded and presumably migratory state that, while still potentially responsive to both light and glutamate stimulation, would not be expected to have incorporated host glutamatergic drive that has been associated with driving CAM kinase II responses and the corresponding cessation of migration and synaptic arbor development [95].

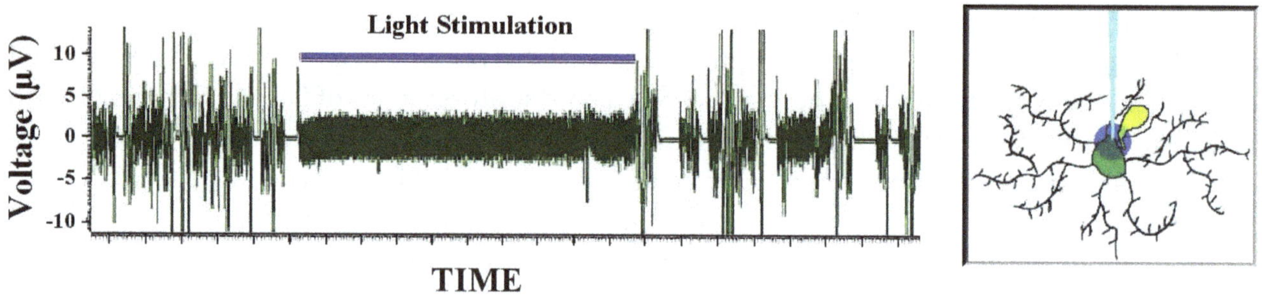

Figure 1. Spontaneous unit activity inhibited by light. Here a spontaneously active unit from within the striatum was inhibited by light. We predict that the connectivity was such that a transplanted (thus light-responsive) unit had adopted a GABAergic transmitter type and when it became activated by local light in sufficient proximity was induced to synaptically suppress the unit it had synapsed upon as depicted in the insert. *Insert Diagram*: Pulled glass electrode depicted descending from top. Darker sphere at electrode tip represents fiber-optic cable-derived blue light stimulation emanating from electrode tip. Small interneuron to electrode right depicts EYFP-expressing transplanted cell presumably sufficiently close to be excited by blue light but not to contribute to recorded *activation* response typical of "direct" stimulation. The recorded medium spiny cell, juxtaposed to the electrode tip, represents the spontaneously-active neuron providing recorded activity that was otherwise insensitive to the blue light barring GABA influence elicited from the sensitive transplanted cell connected to it.

From this study we concluded that when transplants are placed into the less-hospitable intact striatum it is possible that far fewer neurons make synapses with the local host and that when they do at earlier stages, these synaptic connections are far from permanent. It is likely that the unique proximity of the electrode, spontaneously active cell, and photosensitive cell depicted in **Figure 1**, that we hypothesize would elicit the witnessed inhibitory responses, would be serendipitous under the most opportune conditions, particularly considering the scarcity of spontaneously active striatal units within the intact brain (harder to find in general; [93]). Yet the consistency of the findings at 2 weeks and the complete lack at 4 weeks suggests that at least some transplanted units made only temporary synapses that disappeared later either due to cell death or resumption of migration. This may occur when the signals indicating the propensity for circuit interaction by the endogenous host cells are weaker, and there is subsequent reduced effort to formulate more robust and permanent interactions. Therefore, the presumption that once neurons form a synaptic relationship, the newly transplanted cells are somehow

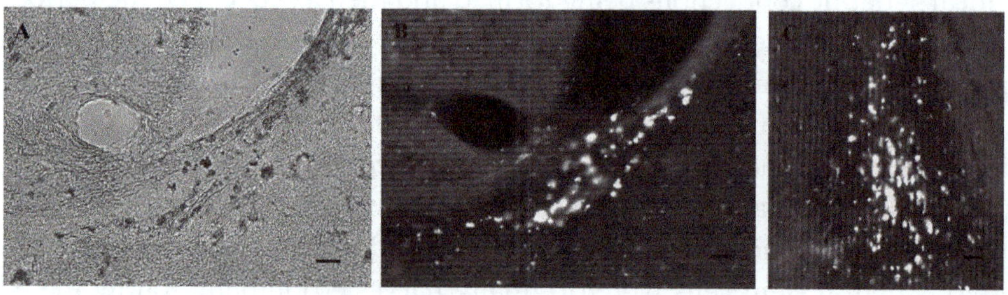

Figure 2. Fluorescent migrating cells at 4 weeks. Shown is a clear mass of cells that had migrated along the ventricles toward the bottom portion of the ventricle seen in both bright field (A) and the fluorescent images of B and C showing migrating transplant-origin cells fluorescing brightly in this location, outside of the recording area of the dorsal striatum. Line segments in each image represent 100 µm. C represents a different region of this clustering from a separate, similarly-treated animal focused at a deeper level of the rostral migratory stream. Bottom of ventricle not seen in C but is just above the upper left corner of image.

safe and likely permanently established is not supported; yet it seems to underlie the persistent sentiment that after certain periods of time, the mere existence of neuronally integrated and transplant-derived neurons in the host tissue represents a *successful* fix for the destruction or deterioration of host tissue. Such reasoning is fallacious and ignores the intricacies and constantly-shifting nature of even seemingly well-established intact neural circuitry.

Others who have transplanted into the intact striatum using lateral ganglionic eminence-derived cells witnessed a correspondingly diminished interaction with the striatal circuit. In fact, following such transplantations, Magavi and Lois [96] found a greater degree of growth into and synaptic integration with orbitofrontal cortex and the claustrum than with either striatal or nigral connections, indicating also the inability of the striatum to attract connections into the homotypic basal ganglia circuit. It is standard procedure that experiments investigating the degree of host incorporation depict dendritic arbors and other signs of likely synaptic input following transplantation, but it would be misleading to indicate that whatever snapshot taken in post-experimentation histology is a fixed and permanent condition. It would run contrary to what we know about natural endogenous synaptic plasticity to believe that any fixed depiction of synaptic status remains a permanent or "set in stone" phenomenon, as we know endogenous synapses are constantly dancing with each other, exchanging connections regularly due to competitive interactions [97]. To compete and participate in this drawn-out request for a place in the circuit, it would be important that sufficient drive is established and, after the driving elements (e.g., corticostriatal or thalamostriatal inputs) are relieved of their targets by prior lesions, there would be a likely increase in terminals seeking destinations, and this is lacking in the intact striatum. It stands to reason that neurons without such drive might continue to migrate until they can position themselves to receive it. Clearly a considerable effort is engaged by both corticostriatal and thalamostriatal afferents to synaptically integrate with striatal grafts that follow target-destructive excitotoxic lesions as well as transplanted neurons that grow far more extensive integrations into the basal ganglia circuitry [84].

As mentioned above, extensive dopaminergic ingrowth occurs from grafts of fetal progenitors into a lesioned striatum, indicating that not only does glutamatergic host innervation likely drive this population, but this population is also modulated by dopamine in a host-controlled manner. Despite this capacity, thus far, most experiments exploring the viability of transplanting cells as a treatment for Parkinson's disease have targeted cells predisposed to become dopaminergic ectopically into the striatum rather than the homotypic substantia nigra. The rationale behind striatal transplantation of these dopaminergic-destined cells rather than transplanting the cells into the substantia nigra region is largely because of the expectation that neurons transplanted into the substantia nigra region would not be able to grow axonal extensions sufficiently through the relatively inhospitable terrain of the adult brain to deliver the needed dopamine into the striatum. Also, striatal transplants would likely provide comparatively more dopamine in the target region. This concept was formulated by Anders Björklund and his collaborators [98, 99] as the idea of dopaminergic tissue transplants for Parkinson's disease was initially proposed. Previously described limitations to extensive axon growth through the adult CNS would clearly support this notion. Thus, the large majority of the experiments exploring replacement transplantations for Parkinsonian circumstances targets the dorsal striatum and would fall into the category of ectopic host destinations.

The question remains largely open how such cells, when they become dopaminergic neurons, will integrate into circuitry, given that they are typically stimulated at their cell body level by glutamatergic signals entering into the substantia nigra. In fact, the substantia nigra seems to receive active control inputs originating from the subthalamic nucleus and the somatosensory/motor cortex, both of which are touted as being capable of initiating rapid responses to salient events [100]. By comparison the cortical drive on striatal neurons tends to be highly converged on any individual medium spiny target from across relatively wide regions of the cortex, an organization that would require high collaboration between multiple regions to activate any single striatal neuron [101]. This common convergence is likely to be partially responsible for the relative silence observed within the striatum while otherwise intact animals are at quiet rest. The chances that cortical input into the striatum would even closely approximate that obtained from the cortical and subthalamic input to the substantia nigra is therefore low to begin with, let alone the serendipity that would be necessary to result in all such transplanted dopaminergic neurons stimulated by the same subset of glutamatergic afferents. This would severely challenge the precision of drive on these transplanted neurons, with terminations more haphazard across the transplanted population, resulting in a much more *constant* degree of afferent stimulation.

Explorations of the corticostriatal input into dopamine-predisposed grafts of fetal mesencephalic tissue have yielded mixed results from inputs that appear to take on the morphologic appearance of nigral cortical input (thick fibers giving off thin collaterals; [102]). Another point raised more recently by Braak and del Tredici [103] is that striatal medium spiny neurons tend to lose their spines over time during the ongoing pathology of Parkinson's disease and that dopaminergic inputs in the intact striatum of otherwise healthy subjects seem to interact in a complicated modulatory manner on spine shafts while the corticostriatal terminals engage their tips. As this arrangement is progressively lost, the ability of dopaminergic grafts to successfully interact with the main projection medium spiny efferents may also be jeopardized. If the drive on grafted dopaminergic neurons in the striatum is not well controlled, the ability to duplicate distinct periods of phasic release that mark events of behavioral significance may be missing from the grafted dopaminergic neurons.

Most synapses engage plastic mechanisms that adopt diminished responses to non-dynamic and unchanging levels of drive in a manner similar to the way sensory systems habituate to consistency. We know that rats given large unilateral 6-OHDA-induced lesions of dopaminergic input to the striatum tend to respond within days to apomorphine stimulation in a manner that depends upon postsynaptic modifications that establish "supersensitivity," and that there are modifications of dopamine receptors related to this occurring for extended periods following the lesion [104]. However, it has also been shown using equivalent lesions in mice that their rotation intensity diminishes over time when their lesioned hemisphere is continuously treated with apomorphine using an osmotic pump, suggesting that these modifications that support the supersensitivity *compensation* are reversible when sufficient dopaminergic stimulation remains persistent [105]. Processing the degree of postsynaptic responsivity to dopamine levels with a behavioral assay is common, since it is likely that adjustments in dopamine receptor sensitivity are continuously occurring in response to the degree of stimulation in a manner that stabilizes responses over time (e.g., [106]). It is interesting to note that, although very popular in the literature, recording diminishing rotation in response to transplantation has been deemed more distinctly inadequate for processing transplants as only a very small boost in dopamine-producing capacity (such as 100–200 surviving transplanted neurons) seems sufficient to eliminate amphetamine-induced rotations by providing both chronic amphetamine-driven dopamine in general to the dorsal striatum [83]. Keeping this in mind, the ongoing adjustments in postsynaptic, and potentially presynaptic responses as well, are likely to reduce the dynamic responsiveness of the transplant-established dopamine system as seen by researchers, cautioning us about the inadequacy of drug-induced rotation in capturing underlying recovery dynamics [107].

The insufficiency of phasic release restoration also likely underlies the inability of Parkinson's patients on L-Dopa replacement therapy to rapidly adjust to ongoing motoric demands [108]. To accomplish a relative surge in dopamine release at a critical behavioral juncture such that the presence of dopamine provides sufficient ongoing support during more emergency situations, such as the need to escape from entrapment or predation, or falling into a body of water and needing to swim, phasic firing of nigrostriatal neurons occurs. The fact that gap junction connections have been found between nigral dopaminergic neurons and that electrophysiological behavior of the nigral population as a whole maintains consistency indicative of such electrotonic coupling [109, 110] suggests that wide ranging locations within the anterior striatal targets receive temporally consistent bursts as a result, in time with the events necessitating dopaminergic modulation. This phasic firing was recorded by Wolfram Schultz from dopamine neurons in the primate ventral tegmental area in his famous experiments that showed the cues responsible for generating increased drive on these mesolimbic neurons shifted from the initial pure reinforcement toward environmental cues *predictive* of the reinforcement and/or the risk associated with the reinforcement [111–113]. It is likely that what engages phasic drive among those neurons that support proper motivation in the arena of learning conditioning is driven in a manner somewhat distinct from the phasic drive on dopamine neurons that serve movement-related calculations within the dorsal part of the striatum. As we approximate human viability of transplantation, it is perhaps fair to mention that the borders of these two dopamine systems within the broader striatum of primates may not be as simple as their general projection parameters, and there is considerable overlap between the ascending dopamine systems (as described in [114]); there has nevertheless been a relatively consistent distinction made in the functional attributes of the projections. The apparent overlap may support the anecdotal events we have heard of where an immobile Parkinson's patient can initiate movement toward the exit of a building should this patient hear warnings of "*fire*" being exclaimed locally, though a stress-related release would be phasic.

Striatal cholinergic interneurons of the large aspiny variety are more likely to be tonically active for larger proportions of time than the main population of medium spiny GABAergic neurons, so their contributions to the ongoing processing within the region can be described as dynamic. These interneurons are controlled in a complicated way by dopamine, glutamate, and local GABA signals. Upon deeper scrutiny, the dopaminergic control of these large aspiny cholinergic neurons has been shown to involve differential employment of glutamate co-released from dopaminergic terminals along with dopamine between dorsal and ventral striata, rendering these regions distinct in how acetylcholine is driven [115]. The common understanding of the interaction between dopamine and acetylcholine in the striatum is that it is inverse, such that phasic bursts of dopamine lead to phasic pauses in ongoing activity among the large aspiny striatal cholinergic neurons. The inverse responsivity to reward in the striatal systems driven by the dopaminergic input akin to what Schultz recorded from was clearly demonstrated by Morris and colleagues [116] in their work that looked at the dopamine responses simultaneously with the cholinergic responses. The complexities of that interaction and the manner in which it may in fact capture an extensive range of guidance information has been thoroughly described (e.g., [117]). Acetylcholine is unique compared with other transmitters in that the enzyme acetylcholinesterase that is abundantly expressed externally breaks the molecule down rapidly and restricts the domain of effectiveness to localized regions. This is relevant to our story because acetylcholine modulates dopamine release at the terminal level [118], adjusting the release that may otherwise be driven by afferent stimulation at the cell body level. In fact this level of local cholinergic control is likely to be driven differently by thalamostriatal versus corticostriatal origins of glutamatergic drive [119], providing those two differential systems unique access to this key transmitter input. On top of this, it has become clear that glutamatergic input also controls local dopamine terminal release in a receptor-dependent manner such that dopamine release may well be modified by both local striatal (reviewed in [120]) and distal nigral/VTA mechanisms. As described before, these inputs find their way in and around the spines expressed by the medium spiny neurons such that glutamatergic inputs to the spine tips get molded by dopaminergic, cholinergic, and GABAergic inputs engaging spine or dendrite shafts (see **Figure 3**) to maintain the proper final output signal that proceeds through the basal ganglia. To be effective, the timing of release would need to be carefully controlled as well as proximity. It is clear that these temporal dynamics contribute to the utility of each differential transmitter contribution, and to the overall effectiveness of the projecting efferents carrying signals to further destinations in the basal ganglia loops, as this aspect of basal ganglia function has been reviewed and explored extensively [121–123].

In the context of the present review, it is relevant to pause and ask ourselves if ectopic transplants of dopaminergic neurons into the striatum, during the course of or following extensive destruction due to Parkinson's disease, can approach the dynamic control present in the otherwise intact system. These transplanted dopaminergic neurons would likely be connected to rather haphazardly by corticostriatal or thalamostriatal glutamatergic, local cholinergic or GABAergic interneurons, and already lack the over-arching control of phasic release that is typically driven at the substantia nigra. The local control features described above have led investigators to suspect that dopamine release within the striatum might be *considerably independent* of nigral control [124], further supported by both anatomical evidence of striatal-derived fibers growing into grafts [125], and electrophysiological evidence showing approximately 50% of grafted mesencephalic cells being activated by frontal cortex stimulation [126]. However, none of these supporting findings suggest any clear resumption of the temporal dynamics of dopamine modulation in a manner that might be expected to fully restore behavioral versatility. Not only this, but such ectopic transplantations would likely lead to a dispersion of neuronal soma due to migration throughout the striatum that, while often seen as a positive attribute given the likely corresponding breadth of dopamine contribution, would also render the temporal release control much more regionally distinct. The previous point about gap junction connectivity between dopaminergic neurons suggests that at least initially, electrophysiological phasic firing is driven in a more unified manner that is more likely to be

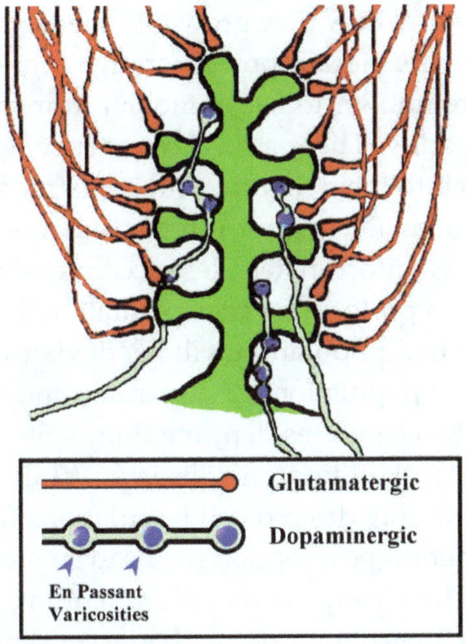

Figure 3. Simplified standard medium spiny dendrite arrangement. The prominent central aspect represents a medium spiny cell dendrite expressing standard dendritic spines. Onto this, many narrow glutamatergic inputs are depicted as synapsing onto the tips of dendritic spines, while dopaminergic input travels upward juxtaposing en-passant varicosities onto spine or dendrite shafts, modulating receptive states in a coordinated manner. Dopaminergic inputs are temporally enhanced by coincident phasic stimulation at the level of the nigra along with electrotonic coupling of nigral neurons. Proximity of cholinergic and GABAergic inputs not shown but each transmitter contribution influences the other either directly or indirectly through their converging influence on the medium spiny striatal efferent.

behavioral-event-related rather than based on local control, with local control as a secondary mechanism. As diffusion of the released dopamine occurs between such contributing neurons, this differential release control would likely establish a new consistent ambient chronic level, lacking a temporal relationship with sensorimotor events that dopamine is meant to modify, providing progressively decreasing phasic relevance to the circuit over time. At this point, if the host system has not adapted in ways that reduce dynamic sensitivities, such dopamine contributions may elicit disruptive effects, such as dyskinesias [127, 128], though other research calls this into question [80, 129]. Certainly the diminished temporal control of striatal dopamine release would be a reason for diminished support of dynamic behavioral control, and might be argued to underlie the longevity of a graft's therapeutic effectiveness.

4. Adaptation of transplanted neural cells to the endogenous host tissue

It is nearly impossible to distinguish between host-to-transplant and transplant-to-host communication because the interactions between both populations are so intimate. However, for the flow of this review, we decided to first address mechanisms of concern regarding modifications engaged by local host cells such as their growth into the transplant and efforts to exert control. Now, we turn our attention to the manner in which transplanted cells likely recognize what they should do and how they grow into the host with an effort to exert control. As indicated previously, there are certain pro-generative regions such as the olfactory bulb and the hippocampus that are known to accommodate transplantation of new neural cells into their architecture more readily. These structures engage a system already established to continue adding new neurons into their circuits with adjustments according to demand regularly throughout adult mammalian lives, while other structures more commonly experiencing disease-driven deterioration are, unfortunately, less accommodating. Certain practical matters come into play when arranging a protocol for transplantation that limits how developmentally committed the transplant-destined population will be, deviating from the ideal circumstance of, for example, generating pure populations of dopamine and cAMP-regulated phosphoprotein (DARPP-32, marker for the classic resident medium spiny type) expressing GABAergic neurons for striatal transplant in Huntington's disease. While it is often an implicit goal to develop purified populations of only desired cell populations for transplantation, the context of "normal" developmental phenotype adoption seems to be modulated quite handily by local glial cells. If not somehow biochemically prevented from doing so, pure stem cell populations also typically develop into mixtures of neurons and glial cells in a manner approximating that expressed developmentally, with more glial cells than neurons, because the signaling molecules responsible for producing this distribution derive from the manner in which neuronal populations distinguish from epithelial populations with both distal and surface interactions [130]. By comparison, the more purified populations of specific neurons raised *in vitro* by various groups [131], would require considerable artificial manipulations compared with natural development.

As described above, previous transplant efforts have utilized populations of cells that have already developed a predisposition toward neuron types that have been responsible for some cells thriving in homotypic versus ectopic target destinations. Thus, when working *in vitro*, complete pre-differentiation and purification of specific neuronal populations requires extensive prior modification, and these efforts seem to benefit from the inclusion of developmentally-consistent proper local glial cell support [132–134]. *In vivo*, this supporting role seems largely adopted by astrocytes that enhance survival [135]. Neuronal differentiation seems to occur in conjunction with an effort to extend neurites and seek connections; a sensible concept given the previously-described importance of being connected to, and making connections in, the developing organism. After culture, the cells in question need to be lifted from their culture conditions and placed into a delivery mechanism (typically a syringe), for transplantation. It has been pointed out that primary neuron cultures might be particularly sensitive to the trypsin dissociation step and suggestions that more gentle procedures, such as papain, for dissociation of these cells have been made in recent scientific communications [136, 137], along with the notion that extensive floating cultures also face challenges. Therefore, researchers frequently opt for transplantation prior to full neurite extension and interconnectedness, even prior to full neuronal commitment, with the presumption that remaining neuronal commitment will occur *in situ*. Transplants often occur with suspensions of dissociated individual cells or of neurospheres (for review of neural sphere transplant contributions see [138]). If final neuronal commitment occurs after transplantation then, to some extent, this process will be guided by environmental cues within the host tissue.

Clearly, to adopt a specific neuronal fate with exclusive neurotransmitter-releasing properties, there are specific genes that must be expressed, as each phenotype would require either exclusive gene expression to produce or post-translationally select specific neuropeptides for release, or to process precursors enzymatically to generate classic neurotransmitters. These genes and immediate products have generated a new phenomenology that captures the immunohistochemical characterization of cell types in modern histology. It has, however, become abundantly clear that gene expression responsible for this is controlled by complicated internal processes that, despite early presumptions to the contrary, are not permanent or irreversible. The more prominent of these involve histone manipulations such as acetylation or methylation of DNA. This leads to the DNA source of specific genes becoming buried within inaccessible Gordian-like knots, which may be unwound to allow for DNA transcription under certain contexts. Current technology maintains the clear capacity to take committed cells and reverse this genetic commitment to generate what is now called "induced pluripotency," essentially restoring a precursor status to cells, even after they have become a more standard somatic type. In order for this induced pluripotency to be remotely possible, as well as subsequent guided induction of specific types of neurons from such cells, some genetic propensities must remain, even in cells that have outwardly adopted noticeably distinct fates. Early explorations of neuronal phenotype commitment involved explorations of the bizarre and seemingly extreme tendency of sympathetic neurons that ended up targeting the sweat glands to *convert* from a noradrenergic to a cholinergic phenotype [139]. Considerable controversy surrounded the search for the target-derived factor that was responsible for inducing this switch, which was clearly necessary given the cholinergic receptor population of the gland, and research centered on a cytokine family molecule [140]. The capacity of neurons to switch transmitter expression or take on more complicated forms of expression during development is broader than this [141], but these examples clearly demonstrate that the mechanisms underlying neuronal phenotype determination remain versatile and responsive to external signals, even after neuronal differentiation. This suggests that precursor cells would harbor an even more versatile capacity to properly respond to host signals and, as such, merge into the circuit in a regionally attentive manner.

The process of becoming a neuron is sensitive to the degree of electrical stimulation in that the corresponding calcium increases tend to facilitate neuronal differentiation [47]. In the case of the earlier stage fetal development following more complex anterior-posterior differentiation of the neural tube and the establishment of prosencephalon, mesencephalon, and rhombencephalon, more distinct neuronal populations begin to emerge due to specific morphogen combinations and temporal sequences of exposure [142, 143], with certain regions producing environmental signals conducive to specific neuronal subtypes. As glutamatergic neurons distinguish from GABAergic neurons within regionally distinct sub-areas of the subventricular source of new neurons, basic helix-loop-helix transcription factors are induced to kick in, such as neurogenins, leading to a glutamatergic fate, and Mash-1 along with the "distal less" homeodomain genes presumably induced into expression by positional signals Dlx1 and Dlx2 that seem to promote a GABAergic fate, with the degree of initial neurogenin or Mash-1 expression a seemingly deciding factor [144]. When cells that are transplanted into the early developing nervous system are evaluated for the expression of regionally specific markers, such as these transcription factors, they seem to express themselves as if they pay little heed to their ectopic location. For example, one experiment demonstrated that only about 6% of the transplanted cells that took up residence in the striatum expressed Dlx immunoreactivity, indicating a GABAergic trajectory, while 37% of the transplanted cells residing in the tectum, a region typically devoid of this marker, expressed this marker [145]. Such data suggest that there may be a longer-term set of guidance steps that feed into promoting the regionally specific neuronal phenotypes that include an earlier need for cell juxtaposition interactions that generate homeodomain predilections prior to the final departure of neurons from the cell cycle. The circumstances seem somewhat different in vitro with populations of neural stem cells, because when growth factors are carefully removed from such populations within N2B27 media (conducive of neuronal differentiation), the large majority of neurons (over 80%) produced adopt the GABAergic phenotype [146]. Another informative embryonic-to-embryonic transplant study that broadens the developmental factors associated with phenotype decisions was performed by Magrassi and colleagues [147]. They found that when ganglionic eminence-derived neurons clustered together as aggregates, they supported each other in maintaining their GABAergic phenotype fate while, by contrast, neurons that migrate into ectopic locations as individuals may adopt alternative fates guided by local signals. The capacity of cells that are predestined to adopt alternative fates based on responding to positional signals has been demonstrated in that they are able to adopt cortical-like morphologies when they migrate into the cortex, presumably as individual neurons [148]. In fact, at this early point in transplantation evaluation, outcome assessments based largely on the morphology of neurons indicated that transplantation into any region seemed to be guided by local cue phenotype induction toward locally appropriate fates (e.g., [149]). These days such assessments are largely considered insufficient, and a more marker-specific immunocytological phenotype determination is encouraged. When these are evaluated with the subventricular-zone-derived adult neural stem cells and their common migration trajectory into the olfactory bulb, it has been suggested that differential phenotypes or phenotype-restrictions might begin to be established quite early, prior to migration to the destination, given the diversity of expressions despite common local cues within the bulb [150]. However, a more recent hypothesis-driven review compiled by Sequerra and colleagues [151] suggests that the capacity for true phenotype guidance from local cues can be quite extensive, such that environmental circumstances can differentiate between glutamatergic and GABAergic phenotypes and manipulations of morphogen expressions, such as sonic hedgehog, by blocking it in ventral locations or ectopically expressing it in dorsal locations can "dorsalize" neuronal phenotypes in ventral sectors or "ventralize" them in dorsal sectors respectively. Transplantation of small numbers of embryonic stem cells into various regions and subsequent specific tracking of resulting neurons indicates that within the intact mouse brain there is a regionally distinct capacity to promote the incorporation of new neurons that is largely progressively lost with age, but when neurons merge into the circuit during more accommodating developmental periods, they typically adopt regionally appropriate functional contributions.

What about the projection potential of transplanted neurons as they attempt to integrate with the host? As described before, Wictorin and his collaborators [84] explored the placement of presumed striatal-predestined rat embryonic ganglionic eminence-derived grafts into the striatum of adult rats following excitotoxic lesions in this same-target location. They witnessed significant growth into the basal ganglia circuitry with the majority of the graft adopting a GABAergic phenotype and projecting *myelinated* axon growth into the host globus pallidus, with only a few projections showing retrograde transport indicating they reached the substantia nigra reticulata. Interestingly in his review, Wictorin [84] also mentions control studies performed in which cerebellar precursor tissue was transplanted into the striatum instead of the ganglionic eminence-derived cells, and that this ectopic transplant resulted in considerably diminished outgrowth and diminished integration with either glutamatergic or dopaminergic host-derived afferent ingrowth. The migration of neurons was even affected when transplants were placed into the developing neonatal striatum in a restricted manner when cerebellar precursor tissue was used instead of striatal precursor tissue, indicating the relevant guidance cues are established early [152]. As might be imagined, hindbrain (rhombencephalon) precursor tissue, transplanted into the adult cerebellum after excitotoxic lesions in that region, adopts several local phenotypes and seems to grow extensively into this region, recapitulating that circuit to an arguably regionally specific, yet similar, degree [153]. This indicates that homotypic versus ectopic concerns are more universal and relevant to multiple regions. Interestingly, human-derived precursor cells transplanted into the rat brain have also been described as growing more extensively into the rat host than do either rat- or mouse-derived precursor cells, though they seemed also to be sensitive to being placed within a homotypic domain (striatal into striatum) versus an ectopic domain (cerebellar into striatum), once again expressing significantly reduced growth into the latter host location [154]. It is intriguing to speculate about how human-derived neural precursors attain a more prominent and extensive host integration into rat host tissue when the signals presumably inspiring growth are likely distinct, though it has been speculated that human cells harbor a propensity to grow for greater distances before target-derived signals are expected while exhibiting a relative insensitivity to growth-inhibiting signals that are produced by the host. The bottom line message of this section is that cell populations seem to acquire, and become limited by, their: (1) neuronal status where they depart from the mitosis cycle, (2) neurotransmitter phenotype that limits their range of influence, and (3) regional predilection that bolsters their contribution to the circuit when they recognize "home" and diminishes contributions from cells delivered elsewhere. This regional predilection has been described above for striatal, or ganglionic eminence-derived neurons, transplanted into the striatum. Apparently, it is also relevant to dopaminergic neuron transplants of fetal ventral mesencephalon, which typically includes both nigral (A9) and ventral tegmental (A10) "type" neurons and for which the ability to successfully re-innervate the striatum is far superior among the nigral type, both anatomically and in terms of behavioral support [155–157]. It seems clear that there are niche components integrated into neuronal phenotypes that extend beyond merely the transmitter they express.

So what does this say about the ectopic dopaminergic cell transplantation into the striatum and the idea that transplant contributions will be more successful if placed within their target region? These efforts do require some background explanation. Parkinson's disease has been understood as mainly a loss of forebrain or more specifically striatal dopamine for most of its history. Although the specific temporal and spatial actions of striatal and greater basal ganglia neurons have been better understood for quite some time, there has been a corresponding lack of attention to the temporal dynamics of the dopamine provisions to that system in the clinical world, presumably because the tools available seem to work without a need for such a concern. The virtue of the most common pharmaceutical treatment, Levodopa, seems to derive largely from ensuring a more consistent dopamine presence. Dopamine agonists, also used as a pharmacological treatment, likely linger outside any strict temporal parameters in that they are likely removed only by diffusion. Animal models benefit from rudimentary delivery mechanisms that also largely appear to maintain dopamine presence with little to no dynamic shifting according to "need," as might be expected of the phasic attributes of an intact dopamine system. Clearly the previously-mentioned movement tests that reveal the insufficient temporal precision of behavioral control with classic treatment has heightened awareness of the concern [108]. Nevertheless it is readily apparent that dopamine cell transplantation for the Parkinson's patient remains largely conceptualized as a more sophisticated delivery system for dopamine that may become increasingly necessary as the ongoing deterioration of dopaminergic neurons diminishes the patient's capacity to convert Levodopa into dopamine. The enzyme aromatic L-amino acid decarboxylase is necessary to complete this conversion step and experimental animal tests indicate that the effects of Levodopa both depend on this action and that serotonergic neurons within the brain, which also harbor this enzyme, may be capable of supporting continued benefit from the drug [158]. Dopamine neuron transplantation into the striatum likely provides improved benefit beyond this serotonergic neuron involvement in that transplanted cells would be capable of growing into greater proximity, and that their terminals would maintain an improved reuptake transport control of the corresponding dopamine released that serotonergic neurons would lack. Nonetheless, for the reasons mentioned in the previous section, the absence of controlled dynamic modification would develop into a problem over time as the greater circuit compensates, and should be attended to as clinical strategies are formulated.

Presumably behavioral support would be improved if derived from dopamine release from more fully reconstructed dopaminergic projections from a grafted nigra into the striatum as there would be improved potential for dynamic temporal control by more "appropriate" afferents. Despite the fact that most reviews of transplants for PD mention this point (e.g., [155]), to our current knowledge, despite several apparent successes in establishing nigra-to-striatum re-innervation from nigral dopaminergic grafts [159–165], there have been no systemic assessments of the afferent control of these grafts established by the host. Clearly the main interest at present with such a grafting strategy is to ensure the dopaminergic reconstruction extends across the inhospitable terrain of the adult brain from the nigra to the striatum. Likely due to the expression of considerable disruptive signals within the adult CNS and the need for more continual support during the growth process, initial efforts to coax this reconstruction from homotypic nigral-placed grafts were unsuccessful in breaching the divide, though even these relatively nigral-restricted grafts did provide some behavioral support [166], likely due to the importance of dendritic dopamine release within the nigra [167]. In fact, the neuronal populations upon which the dendritic dopamine release likely plays its role are GABAergic neurons in the reticulata, and efforts to transplant GABA-producing neurons into this region have also demonstrated some behavioral benefit, presumably by somehow expanding the repertoire of this basal ganglia output region [83, 168]. Such an effect speaks volumes, questioning the precision of the disinhibitory feedback loop formed by striatal efferents to the nigra reticulata and on to the ventrolateral and ventromedial thalamus, understood to form the basis of motor program selection provided by the basal ganglia [169]. These GABAergic transplants into the nigra also may contribute benefit by increasing the local suppression of noise as described previously for the seemingly noisy striatum. As efforts expanded, it became clear that considerable neurotrophic support was necessary and this was either provided by "bridge" tissue grafts that might be likely to release such compounds, such as Schwann cell type cells, or the local cells were induced to release these compounds by viral transgenic expression (e.g., [82, 160, 170]). This strategy renders the CNS territory through which the new dopaminergic fibers must grow more hospitable, presumably also providing retrograde support signals, inspiring continued growth, and staving off the previously-described cell death that results from the lack of connectedness during this growth journey.

It is notable that while many of these strategies were being tested, a well-recognized age dependency was revealed in that even significant dopamine-depleting lesions performed on young and neonatal animals yielded only mild or dramatically diminished behavioral deficits [171, 172]. At the same time, these animals, when grown to adults, still depended upon dopamine for their locomotor behavior, albeit in an altered way [173], and produced sufficient but diminished levels of striatal dopamine to accomplish this [174]. Perhaps the enhanced plasticity supporting this maintenance of dopamine-dependent behavioral control was derived from the natural expression of neurotrophic factors that maintain a higher presence during early postnatal periods of development [175]. A general protection of dopaminergic neurons has been shown to derive from glial-derived neurotrophic factor (GDNF) in particular [176]. In fact, it has been determined that developing nigral dopaminergic neurons depends considerably on GDNF for their survival and maintenance by the establishment of a conditional GDNF knock-out mouse that exhibits clear dopaminergic disruption-related hypokinesia and diminished tyrosine hydroxylase among dopaminergic neurons once GDNF production is blocked during adulthood [177]. The age-dependency factor, regarding the dopamine system, has also been demonstrated in the ability to incorporate dopaminergic transplants. Efforts to unilaterally transplant dopaminergic fetal grafts into the substantia nigra on postnatal days 3, 10, and 20 into rats that had received bilateral 6-OHDA lesions on postnatal day 1 resulted in the intriguing finding that transplants given on postnatal days 3 and 10 showed evidence of nigrostriatal regrowth or fuller incorporation into that circuit, while those receiving transplants on postnatal day 20 did not [178]. It seems GDNF and BDNF may cooperate, to some extent, in supporting dopaminergic cells, as BDNF has also been used successfully to promote a sparse re-innervation of the striatum from a nigral-targeted graft [179]. The neurotrophic factors that seem to play supportive roles expand considerably when observed in the light of what supports the original production of the medial forebrain bundle during development [180].

Coaxing the growth-trajectory environment to also express adhesion molecules that new growth cones might grow along has also been considered (e.g., [170]). The sorts of glial cells or other tissue, which are often added to the equation of a "bridge," are generally not those known to be disruptive to axon growth such as astrocytes and oligodendrocytes. In fact when the medial forebrain bundle pathway is observed for regrowth following axotomy, sprouting of new axons is considerably enhanced by removing glial cells from the growth path by use of a glial toxin [181]. Among the putative interfering variables to this sort of existing cell regrowth are heparan sulfate proteoglycans, chondroitin sulfate proteoglycans, and keratan sulfate proteoglycans that are derived from activated astrocytes that surround lesions [182]. Developing dopaminergic neurons of the substantia nigra must sprout axons that grow anteriorly for substantial lengths to reach their target termination zones. Also, anatomists have recognized a substantial formation of synapses *en passant* among these and other monoaminergic neuron types, suggesting multiple way stations occur within target structures prior to establishing classic terminal boutons, each subject to various degrees of local control [183]. Their extensive growth trajectory requires growth-promoting and cell-death-diminishing signal molecules during axon extension, particularly when transplants are placed during adulthood when the road is longer. Thus, regrowth from such posterior-ventral origins likely depend on the presence of cellular *guideposts* along the way that might break up the full growth required of the nigrostriatal tract into growth stints that are supported by retrograde feedback signals, as well as the removal of potentially interfering substances derived from activated glia. The involvement of glia in the diminished propensity to grow extensive connections from posterior regions may also depend on the manner in which the original lesion is created. It may be that the neurotoxins used in animal models to induce dopamine-depleting lesions (e.g., 6-OHDA, MPTP) exacerbate glia, resulting in more activation of astrocytes and thereby interfering with regrowth (see [184, 185]). However in most idiopathic cases of Parkinson's disease, there is a distinct lack of reactive astrocytes during the course of deterioration or afterward [186, 187], indicating that the contributions of chondroitin sulfate and other growth-interfering responses might be lower in this condition, despite a clear insufficiency of dopaminergic regrowth. Nevertheless, the indication that reactive astrocytes may linger for up to 90 days following 6-OHDA administration [185] is intriguing when the rat 6-OHDA treated model system is considered because usually transplantation is performed prior to that time in those animal models.

Homotypic transplant placement may also be promoted in the context of dopaminergic cells, given that their qualities may be guided more substantially by local cues, as well as gaining from local afferent control. During development, the local ventral midbrain environment seems to contribute considerable epigenetic guidance to newly generated neurons in the form of morphogens. One of these morphogens that has been classically associated with ventral development beginning at the neural tube stage is sonic hedgehog (for review see [188]). The two prominent locally secreted factors that drive dopaminergic phenotype development are fibroblast growth factor 8 (FGF-8) and sonic hedgehog [175], leading to internal genetic expression of Nurr1 and Ptx3 transcription factors that further establish phenotype delineation. This is likely why those two secreted factors are used in protocols that guide the development of dopaminergic phenotypes from more pluripotent precursors *in vitro* (e.g., [189, 190]). When ventral mesencephalic-derived embryonic stem cells are left to develop freely in culture, many of them develop as dopaminergic, but there is also a mixture of phenotypes that might be expected from the ventral midbrain or hindbrain such as serotonergic and GABAergic neurons. Efforts to improve the yield of dopaminergic phenotypes have produced multiple proposed protocols involving different steps that replicate different aspects of developmental phenotype adoption. For example, one of these uses the Wnt signaling to influence developing neurons at the location of the developing nigra. Wnt signaling seems to be established to differential degrees in the developing nervous system, in large part by cell to cell contact information and signal gradients that get established during the course of progressive commitment in gene expression. Specifically, inducing the transcription factor known as Wnt5a via transfection, following sonic hedgehog and FGF-8 exposure, seems to generate greater dopaminergic phenotype yields than sonic hedgehog and FGF-8 alone [191]. In addition, bone marrow derived stem cells seem to require a neuronal-enhancing, region-specific environment characterized by low oxygen, retinoic acid, and continuous neurotrophin-3 stimulation, as these in combination with the aforementioned sonic hedgehog and FGF-8 stimulation seem to enhance dopaminergic phenotype expression further [192]. All this indicates that there are specific local environments that would induce phenotype commitment based on regionally-specific combinations of factors that are provided in the appropriate sequence during development, and these remain in a sort of residual form still capable of supporting, albeit at a more limited degree of commitment, in the adult structure. The capacity of dopaminergic neurons grafted into the nigra to acquire afferent control remains understudied, but this capacity would likely be higher than that of ectopic transplants into the striatum. If gap junction connections could also be established with the local endogenous dopamine neurons of the nigra, this could enhance temporal pattern production substantially. Of course, if there are ongoing deterioration-inducing challenges among the Parkinsonian endogenous dopamine neurons this could induce the closure of gap junction connections, due to sensed pH or calcium changes, as a protective response [193]. However, given the circumscribed positioning of the dopaminergic neurons within the nigra following the transplant, it would seem a far more straightforward incorporation process regarding afferent stimulation in general than what would otherwise be required within the striatum.

Multiple placement transplants have been performed using animal models that have shown more substantial support for behavior. Experiments performed by Mukhida and colleagues showed considerable improvement in behavioral control with dopaminergic-destined fetal ventral mesencephalic transplants into the striatum, substantia nigra, and subthalamic nucleus that seemed to improve behavioral recovery better than the typical single transplant alone [194]. Clearly there may be a benefit to such extended transplantation but there are two major issues drawing the practicality of such strategies into question. First, transplantation of cells into one area in human patients is already a significant procedure, fraught with considerable risk and expense. The idea of multiple sites of transplantation would need to be justified by not only significant movement restoration but also in long-term viability beyond the 5-week, post-transplantation assessments commonly used. Second, given the concerns raised in this review, each ectopic transplant performed is likely to both provide some distortion in the temporal dynamics of delivery and also would perhaps block the more successful growth and penetration of the homotypic aspect. How well would new nigrostriatal terminals grow into the striatum if there are already local striatal dopaminergic terminals competing for CNS real estate in the same region? Given the clinical limitations and the likely extended growth time that would be required for nigrostriatal restoration, it may be prudent to consider formulating temporary neurons that could be progressively eliminated as fibers reach the striatum that could maintain a "substitute" dopamine presence. The concern with dual transplants (both in the nigra and the striatum) is that striatal transplants would likely diminish the growth or synaptogenesis drive among incoming nigrostriatal growth cones in a manner similar to what seems to occur among striatal neurons transplanted into the intact striatum (establishing limited interactions with the host as a result). At this point, developing transgenic transplantable cells with pharmacologically inducible properties may be able to accomplish this temporary substitute goal. Initial inefficient support might be maintained during the growth process and this might be progressively and selectively removed as dopaminergic growth from homotypic regions reaches the area.

5. Concluding remarks

Plastic adaptation was described above as representing a multitude of cellular responses that occur with the apparent role of maintaining cellular homeostasis, yet within the nervous system also support the maintenance of a sort of dynamic status quo in which compensatory changes adjust the actions or response capacities of local healthy neurons in support of a superseding circuit-associated need. We understand that various CNS circuits establish the capacity to process a wide range of information with various degrees of versatility that presumably evolved to provide stability in some areas of common reliance and flexibility in areas where learning functions occur regularly and synaptic adjustments are correspondingly at higher demand. Neurons appear to undergo adaptations as they attempt to enter a circuit, and the environmental guidance for the control contributed by new additions extends to various degrees backward into the history of the newly added cells in question as it signals what it can provide and encourages host connections while it negotiates for acceptance into the host circuit and the privilege of contributing. As neurons do this during development, their relative pluripotency diminishes toward the eventual niche they enter into and it is highly likely that new neuronal contributions transplanted into these circumstances go through similar steps as they adapt to the roles they play. The long-term viability of additions requires that a utility anticipated by the circuit is fulfilled or the host circuit may adapt the addition out of relevance like an efficient social system isolates and eventually eliminates an influence perceived as disruptive. As an example, a long-term neurotransmitter lingering without dynamic change could come from leaky or malfunctioning neurons, so it would benefit a circuit to recognize this and diminish postsynaptic responses until the signal once again exceeds noise. Synaptic negotiation during development of the mammalian neuromuscular system, which has been more accessible and easier to manipulate with experiments, shows a series of back and forth messages that eventually culminate in the muscle fiber accepting one motoneuron terminal and rejecting other applications for the job (see [195] for detailed discussion of this process). It is likely that whether neurons incorporate into CNS circuits depends upon their capacity to apply themselves and on whether the corresponding job has already been taken, as indicated by the diminished success of transplants into adult intact CNS structures achieving synaptic incorporation. While it is possible for neuronal precursors to be conditioned in a manner that promotes certain wanted phenotypes, the ability to properly incorporate into a workable circuit is challenged when they are placed into an ectopic environment as described above. To draw an analogy to human socialization, it's as if the cells in question either have, or are given, an agenda that may or may not merge with the agenda of the local host circuit. The mechanisms in place that promote apoptosis, in this context, are a useful and positive contribution to the overall circuit despite the fact that the death of cells seems unfortunate. Neurons in various deteriorative diseases adopt abnormal activities. In fact, the whole basis of deep brain stimulation, as derived from earlier therapies for Parkinson's disease, was to render excessive and aberrant activity quiescent (see [196, 197]). It is important that our clinical efforts consider the adaptive nature of the host tissue, into which we desire our transplants to be incorporated as this strategy will meet with greater long-term success and fewer potentially disruptive side-effects that generate additional, unwanted measures into the equation if these concerns are not accounted for from the outset.

Acknowledgements

Support for this work was provided by the Central Michigan Neuroscience Program, the Central Michigan University Office of Research and Sponsored Programs, the John G. Kulhavi Professorship, and the Field Neurosciences Institute.

Author details

Michael I. Sandstrom[1*], Kevin A. Anderson[1], Naveen Jayaprakash[2], Parnit K. Bhupal[1] and Gary L. Dunbar[1,3]

*Address all correspondence to: sands1m@cmich.edu

1 Neuroscience and Experimental Psychology Programs, Central Michigan University, Mount Pleasant, MI, USA

2 Biomedical Science, Marquette University, Milwaukee, WI, USA

3 Field Neurosciences Institute, Saginaw, MI, USA

References

[1] Mazzini L, Ferrero I, Luparello V, Rustichelli D, Gunetti M, Mareschi K, Testa L, Stecco A, Tarletti R, Miglioretti M, Fava E, Nasuelli N, Cisari C, Massara M, Vercelli R. Mesenchymal stem cell transplantation in amyotrophic lateral sclerosis: A phase I clinical trial. Experimental Neurology. 2010;**223**(1):229-237. DOI: 10.1016/j.expneurol.2009.08.007

[2] Lindvall O, Kokaia Z. Stem cells for the treatment of neurological disorders. Nature. 2006; **441**:1094-1096. DOI: 10.1038/nature04960

[3] Mezey E, Key S, Vogelsang G, Szalayova I, Lange D, Crain B. Transplanted bone marrow generates new neurons in human brains. Proceedings of the National Academy of Sciences of the United States of America. 2003;**100**(3):1364-1369. DOI: 10.1073/pnas.0336479100

[4] Rossignol J, Fink K, Davis K, Clerc S, Crane A, Matchynski J, Lowrance S, Bombard M, Derkorver N, Lescaudron L, Dunbar GL. Transplants of adult mesenchymal and neural stem cells provide neuroprotection and behavioral sparing in a transgenic rat model of Huntington's disease. Stem Cells. 2014;**32**(2):500-509. DOI: 10.1002/stem.1508

[5] Lescaudron L, Unni D, Dunbar GL. Autologous adult bone marrow stem cell transplantation in an animal model of Huntington's disease: Behavioral and morphological outcomes. International Journal of Neuroscience. 2003;**113**(7):945-956. DOI: 10.1080/00207450390207759

[6] Kim J-H, Auerbach JM, Rodríguez-Gómez JA, Velasco I, Gavin D, Lumelsky N, Lee S-H, Nguyen J, Sánchez-Pernaute R, Bankiewicz K, McKay R. Dopamine neurons derived from embryonic stem cells function in an animal model of Parkinson's disease. Nature. 2002; **418**:50-56. DOI: 10.1038/nature00900

[7] Li W, Englund E, Widner H, Mattsson B, van Westen D, Latt J, Rehncrona S, Brundin P, Björklund A, Lindvall O, Li JY. Extensive graft-derived dopaminergic innervation is maintained 24 years after transplantation in the degenerating parkinsonian brain. Proceedings of the National Academy of Sciences of the United States of America. 2016;**113**(23):6544-6549. DOI: 10.1073/pnas.1605245113

[8] Björklund A, Dunnett SB, Brundin P, Stoessl AJ, Freed CR, Breeze RE, Levivier M, Peschanski M, Studer L, Barker R. Neural transplantation for the treatment of Parkinson's disease. The Lancet Neurology. 2003;**2**:437-445. DOI: 10.1016/S1474-4422(03)00442-3

[9] Freeman TB, Olanow CW, Hauser RA, Nauert GM, Smith DA, Borlongan CV, Sanberg PR, Holt DA, Kordower JH, Vingerhoets FJ, Snow BJ, Calne D, Gauger LL. Bilateral fetal nigral transplantation into the postcommissural putamen in Parkinson's disease. Annals of Neurology. 1995;**38**(3):379-388. DOI: 10.1002/ana.410380307

[10] Napoli E, Borlongan CV. Cell therapy in Parkinson's disease: Host repair machinery gets a boost from stem cell grafts. Stem Cells. 2017;**35**(6):1443-1445. DOI: 10.1002/stem.2636

[11] Walczak P, Chen N, Eve D, Hudson J, Zigova T, Sanchez-Ramos J, Sanberg PR, Sanberg CD, Willing AE. Long-term cultured human umbilical cord neural-like cells transplanted into the striatum of NOD SCID mice. Brain Research Bulletin. 2007;**74**(1-3):155-163. DOI: 10.1016/j.brainresbull.2007.06.015

[12] Conti L, Reitano E, Cattaneo E. Neural stem cell systems: Diversities and properties after transplantation in animal models of diseases. Brain Pathology. 2006;**16**(2):143-154. DOI: 10.1111/j.1750-3639.2006.00009.x

[13] Rokni U, Richardson AG, Bizzi E, Seung HS. Motor learning with unstable neural representations. Neuron. 2007;**54**(4):653-666. DOI: 10.1016/j.neuron.2007.04.030

[14] Hyman SE. Addiction: A disease of learning and memory. American Journal of Psychiatry. 2005;**162**(8):1414-1422. DOI: 10.1176/appi.ajp.162.8.1414

[15] Baker-Andresen D, Ratnu VS, Bredy TW. Dynamic DNA methylation: A prime candidate for genomic metaplasticity and behavioral adaptation. Trends in Neurosciences. 2013;**36**(1):3-13. DOI: 10.1016/j.tins.2012.09.003

[16] Day JJ, Sweatt JD. Epigenetic mechanisms in cognition. Neuron. 2011;**70**(5):813-829. DOI: 10.1016/j.neuron.2011.05.019

[17] Tsankova N, Rentha W, Kumar A, Nestler EJ. Epigenetic regulation in psychiatric disorders. Nature Reviews Neuroscience. 2007;**8**:355-367. DOI: 10.1038/nrn2132

[18] Renthal W, Maze I, Krishnan V, Covington HE III, Xiao G, Kumar A, Russo SJ, Graham A, Tsankova N, Kippin TE, Kerstetter KA, Neve RL, Haggarty SJ, McKinsey TA, Bassel-Duby R, Olson EN, Nestler EJ. Histone deacetylase 5 epigenetically controls behavioral adaptations to chronic emotional stimuli. Neuron. 2007;**56**(3):517-529. DOI: 10.1016/j.neuron.2007.09.032

[19] Ganguly K, Poo M. Activity-dependent neural plasticity from bench to bedside. Neuron. 2013;**80**(3):729-741. DOI: 10.1016/j.neuron.2013.10.028

[20] Abbott LF, Nelson SB. Synaptic plasticity: Taming the beast. Nature Neuroscience. 2000;**3**: 1178-1183. DOI: 10.1038/81453

[21] Ziles K. Neuronal plasticity as an adaptive property of the central nervous system. Annals of Anatomy - Anatomischer Anzeiger. 1992;**174**(5):383-391. DOI: 10.1016/S0940-9602(11)80255-4

[22] Klein WL, Sullivan J, Skorupa A, Aguilar JS. Plasticity of neuronal receptors. The FASEB Journal. 1989;**3**(10):2132-2140. DOI: 10.1096/fj.1530-6860

[23] Hou ST, Jiang SX, Smith RA. Permissive and repulsive cues and signaling pathways of axonal outgrowth and regeneration. International Review of Cell and Molecular Biology. 2008;**267**:125-181. DOI: 10.1016/S1937-6448(08)00603-5

[24] Yu LMY, Leipzig ND, Shoichet MS. Promoting neuron adhesion and growth. Materials Today. 2008;**11**(5):36-43. DOI: 10.1016/S1369-7021(08)70088-9

[25] Chen DF, Tonegawa S. Why do mature CNS neurons of mammals fail to re-establish connections following injury—functions of Bcl-2. Cell Death and Differentiation. 1998; **5**(10):816-822. DOI: 10.1038/sj.cdd.4400431

[26] Silver J. Inhibitory molecules in development and regeneration. Journal of Neurology. 1994;**242**(Suppl.1):S22-S24. DOI: 10.1007/BF00939236

[27] Hidalgo A. Neuron-glia interactions during axon guidance in Drosophila. Biochemical Society Transactions. 2003;**31**(1):50-55. DOI: 10.1042/bst0310050

[28] Bovolenta P, Mason C. Growth cone morphology varies with position in the developing mouse visual pathway from retina to first targets. Journal of Neuroscience. 1987; **7**(5):1447-1460

[29] Li GN, Liu J, Hoffman-Kim D. Multi-molecular gradients of permissive and inhibitory cues direct neurite outgrowth. Annals of Biomedical Engineering. 2008;**36**(6):889-904. DOI: 10.1007/s10439-008-9486-z

[30] Panicker MM, Rao M. Stem cells and neurogenesis. Chapter 18 In: Marshak DR, Gardner RL, Gottlieb D, editors. Stem Cell Biology. Cold Spring Harbor Monograph Series. Cold Spring Harbor, New York: Cold Spring Harbor Laboratory Press. Vol. 40. 2001. pp. 399-438. DOI: 10.1101/087969673.40.399

[31] Scherson T, Serbedzija G, Fraser S, Bronner-Fraser M. Regulative capacity of the cranial neural tube to form neural crest. Development. 1993;**118**:1049-1062

[32] Uylings HBM. Development of the human cortex and the concept of "critical" or "sensitive" periods. Language Learning. 2006;**56**:59-90. DOI: 10.1111/j.1467-9922.2006.00355.x

[33] Henderson C. Role of neurotrophic factors in neuronal development. Current Opinion in Neurobiology. 1996;**6**:64-70. DOI: 10.1016/s0959-4388(96)80010-9

[34] Rabinowicz T, de Courten-Myers GM, Petetot JM-C, Xi G, de los Reys E. Human cortex development: Estimates of neuronal numbers indicate major loss late during gestation. Journal of Neuropathology and Experimental Neurology. 1996;**55**(3):320-328. DOI: 10.1097/00005072-199603000-00007

[35] Lardi-Studler B, Fritschy J-M. Matching of pre- and postsynaptic specializations during synaptogenesis. The Neuroscientist. 2007;**13**(2):115-126. DOI: 10.1177/1073858406296803

[36] Garner CC, Zhai RG, Gundelfinger ED, Ziv NE. Molecular mechanisms of CNS synaptogenesis. Trends in Neurosciences. 2002;**25**(5):243-250. DOI: 10.1016/S0166-2236(02)02152-5

[37] Kwon H-B, Kozorovitskiy Y, Oh W-J, Peixto RT, Akhtar N, Saulnier JL, Gu C, Sabatini BL. Neuroligin-1-dependent competition regulates cortical synaptogenesis and synapse number. Nature Neuroscience. 2012;**15**:1667-1674. DOI: 10.1038/nn.3256

[38] Peng HB, Yang J-F, Dai Z, Lee CW, Hung HW, Feng ZH, Ko C-P. Differential effects of neurotrophins and Schwann cell-derived signals on neuronal survival/growth and synaptogenesis. Journal of Neuroscience. 2003;**23**(12):5050-5060

[39] van Ooyen A, Willshaw DJ. Competition for neurotrophic factor in the development of nerve connections. Proceedings of the Royal Society B - Biological Sciences. 1999;**266**(1422): 883-892. DOI: 10.1098/rspb.1999.0719

[40] Kaiser M, Hilgetag CC, van Ooyen A. A simple rule for axon outgrowth and synaptic competition generates realistic connection lengths and filling fractions. Cerebral Cortex. 2009; **19**(12):3001-3010. DOI: 10.1093/cercor/bhp071

[41] Gulledge AT, Kampa BM, Stuart GJ. Synaptic integration in dendritic trees. Journal of Neurobiology. 2005;**64**(1):75-90. DOI: 10.1002/neu.20144

[42] Lippman J, Dunaevsky A. Dendritic spine morphogenesis and plasticity. Journal of Neurobiology. 2005;**64**(1):47-57. DOI: 10.1002/neu.20149

[43] Spruston N, Stuart G, Hausser M. Dendritic integration. In: Stuart G, Spruston N, Hausser M, editors. Dendrites. New York: Oxford University Press; 1999. pp. 231-270. Ch10

[44] Wefelmeyer W, Puhl CJ, Burrone J. Homeostatic plasticity of subcellular neuronal structures: From inputs to outputs. Trends in Neurosciences. 2016;**39**(10):656-667. DOI: 10.1016/j.tins.2016.08.004

[45] Katsuki T, Joshi R, Ailani D, Hiromi Y. Compartmentalization within neurites: Its mechanisms and implications. Developmental Neurobiology. 2011;**71**(6):458-473. DOI: 10.1002/dneu.20859

[46] Kuba H, Oichi Y, Ohmori H. Presynaptic activity regulates Na^+ channel distribution at the axon initial segment. Nature. 2010;**465**:1075-1078. DOI: 10.1038/nature09087

[47] Yamada M, Tanemura K, Okada S, Iwanami A, Nakamura M, Mizuno H, Ozawa M, Ohyama-Goto R, Kitamura N, Kawano M, Tan-Takeuchi K, Ohtsuka C, Miyawaki A, Takashima A, Ogawa M, Toyama Y, Okano H, Kondo T. Electrical stimulation modulates fate determination of differentiating embryonic stem cells. Stem Cells. 2007;**25**(3):562-570. DOI: 10.1634/stemcells.2006-0011

[48] Babu H, Ramirez-Rodriguez G, Fabel K, Bischofberger J, Kemperman G. Synaptic network activity induces neuronal differentiation of adult hippocampal precursor cells through BDNF signaling. Frontiers in Neuroscience. 2009;**30**:49. DOI: 10.3389/neuro.22.001.2009

[49] Cho T, Ryu JK, Taghibiglou C, Ge Y, Chan AW, Liu L, Lu J, McLarnon JG, Wang YT. Long-term potentiation promotes proliferation/survival and neuronal differentiation of neural stem/progenitor cells. PLoS One. 2013;**8**(10):e76860. DOI: 10.1371/journal.pone.0076860

[50] Jontes JD, Smith SJ. Filopodia, spines, and the generation of synaptic diversity. Neuron. 2000;**27**(1):11-14. DOI: 10.1016/S0896-6273(00)00003-9

[51] Personius KE, Balice-Gordon RJ. Activity-dependent editing of neuromuscular synaptic connections. Brain Research Bulletin. 2000;**53**(5):513-522. DOI: 10.1016/S0361-9230(00)00384-1

[52] Bibel M, Barde Y-A. Neurotrophins: Key regulators of cell fate and cell shape in the vertebrate nervous system. Genes & Development. 2000;**14**:2919-2937. DOI: 10.1101/gad.841400

[53] Gordon N. Apoptosis (programmed cell death) and other reasons for elimination of neurons and axons. Brain and Development. 1995;**17**(1):73-77. DOI: 10.1016/0387-7604(94)00109-B

[54] Temple S. The development of neural stem cells. Nature. 2001;**414**:112-117. DOI: 10.1038/35102174

[55] Soares S, Sotelo C. Adult neural stem cells from the mouse subventricular zone are limited in migratory ability compared to progenitor cells of similar origin. Neuroscience. 2004;**128**(4):807-817. DOI: 10.1016/j.neuroscience.2004.07.031

[56] Zhang Y, Klassen HJ, Tucker BA, Perez M-TR, Young MJ. CNS progenitor cells promote a permissive environment for neurite outgrowth via a matrix metalloproteinase-2-dependent mechanism. Journal of Neuroscience. 2007;**27**(17):4499-4506. DOI: 10.1523/JNEUROSCI.0200-07.2007

[57] Shetty AK, Hattiangady B. Postnatal age governs the extent of differentiation of hippocampal CA1 and CA3 subfield neural stem/progenitor cells into neurons and oligodendrocytes. International Journal of Developmental Neuroscience. 2013;**31**(7):646-656. DOI: 10.1016/j.ijdevneu.2013.05.006

[58] Van Zant G, Liang Y. Concise review: Hematopoietic stem cell aging, life span, and transplantation. STEM CELLS Translational Medicine. 2012;**1**:651-657. DOI: 10.5966/sctm.2012-0033

[59] Akiyama M, Hoshi Y, Sakurai S. Changes of telomere length in children after hematopoietic stem cell transplantation. Bone Marrow Transplantation. 1998;**21**:167-171. DOI: 10.1038/sj.bmt.1701060

[60] Stein DG, Brailowsky S, Will B. Brain Repair. New York: Oxford University Press; 1995. 147 p

[61] Blurton-Jones M, Kitazawa M, Martinez-Coria H, Castello NA, Muller F-J, Loring JF, Yamasaki TR, Poon WW, Green KN, LeFeria FM. Neural stem cells improve cognition via BDNF in a transgenic model of Alzheimer disease. Proceedings of the National Academy of Sciences. 2009;**106**(32):13594-13599. DOI: 10.1073/pnas.0901402106

[62] Alberts JL, Linder SM, Penko AL, Lowe MJ, Phillips M. It is not about the bike, it is about the pedaling: Forced exercise and Parkinson's disease. Exercise and Sport Sciences Reviews. 2011;**39**(4):177-188. DOI: 10.1097/JES.0b013e31822cc71a

[63] Mayer E, Brown VJ, Dunnett SB, Robbins TW. Striatal graft-associated recovery of a lesion-induced performance deficit in the rat requires learning to use the transplant. European Journal of Neuroscience. 1992;**4**:119-126 https://doi.org/10.1111/j.1460-9568.1992.tb00858.x

[64] Barker RA, Widner H. Immune problems in central nervous system cell therapy. NeuroRX. 2004;**1**(4):472-481. DOI: 10.1602/neurorx.1.4.472

[65] Ideguchi M, Shinoyama M, Gomi M, Hayashi H, Hashimoto N, Takahashi J. Immune or inflammatory response by the host brain suppresses neuronal differentiation of transplanted ES cell-derived neural precursor cells. Journal of Neuroscience Research. 2008;**86**(9):1936-1943. DOI: 10.1002/jnr.21652

[66] Di Filipo M, Sarchielli P, Picconi B, Calabresi P. Neuroinflammation and synaptic plasticity: Theoretical basis for a novel, immune-centred, therapeutic approach to neurological disorders. Trends in Pharmacological Sciences. 2008;**29**(8):402-412. DOI: 10.1016/j.tips.2008.06.005

[67] Xanthos DN, Sandkuhler J. Neurogenic neuroinflammation: Inflammatory CNS reactions in response to neuronal activity. Nature Reviews Neuroscience. 2014;**15**:43-53. DOI: 10.1038/nrn3617

[68] Alvarez-Buylla A, Garcia-Verdugo JM. Neurogenesis in adult subventricular zone. Journal of Neuroscience. 2002;**22**(3):629-634

[69] Gould E, Beylin A, Tanapat P, Reeves A, Shors TJ. Learning enhances adult neurogenesis in the hippocampal formation. Nature Neuroscience. 1999;**2**:260-265. DOI: 10.1038/6365

[70] Lledo P-M, Saghatelyan A. Integrating new neurons into the adult olfactory bulb: Joining the network, life-death decisions, and the effects of sensory experience. Trends in Neurosciences. 2005;**28**(5):248-254. DOI: 10.1016/j.tins.2005.03.005

[71] Christie KJ, Turnley AM. Regulation of endogenous neural stem/progenitor cells for neural repair-factors that promote neurogenesis and gliogenesis in the normal and damaged brain. Frontiers in Cellular Neuroscience. 2013;**6**:70. DOI: 10.3389/fncel.2012.00070

[72] Johnson MA, Ables JL, Eisch AJ. Cell-intrinsic signals that regulate adult neurogenesis in vivo: Insights from inducible approaches. BMB Reports. 2009;**42**(5):245-259. DOI: 10.5483/bmbrep.2009.42.5.245

[73] Luzzati F, DeMarchis S, Parlato R, Gribaudo S, Schutz G, Fasolo A, Peretto P. New striatal neurons in a mouse model of progressive striatal degeneration are generated in both the subventricular zone and the striatal perenchyma. PLoS One. 2011;**6**(9):e25088. DOI: 10.1371/journal.pone.0025088

[74] Pahuja R, Seth K, Shukla A, Shukla RK, Bhatnagar P, Chauhan LKS, Saxena PN, Arun J, Chaudhari BP, Patel DK, Singh SP, Shukla R, Khanna VK, Kumar P, Chaturvedi RK, Gupta KC. Trans-blood brain barrier delivery of dopamine-loaded nanoparticles reverses functional deficits in Parkinsonian rats. ACS Nano. 2015;**9**(5):4850-4871. DOI: 10.1021/nn506408v

[75] Chen S, Xianwen C, Dehua X, Zhenguo L, Lingfei X, Smith SW, Zhongcheng Z. Behavioral correction of Parkinsonian rats following the transplantation of immortalized fibroblasts genetically modified with TH and GCH genes. Parkinsonism & Related Disorders. 2003; **9**(2):91-97. DOI: 10.1016/S1353-8020(03)00020-8

[76] Zoli M, Agnati LF. Wiring and volume transmission in the central nervous system: The concept of closed and open synapses. Progress in Neurobiology. 1996;**49**(4):363-380. DOI: 10.1016/0301-0082(96)00020-2

[77] Zolia M, Torria C, Farraria R, Janssonb A, Zinia I, Fuxeb K, Agnatia LF. The emergence of the volume transmission concept. Brain Research Reviews. 1998;**26**(2-3):136-147. DOI: 10.1016/S0165-0173(97)00048-9

[78] Pritzel M, Isacson O, Brundin P, Wiklund L, Björklund A. Afferent and efferent connections of striatal grafts implanted into the ibotenic acid lesioned neostriatum in adult rats. Experimental Brain Research. 1986;**65**:112-126. DOI: 10.1007/bf00243834

[79] Freed CR, Greene PE, Breeze RE, Tsai WY, DuMouchel W, Kao R, Dillon S, Winfield H, Culver S, Trojanowski JQ, Eidelberg D, Fahn S. Transplantation of embryonic dopamine neurons for severe Parkinson's disease. New England Journal of Medicine. 2001;**344**(10):710-719. DOI: 10.1056/NEJM200103083441002

[80] Lee CS, Cenci MA, Schulzer M, Björklund A. Embryonic ventral mesencephalic grafts improve levodopa-induced dyskinesia in a rat model of Parkinson's disease. Brain. 2000; **123**(Pt. 7):1365-1379 https://doi.org/10.1093/brain/123.7.1365

[81] Fraichard A, Chassande O, Bilbaut G, Dehay C, Savatier P, Samarut J. In vitro differentiation of embryonic stem cells into glial cells and functional neurons. Journal of Cell Science. 1995;**108**:3181-3188

[82] Kauhausen J, Thompson LH, Parish CL. Cell intrinsic and extrinsic factors contribute to enhance neural circuit reconstruction following transplantation in parkinsonian mice. The Journal of Physiology. 2013;**591**(1):77-91. DOI: 10.1113/jphysiol.2012.243063

[83] Winkler JD, Kirik D, Björklund A, Dunnett SB. Transplantation in the rat model of Parkinson's disease: Ectopic versus homotopic graft placement. In: Functional Neural

Transplantation II. Novel Cell Therapies for CNS Disorders. Progress in Brain Research. 2000;**127**:233-265. DOI: 10.1016/s0079-6123(00)27012-x Ch11

[84] Wictorin K. Anatomy and connectivity of intrastriatal striatal transplants. Progress in Neurobiology. 1992;**38**:611-639. DOI: 10.1016/0301-0082(92)90044-f

[85] Labandeira-Garcia JL, Wictorin K, Cunningham ET Jr, Björklund A. Development of intrastriatal striatal grafts and their afferent innervation from the host. Neuroscience. 1991; **42**:407-426. DOI: 10.1016/0306-4522(91)90385-2

[86] Xu ZC, Wilson CJ, Emson PC. Synaptic potentials evoked in spiny neurons in rat neostriatal grafts by cortical and thalamic stimulation. Journal of Neurophysiology. 1991;**65**: 477-493

[87] Rutherford A, Garcia-Munoz M, Dunnett SB, Arbuthnott GW. Electrophysiological demonstration of host cortical inputs to striatal grafts. Neuroscience Letters. 1987;**83**:275-281

[88] Sirinathsinghji DJS, Dunnett SB, Isacson O, Clark DJ, Kendrick K, Björklund A. Striatal grafts in rats with unilateral neostriatal lesions II. In vivo monitoring of GABA release in globus pallidus and substantia nigra. Neuroscience. 1988;**24**:803-811. DOI: 10.1016/ 0306-4522(88)90068-1

[89] Miller BR, Walker AG, Shah AS, Barton SJ, Rebec GV. Dysregulated information processing by medium-spiny neurons in striatum of freely behaving mouse models of Huntington's disease. Journal of Neurophysiology. 2008;**100**(4):2205-2216. DOI: 10.1152/jn.90606.2008

[90] Plotkin JL, Surmeier DJ. Corticostriatal synaptic adaptations in Huntington's disease. Current Opinion in Neurobiology. 2015;**33**:53-62. DOI: 10.1016/j.conb.2015.01.020

[91] Estrada-Sanchez AM, Rebec GV. Corticostriatal dysfunction and glutamate transporter 1 (GLT1) in Huntington's disease: Interactions between neurons and astrocytes. Basal Ganglia. 2012;**2**(2):57-66. DOI: 10.1016/j.baga.2012.04.029

[92] Miller BR, Dorner J, Brunner KD, Gaither TW, Klein EL, Barton SJ, Rebec GV. Up-regulation of GLT1 reverses the deficit in cortically evoked striatal ascorbate efflux in the R6/2 mouse model of Huntington's disease. Journal of Neurochemistry. 2012;**121**(4):629-638. DOI: 10.1111/j.1471-4159.2012.07691.x

[93] Sandstrom M, Rebec GV. Characterization of striatal activity in conscious rats: Contribution of NMDA and AMPA/kainate receptors to both spontaneous and glutamate-driven firing. Synapse. 2003;**47**:91-100

[94] Liu G, Rao Y. Neuronal migration from the forebrain to the olfactory bulb requires a new attractant persistent in the olfactory bulb. Journal of Neuroscience. 2003;**23**(16):6651-6659

[95] Wu GY, Cline HT. Stabilization of dendritic arbor structure in vivo by CaMKII. Science. 1998;**279**(5348):222-226. DOI: 10.1126/science.279.5348.222

[96] Magavi SSP, Lois C. Transplanted neurons form both normal and ectopic projections in the adult brain. Developmental Neurobiology. 2008;**68**(14):1527-1537. DOI: 10.1002/dneu.20677

[97] Craig AM, Lichtman JW. Synapse formation and maturation. In: Cowan WM, Sudhof TC, Stevens CF, editors. Synapses. Baltimore: Johns Hopkins University Press; 2001. pp. 571-612. Ch12

[98] Gage FH, Dunnett SB, Stenevi U, Björklund A. Aged rats: Recovery of motor impairments by intrastriatal nigral grafts. Science. 1983;**221**(4614):966-969. DOI: 10.1126/science.6879196

[99] Björklund A, Dunnett SB, Stenevi U, Lewis ME, Iverson SD. Reinnervation of the denervated striatum by substantia nigra transplants: Functional consequences as revealed by pharmacological and sensorimotor testing. Brain Research. 1980;**199**(2):307-333. DOI: 10.1016/0006-8993(80)90692-7

[100] Watabe-Uchida M, Zhu L, Ogawa S, Vamanrao A, Uchida N. Whole brain mapping of direct inputs to midbrain dopamine neurons. Neuron. 2012;**74**(5):858-873. DOI: 10.1016/j.neuron.2012.03.017

[101] Parent A, Hazrati L-N. Functional anatomy of the basal ganglia I. The cortico-basal ganglia-thalamo-cortical loop. Brain Research Reviews. 1995;**20**:91-127. DOI: 10.1016/0165-0173(94)00007-C

[102] Doucet G, Murata Y, Brundin P, Bosler O, Mons N, Geffard M, Ouimet CC, Björklund A. Host afferents into intrastiatal transplants of fetal ventral mesencephalon. Experimental Neurology. 1989;**106**(1):1-19. DOI: 10.1016/0014-4886(89)90139-8

[103] Braak H, Del Tredici K. Assessing fetal nerve cell grafts in Parkinson's disease. Nature Medicine. 2008;**14**(5):483-485. DOI: 10.1038/nm1768

[104] Neve KA, Kozlowski MR, Marshall JF. Plasticity of neostriatal dopamine receptors after nigrostriatal injury: Relationship to recovery of sensorimotor functions and behavioral supersensitivity. Brain Research. 1982;**244**(1):33-44. DOI: 10.1016/0006-8993(82)90901-5

[105] Winkler JD, Weiss B. Reversal of supersensitive apomorphine-induced rotational behavior in mice by continuous exposure to apomorphine. Journal of Pharmacology and Experimental Therapeutics. 1986;**238**(1):242-247

[106] Turrigiano G. Homeostatic synaptic plasticity: Local and global mechanisms for stabilizing neuronal function. Cold Spring Harbor Perspectives in Biology. 2017;**4**. Article a005736. DOI: 10.1101/cshperspect.a005736

[107] Castañeda E, Fleming S, Paquette MA, Boat K, Moffett J, Stachowiak EK, Bloom DC, Stachowiak MK. Assessment of recovery in the hemiparkinson rat: Drug-induced rotation is inadequate. Physiology and Behavior. 2005;**84**(4):525-535. DOI: 10.1016/j.physbeh.2005.01.019

[108] Tunik E, Feldman AG, Poizner H. Dopamine replacement therapy does not restore the ability of Parkinsonian patients to make rapid adjustments in motor strategies according to changing sensorimotor contexts. Parkinsonism & Related Disorders. 2007;**13**(7):425-433. DOI: 10.1016/j.parkreldis.2007.02.003

[109] Vandecasteele M, Glowinski J, Venance L. Electrical synapses between dopaminergic neurons of the substantia nigra pars compacta. Journal of Neuroscience. 2005;**25**(2):291-298. DOI: 10.1523/jneurosci.4167-04.2005

[110] Grace AA, Bunney BS. Intracellular and extracellular electrophysiology of nigral dopaminergic neurons - 3. Evidence of electrotonic coupling. Neuroscience. 1983;**10**(2):333-336. DOI: 10.1016/0306-4522(83)90137-9

[111] Schultz W. Dopamine signals for reward value and risk: Basic and recent data. Behavioral and Brain Functions. 2010;**6**:24. DOI: 10.1186/1744-9081-6-24

[112] Hillerman JR, Schultz W. Dopamine neurons report an error in the temporal prediction of reward during learning. Nature Neuroscience. 1998;**1**:304-309. DOI: 10.1038/1124

[113] Schultz W, Dayan P, Montague RR. A neural substrate of prediction and reward. Science. 1997;**275**:1593-1599. DOI: 10.1126/science.275.5306.1593

[114] Haber SN, Fudge JL, McFarland NR. Striatonigrostriatal pathways in primates form an ascending spiral from the shell to the dorsolateral striatum. Journal of Neuroscience. 2000;**20**(6):2369-2382

[115] Chuhma N, Mingote S, Moore H, Rayport S. Dopamine neurons control striatal cholinergic neurons via regionally heterogeneous dopamine and glutamate signaling. Neuron. 2014;**81**:901-912. DOI: 10.1016/j.neuron.2013.12.027

[116] Morris G, Arkadir D, Nevet A, Vaadia E, Bergman H. Coincident but distinct messages of midbrain dopamine and striatal tonically active neurons. Neuron. 2004;**43**:133-143. DOI: 10.1016/j.neuron.2004.06.012

[117] Cragg SJ. Meaningful silences: How dopamine listens to the ACh pause. Trends in Neurosciences. 2006;**29**(3):125-131. DOI: 10.1016/j.tins.2006.01.003

[118] Threlfell A, Cragg SJ. Dopamine signaling in dorsal versus ventral striatum: The dynamic role of cholinergic interneurons. Frontiers in Systems Neuroscience. 2011;**5**. Article 11. DOI: 10.3389/fnsys.2011.00011

[119] Threlfell S, Lalic T, Platt NJ, Jennings KA, Deisseroth K, Cragg SJ. Striatal dopamine release is triggered by synchronized activity in cholinergic interneurons. Neuron. 2012;**75**(1):58-64. DOI: 10.1016/j.neuron.2012.04.038

[120] Cachope R, Cheer JF. Local control of striatal dopamine release. Frontiers in Behavioral Neuroscience. 2014;**8**. Article 188. DOI: 10.3389/fnbeh.2014.00188

[121] Cui G, Jun SB, Jin X, Pham MD, Vogel SS, Lovinger DM, Costa RM. Concurrent activation of striatal direct and indirect pathways during action initiation. Nature. 2013;**494**:238-242. DOI: 10.1038/nature11846

[122] Plamen G, Darbin O, Wichmann T. Oscillations in the basal ganglia under normal conditions and in movement disorders. Movement Disorders. 2006;**21**(10):1566-1577. DOI: 10.1002/mds.21033

[123] Grillner S, Hellgren J, Menard A, Saitoh K, Wikstrom MA. Mechanisms for selection of basic motor programs - Roles for the striatum and pallidum. Trends in Neurosciences. 2005;**28**(7):364-370. DOI: 10.1016/j.tins.2005.05.004

[124] Björklund A, Lindvall O. Cell replacement therapies for central nervous system disorders. Nature Neuroscience. 2000;**3**(6):537-544. DOI: 10.1038/75705

[125] Chkirate M, Vallee A, Doucet G. Host striatal projections into fetal ventral mesencephalic tissue grafted to the striatum of immature or adult rat. Experimental Brain Research. 1993;**94**(2):357-362. DOI: 10.1007/BF00230306

[126] Fisher LJ, Young SJ, Tepper JM, Groves PM, Gage FH. Electrophysiological characteristics of cells within mesencephalon suspension grafts. Neuroscience. 1991;**40**(1):109-122. DOI: 10.1016/0306-4522(91)90178-q

[127] Hagell P, Cenci MA. Dyskinesias and dopamine cell replacement in Parkinson's disease: A clinical perspective. Brain Research Bulletin. 2005;**68**(1-2):4-15. DOI: 10.1016/j.brainresbull.2004.10.013

[128] Ma Y, Feigin A, Dhawan V, Fukuda M, Shi Q, Greene P, Breeze R, Fahn S, Freed C, Eidelberg D. Dyskinesia after fetal cell transplantation for parkinsonism: A PET study. Annals of Neurology. 2002;**52**(5):628-634. DOI: 10.1002/ana.10359

[129] Carta M, Carlsson T, Munoz A, Kirik D, Björklund A. Role of serotonin neurons in the induction of levodopa- and graft-induced dyskinesias in Parkinson's disease. Movement Disorders. 2010;**25**(Supplementary 1):S174-S179. DOI: 10.1002/mds.22792

[130] Gotz M, Huttner WB. The cell biology of neurogenesis. Nature Reviews Molecular Cell Biology. 2005;**6**(10):777-788. DOI: 10.1038/nrm1739

[131] Lee S-H, Lumelsky N, Studer L, Auerbach JM, McKay RD. Efficient generation of midbrain and hindbrain neurons from mouse embryonic stem cells. Nature Biotechnology. 2000;**18**:675-679. DOI: 10.1038/76536

[132] Song H, Stevens CF, Gage FH. Astroglia induce neurogenesis from adult neural stem cells. Nature. 2002;**417**:39-44. DOI: 10.1038/417039a

[133] Pfreiger FW, Barres BA. Synaptic efficacy enhanced by glial cells in vitro. Science. 1997; **277**(12):1684-1687. DOI: 10.1126/science.277.5332.1684

[134] O'Malley EK, Seiber B-A, Black IB, Dreyfus CF. Mesencephalic type I astrocytes mediate the survival of substantia nigra dopaminergic neurons in culture. Brain Research. 1992; **582**(1):65-70. DOI: 10.1016/0006-8993(92)90317-3

[135] Barres BA. The mystery and magic of glia: A perspective on their roles in health and disease. Neuron. 2008;**60**(3):430-440. DOI: 10.1016/j.neuron.2008.10.013

[136] Belland ER. Researchgate.net Blog Response to "Can anyone help me with pure primary neuronal culture?". 2014. Available from: https://www.researchgate.net/post/Can_anyone_help_me_with_pure_primary_neuronal_culture [Accessed: 31-07-2017]

[137] Wu H-Y, Geddes J, Opperman K, Kaboord B. Thermofisher Scientific Protein Biology Application Notes. An Efficient Method for the Isolation of Highly Functional Primary Neurons. 2014. Available from: https://www.thermofisher.com/us/en/home/life-science/protein-biology/protein-biology-learning-center/protein-biology-resource-library/protein-biology-application-notes/efficient-method-isolation-highly-functional-primary-neurons.html [Accessed: 31-07-2017]

[138] Reynolds BA, Rietze RL. Neural stem cells and neurospheres—Re-evaluating the relationship. Nature Methods. 2005;**2**:333-336. DOI: 10.1038/nmeth758

[139] Landis SC, Keefe D. Evidence for neurotransmitter plasticity in vivo: Developmental changes in properties of cholinergic sympathetic neurons. Developmental Biology. 1983;**98**(2):349-372. DOI: 10.1016/0012-1606(83)90365-2

[140] Habecker BA, Symes AJ, Stahl N, Francis NJ, Economides A, Fink JS, Yancopaulos GD, Landis SC. A sweat-gland differentiation activity acts through known cytokine signaling pathways. Journal of Biological Chemistry. 1997;**272**(48):30421-30428. DOI: 10.1074/jbc.272.48.30421

[141] Spitzer NC. Neurotransmitter switching? No surprise. Neuron. 2015;**86**(5):1131-1144. DOI: 10.1016/j.neuron.2015.05.028

[142] Borodinsky LN, Belgacem YH. Crosstalk among electrical activity, trophic factors, and morphogenetic proteins in the regulation of neurotransmitter phenotype specification. Journal of Chemical Neuroanatomy. 2016;**73**:3-8. DOI: 10.1016/j.jchemneu.2015.12.001

[143] Borodinsky LN, Belgacem YH, Swapna I, Sequerra EB. Dynamic regulation of neurotransmitter specification: Relevance to nervous system homeostasis. Neuropharmacology. 2014;**78**:75-80. DOI: 10.1016/j.neuropharm.2012.12.005

[144] Roybon L, Mastracci TL, Ribeiro D, Sussel L, Brundin P, Li J-Y. GABAergic differentiation induced by Mash1 is compromised by bHLH proteins neurogenin2, NeuroD1, and NeuroD2. Cerebral Cortex. 2009;**20**(5):1234-1244. DOI: 10.1093/cercor/bhp187

[145] Wernig M, Benninger F, Schmandt T, Rade M, Tucker KI, Bussow H, Beck H, Brustle O. Functional integration of embryonic stem cell-derived neurons in vivo. Journal of Neuroscience. 2004;**24**(22):5258-5268. DOI: 10.1523/jneurosci.0428-04.200

[146] Burney MJ, Johnston C, Wong K-Y, Teng S-W, Beglopoulos V, Stanton LW, Williams BP, Bithell A, Buckley NJ. An epigenetic signature of developmental potential in neural stem cells and early neurons. Stem Cells. 2013;**31**(9):1868-1880. DOI: 10.1002/stem.1431

[147] Magrassi L, Ehrlich ME, Butti G, Pezzotta S, Govoni S, Cattaneo E. Basal ganglia precursors found in aggregates following embryonic transplantation adopt a striatal phenotype in hetrotopic locations. Development. 1998;**125**:2847-2855

[148] Fishell G. Striatal precursors adopt cortical identities in response to local cues. Development. 1995;**121**:803-812

[149] Shihabuddin LS, Hertz JA, Holets VR, Whittemore SR. The adult CNS retains the potential to direct region-specific differentiation of a transplanted neuronal precursor cell line. Journal of Neuroscience. 1995;**15**(10):6666-6678

[150] Merkle FT, Mirzadeh Z, Alvarez-Buylla A. Mosaic organization of neural stem cells in the adult brain. Science. 2007;**317**:381-384. DOI: 10.1126/science.1144914

[151] Sequerra EB, Costa MR, Menezes JRL, Hedin-Periera C. Adult neural stem cells: Plastic or restricted neuronal fates? Development. 2013;**140**:3303-3309. DOI: 10.1242/dev.093096

[152] Wictorin K, Lagenaur CF, Lund RD, Björklund A. Efferent projections to the host brain from intrastriatal striatal mouse-to-rat grafts: Timecourse and tissue-type specificity as revealed by a mouse specific neuronal marker. European Journal of Neuroscience. 1991;**3**(1):86-101. DOI: 10.1111/j.1460-9568.1991.tb00814.x

[153] Kritsanasrinuan N, Kotchabhakdi N, Therapanchareon V. Development of embryonic rhombencephalon transplanted into adult rat cerebellum. Journal of the Science Society of Thailand. 1993;**19**:129-142

[154] Wictorin K, Brundin P, Gustavii B, Lindvall O, Björklund A. Reformation of long axon pathways in adult rat CNS by human forebrain neuroblasts. Nature. 1990;**347**:556-558. DOI: 10.1038/347556a0

[155] Gaillard A, Jaber M. Rewiring the brain with cell transplantation in Parkinson's disease. Trends in Neurosciences. 2011;**34**(3):124-133. DOI: 10.1016/j.tins.2011.01.003

[156] Grealish S, Jonsson ME, Li M, Kirik D, Björklund A, Thompson LH. The A9 dopamine neuron component in grafts of ventral mesencephalon is an important determinant for recovery of motor function in a rat model of Parkinson's disease. Brain. 2010;**133**(Pt2): 482-495. DOI: 10.1093/brain/awp328

[157] Björklund A, Dunnett SB. Dopamine neuron systems in the brain: An update. Trends in Neurosciences. 2007;**30**:194-202. DOI: 10.1016/j.tins.2007.03.006

[158] Lopez A, Munoz A, Guerra MJ, Labandeira-Garcia JL. Mechanisms of the effects of exogenous levodopa on the dopamine-denervated striatum. Neuroscience. 2001;**103**(3):639-651. DOI: 10.1016/s0306-4522(00)00588-1

[159] Gaillard A, Decressac M, Frappe I, Fernagut PO, Prestoz L, Besnard S, Jaber M. Anatomical and functional reconstruction of the nigrostriatal pathway by intranigral transplants. Neurobiology of Disease. 2009;**35**:477-488. DOI: 10.1016/j.nbd.2009.07.003

[160] Wilby MJ, Sinclair SR, Muir EM, Zietlow R, Adcock KH, Horellou P, Rogers JH, Dunnett SB, Fawcett JW. A glial cell line-derived neurotrophic factor-secreting clone of the Schwann cell line SCTM41 enhances survival and fiber outgrowth from embryonic nigral neurons grafted to the striatum and to the lesioned substantia nigra. Journal of Neuroscience. 1999;**19**(6):2301-2312

[161] Brecknell JE, Du JS, Muir E, Fidler PS, Hlavin ML, Dunnett SB, Fawcett JW. Bridge grafts of fibroblast growth factor-4-secreting schwannoma cells promote functional axonal regeneration in the nigrostriatal pathway of the adult rat. Neuroscience. 1996;**74**(3):775-784. DOI: 10.1016/0306-4522(96)00167-4

[162] Isacson O, Deacon TW. Specific guidance factors persist in the adult brain as demonstrated by pig neuroblasts transplanted to the rat. Neuroscience. 1996;**74**:827-837. DOI: 10.1016/0306-4522(96)00305-3

[163] Wang Y, Tien LT, Lapchack PA, Hoffer BJ. GDNF triggers fiber outgrowth of fetal ventral mesencephalic grafts from nigra to striatum in 6-OHDA-lesioned rats. Cell Tissue Research. 1996;**286**(2):225-233

[164] Wictorin K, Brundin P, Sauer H, Lindvall O, Björklund A. Long distance directed axonal growth from human dopaminergic mesencephalic neuroblasts implanted along the nigrostriatal pathway in 6-hydroxydopamine lesioned adult rats. Journal of Comparative Neurology. 1992;**323**(4):475-494. DOI: 10.1002/cne.903230403

[165] Dunnett SB, Rogers DC, Richards SJ. Nigrostriatal reconstruction after 6-OHDA lesions in rats: Combination of dopamine-rich nigral grafts and nigrostriatal "bridge" grafts. Experimental Brain Research. 1989;**75**(3):523-535. DOI: 10.1007/bf00249903

[166] Nikkhah G, Bentlage C, Cunningham MG, Björklund A. Intranigral fetal dopamine grafts induce behavioral compensation in the rat Parkinson model. Journal of Neuroscience. 1994;**14**(6):3449-3461

[167] Cheramy A, Leviel V, Glowinski J. Dendritic release of dopamine in the substantia nigra. Nature. 1981;**289**(5798):537-542. DOI: 10.1038/289537a0

[168] Winkler JD, Bentlage C, Nikkhah G, Samii M, Björklund A. Intra-nigral transplants of GABA-rich striatal tissue induce behavioral recovery in the rat Parkinson model and promote the effects obtained by intrastriatal dopaminergic transplants. Experimental Neurology. 1999;**155**(2):165-186. DOI: 10.1006/exnr.1998.6916

[169] Chevalier G, Deniau JM. Disinhibition as a basic process in the expression of striatal functions. Trends in Neurosciences. 1990;**13**(7):277-280. DOI: 10.1016/0166-2236(90)90109-n

[170] Zhang C, Jin Y, Ziemba KS, Fletcher AM, Ghosh B, Truit E, Yurek DM, Smith GM. Long distance directional growth of dopaminergic axons along pathways of netrin-1 and GDNF. Experimental Neurology. 2013;**250**:156-164. DOI: 10.1016/j.expneurol.2013.09.022

[171] Bruno JP, Sandstrom MI, Arnold HM, Nelson CL. Age-dependent neurobehavioral plasticity following forebrain dopamine depletions. Developmental Neuroscience. 1998;**20**(2-3): 164-179. DOI: 10.1159/000017311

[172] Erinoff L, Macphail RC, Heller A, Seiden LS. Age-dependent effects of 6-hydroxydopamine on locomotor activity in the rat. Brain Research. 1979;**164**(1-2):195-205. DOI: 10.1016/0006-8993(79)90015-5

[173] Johnson BJ, Bruno JP. D1 and D2 receptor contributions to ingestive and locomotor behavior are altered after dopamine depletions in neonatal rats. Neuroscience Letters. 1990; **118**(1):120-123. DOI: 10.1016/0304-3940(90)90263-9

[174] Castañeda E, Wishaw IQ, Lermer L, Robinson TE. Dopamine depletion in neonatal rats: Effects on behavior and striatal dopamine release assessed by intracerebral microdialysis during adulthood. Brain Research. 1990;**508**(1):30-39. DOI: 10.1016/0006-8993(90)91113-U

[175] Abe M, Kimoto H, Eto R, Sasaki T, Kato H, Kasahara J, Araki T. Postnatal development of neurons, interneurons, and glial cells in the substantia nigra of mice. Cellular and Molecular Neurobiology. 2010;**30**(6):917-928. DOI: 10.1007/s10571-010-9521-0

[176] Tomac A, Lindqvist E, Lin LF, Ogren SO, Young D, Hoffer BJ, Olson L. Protection and repair of the nigrostriatal dopaminergic system by GDNF in vivo. Nature. 1995;**373**(6512):335-339. DOI: 10.1038/373335a0

[177] Pascual A, Hildago-Figueroa M, Biruat JI, Pintado CO, Gomez-Diaz R, Lopez-Barneo J. Absolute requirement of GDNF for adult catecholaminergic neuron survival. Nature Neuroscience. 2008;**11**:755-761. DOI: 10.1038/nn.2136

[178] Bentlage C, Nikkhah G, Cunningham MG, Björklund A. Reformation of the nigrostriatal pathway by fetal dopaminergic micrografts into the substantia nigra is critically dependent on the age of the host. Experimental Neurology. 1999;**159**(1):177-190. DOI: 10.1006/exnr.1999.7110

[179] Somoza R, Juri C, Baes M, Wyneken U, Rubio FJ. Intranigral transplantation of epigenetically induced BDNF-secreting human mesenchymal stem cells: Implications for cell-based therapies in Parkinson's disease. Biology of Blood and Marrow Transplantation. 2010;**16**(11):1530-1540. DOI: 10.1016/j.bbmt.2010.06.006

[180] Aubert I, Ridet J-L, Gage FH. Regeneration in the adult mammalian CNS: Guided by development. Current Opinion in Neurobiology. 1995;**5**(5):625-635. DOI: 10.1016/0959-4388(95)80068-9

[181] Moon LDF, Brecknell JE, Franklin RJM, Dunnett SB, Fawcett JW. Robust regeneration of CNS axons through a track depleted of CNS glia. Experimental Neurology. 2000;**161**(1):49-66. DOI: 10.1006/exnr.1999.7230

[182] Moon LDF, Asher RA, Rhodes KE, Fawcett JW. Relationship between sprouting axons, proteoglycans, and glial cells following unilateral nigrostriatal axotomy in the adult rat. Neuroscience. 2002;**109**(1):101-117. DOI: 10.1016/S0306-4522(01)00457-2

[183] Prensa L, Parent A. The nigrostriatal pathway in the rat: A single-axon study of the relationship between dorsal and ventral tier nigral neurons and the striosome/matrix striatal compartments. Journal of Neuroscience. 2001;**21**(18):7247-7260

[184] McNaught KSP, Jenner P. Altered glial function causes neuronal death and increases neuronal susceptibility to 1-methyl-4-phenylpiridinium- and 6-hydroxydopamine-induced

toxicity in astrocytic/ventral mesencephalic co-cultures. Journal of Neurochemistry. 1999;**73**(6):2469-2476. DOI: 10.1046/j.1471-4159.1999.0732469.x

[185] Haruhiko A, McGeer PL. Microglial response to 6-hydroxydopamine-induced substantia nigra lesions. Brain Research. 1989;**489**(2):247-253. DOI: 10.1016/0006-8993(89)90857-3

[186] Mirza B, Hadberg H, Thomsen P, Moos T. The absence of reactive astrocytosis is indicative of a unique inflammatory process in Parkinson's disease. Neuroscience. 1999;**95**(2):425-432. DOI: 10.1016/S0306-4522(99)00455-8

[187] Forno LS, DeLanney LE, Irwin I, Di Monte D, Langston JW. Astrocytes and Parkinson's disease. Progress in Brain Research. 1992;**94**:429-436. DOI: 10.1016/s0079-6123(08)61770-7

[188] Dessaud E, McMahon AP, Briscoe J. Pattern formation in the vertebrate neural tube: A sonic hedgehog morphogen-regulated transcriptional network. Development. 2008;**135**:2489-2503. DOI: 10.1242/dev.009324

[189] Perrone-Capano C, Di Porzio U. Genetic and epigenetic control of midbrain dopaminergic neuron development. International Journal of Developmental Biology. 2000;**44**:679-687

[190] Trzaska KA, King CC, Li K-Y, Kuzhikandathil EV, Nowycky MC, Ye J-H, Rameshwar P. Brain-derived neurotrophic factor facilitates maturation of mesenchymal stem cell-derived dopamine progenitors to functional neurons. Journal of Neurochemistry. 2009; **110**:1058-1069. DOI: 10.1111/j.1471-4159.2009.06201.x

[191] Parish CL, Castelo-Branco G, Rawal N, Tonnesen J, Sorensen AT, Salto C, Kokaia M, Lindvall O, Arenas E. Wnt5a-treated midbrain neural stem cells improve dopamine cell replacement therapy in parkinsonian mice. Journal of Clinical Investigation. 2008;**118**(1): 149-160 https://doi.org/10.1172/jci32273

[192] Tatard VM, D'Ippolito G, Diabira S, Valeyev A, Hackman J, McCarthy M, Bouckenooghe T, Menei P, Montero-Menei CN, Schiller PC. Neurotrophin-directed differentiation of human adult marrow stromal cells to dopaminergic-like neurons. Bone. 2007;**40**(2):360-373. DOI: 10.1016/j.bone.2006.09.013

[193] Paracchia C. Chemical gating of gap junction channels: Roles of calcium, pH and calmodulin. Biochimica et Biophysica Acta (BBA – Biomembranes). 2004;**1662**:61-80. DOI: 10.1016/j.bbamem.2003.10.020

[194] Mukhida K, Baker KA, Sadi D, Mendez I. Enhancement of sensorimotor behavioral recovery in hemiparkinsonian rats with intrastriatal, intranigral, and intrasubthalamic nucleus dopaminergic transplants. Journal of Neuroscience. 2001;**21**(10):3521-3530

[195] Narayanan K, Lichtman JW. The role of neuronal identity in synaptic competition. Nature. 2003;**424**:426-430. DOI: 10.1038/nature01836

[196] Lozano AM, Snyder BJ, Hamani C, Huchison WD, Dostrovsky JO. Basal ganglia physiology and deep brain stimulation. Movement Disorders. 2010;**25**(51):571-575. DOI: 10.1002/mds.22714

[197] Benabid AL. Deep brain stimulation for Parkinson's disease. Current Opinion in Neurobiology. 2003;**13**(6):696-706. DOI: 10.1016/j.conb.2003.11.001

5

Sleep Disorders in Multiple Sclerosis

Montserrat González Platas and
María Yaiza Pérez Martin

Abstract

Patients with multiple sclerosis (MS) have multiple causes of poor sleep and potential triggers may relate to MS-related symptoms, co-morbidities and adverse effects from medication. Sleep disorders may occur independently of demographic factors, gender and clinical condition. The real frequency of sleep disturbances in MS and their impact on the patients' quality of life are unknown. The prevalence of sleep problems in the population with MS ranges between 47 and 62% and is more frequent in women, as well as having a higher risk of mortality. High psychological burden has been associated with poor sleep and with increased risk of co-morbid conditions such as heart disease, obesity, dyslipidemia and diabetes, which may have a profound impact on long-term health. The poor sleeping patients with MS were more likely to report fatigue and sleepiness. Insomnia is present in mood disorders, restless leg syndrome (RLS), pain, nocturia and obstructive sleep apnea (OSA), in patients with MS. All the symptoms are intermixed, and it is not possible to discern the precipitating factor or the perpetuating factor. Clinicians should routinely ask about sleep when forming a comprehensive care plan for patients with MS. Sleep specialty referrals should be considered for management of conditions that require polysomnography (PSG) diagnosis.

Keywords: sleep disorders, insomnia, sleepiness, fatigue, respiratory disorders during sleep, cognitive impairment, cognitive behavioral therapy, multiple sclerosis

1. Introduction

Multiple sclerosis (MS) is a chronic autoimmune disease of the central nervous system that is increasingly prevalent in young adults. Patients with MS have multiple causes of poor sleep, and potential triggers may be related to MS-related symptoms, co-morbidities and adverse effects from drug therapy.

Major sleep disorders have been reported to be associated with numerous co-morbid conditions, including heart disease, obesity, stroke and diabetes [1].

The poor sleepers among patients with MS are more likely to report fatigue (one of the most frequent symptoms in MS) and pain (a co-morbid condition to MS-related fatigue but is confounded by depression and medication for treating pain or pain-induced sleep disorder) [1].

All the symptoms are intermixed, and it is not possible to discern the precipitating factor and the perpetuating factor. In this respect, sleepiness and fatigue may converge in some situations [1].

Insomnia is present in mood disorders (depression and anxiety), restless leg syndrome (RLS), pain, nocturia and others [1]. RLS is also an important cause of pain in patients with MS. Sleep disorders may occur independently of demographic factors such as gender and clinical-demographic factors. High psychological burden has been said to be independently associated with poor sleep patients with increased risk of co-morbid conditions such as heart disease, obesity and diabetes, which may have a profound impact on long-term health. The reverse situation is also possible.

The frequency of sleep disturbances in MS and their impact on the patients' quality of life are unknown. The prevalence of sleep problems in the MS population ranges from 47 to 62%, with a higher prevalence in women [2–5]. Sex hormones and genetic mechanisms, psychosocial factors, certain physical factors that disrupt sleep, such as pain or bladder dysfunction may contribute to sleep differences between women and men [5].

Obstructive sleep apnea (OSA), RLS and chronic insomnia in particular are frequent problems in the MS population, and play a key role in the development of debilitating fatigue and other poor functional outcomes in MS. Yet, despite their impact, sleep disorders in MS remain critically under-recognized in most clinical settings. A recommended approach to the fatigued patient with MS is also highlighted [6].

Sleep disorders during the course of MS may be secondary to numerous symptoms arising from the disease itself or can be primary with a common biological link. In either of the two cases, a bidirectional relationship exists between these co-morbid conditions [7].

Sleep disturbances have been associated with increased risk of mortality, cardiac disease, obesity and diabetes [8] and can contribute to the depression, pain and fatigue symptoms that are commonly seen in MS patients, which are often disabling [3, 9].

Sleep disorders are under-recognized in persons with MS. These sleep disorders can contribute significantly to fatigue, other daytime dysfunction and poor quality of life. A systematic, practical approach that takes into account clinical features of MS is recommended to enhance recognition of these conditions and facilitate appropriate treatment. Clinicians caring for patients with MS should routinely screen for sleep disturbances and initiate diagnostic workups, if clinically indicated.

Sleep specialty referrals should be considered for management of conditions that require polysomnography (PSG) diagnosis, for complex patients who present a diagnostic challenge and for patients who do not respond to first-line treatments. Clinicians should also routinely ask about sleep when forming a comprehensive care plan for patients with MS.

2. Effect or influence of multiple sclerosis in sleep disorders

2.1. Insomnia

Sleeplessness or insomnia is an inability to fall asleep or to stay asleep as long as desired. Insomnia is described as a complaint of prolonged sleep-onset latency, disturbance of sleep maintenance or the experience of non-refreshing sleep [10]. Episodic insomnia can usually be traced to an acute psychological stressor or an environmental change. Chronic insomnia may be related to a combination of factors including depression, poor sleep hygiene, learned sleeplessness, sleep-disordered breathing, nocturia, drugs or extrinsic factors such as noise [6, 11].

Patients with MS face a high risk of insomnia of around 40% [6] compared to roughly 10–15% in the general population [12]. Awakening too early in the morning is the most common symptom (58%) [13].

Primary symptoms of MS that can condition the onset of insomnia are neurogenic bladder (nocturia), spasticity, sexual dysfunction, neuropathic pain, paroxysmal phenomena, depression and anxiety [7].

Insomnia affects daytime activities, because of fatigue, mood disturbances (depression and anxiety), attention, concentration and memory impairment [7]. Higher fatigue scores have also been found to correlate with insomnia, especially middle insomnia [13].

2.1.1. Diagnostic approach

Patients with insomnia may complain of difficulty falling asleep, difficulty staying asleep or waking up sooner than desired [10]. There are screening tools to identify such patients.

The Pittsburgh Sleep Quality Index (PSQI) measures seven domains: subjective sleep quality, latency, duration, habitual efficiency, disturbances, use of sleep medication and daytime dysfunction over the last month. Each of these seven domains is self-rated by the individuals. The score of each question is based on a scale from 0 to 3, in which a score of 3 demonstrates the negative extreme on the Likert Scale. A global sum of 5 or greater indicates a poor sleeper (sensitivity of almost 100% for insomnia) [14, 15].

Insomnia Severity Index (ISI): a seven item questionnaire designed to assess the nature, severity, and impact of insomnia in adults. Scores >15 reflect moderate clinical insomnia. It is also a useful tool to monitor the effects of insomnia interventions [6].

Athens Insomnia Scale (AIS): a psychometric instrument designed for quantifying sleep difficulty. It consists of eight items: the first five pertain to sleep induction, awakenings during the night, final awakening, total sleep duration and sleep quality; while the last three refer to well-being, functioning capacity and sleepiness during the day. Either the entire eight-item scale (AIS-8) or the brief five-item version (AIS-5), which contains only the first five items, can be used. The score of each question is based on a scale from 0 to 3, where a score of 3 indicates the negative or normal extreme on the Likert Scale. A cut-off score of ≥6 on the AIS is used to establish the diagnosis of insomnia [16].

2.1.2. Management

After detecting insomnia, amelioration of any precipitating causes of insomnia is a cardinal step in its management. Medications or substances that may contribute to insomnia should be reduced or discontinued, if possible, there should be a check on which drugs the patient is taking (medications used to alleviate MS-related symptoms, including over-the-counter medications).

Selective serotonin reuptake inhibitors, while helpful for depressive symptoms, may worsen insomnia.

Stimulants and wake-promoting agents, which are commonly used for fatigue, may interfere with sleep initiation if taken during the late afternoon or early evening hours.

Antihistamines, which are used as sleep aids by up to 25% of patients with MS, have the potential to worsen RLS, and thereby worsen sleep-onset insomnia [6].

Co-morbid symptoms must be identified and treated: neuropathic pain (tricyclic antidepressants and the α-2-δ ligand pregabalin), spasticity (baclofen or tizanidine) and urinary urgency (anticholinergics) [6].

Cognitive behavioral therapy (CBT) is an innovative psychotherapy approach. CBT treatment could reduce anxiety and depression by changing thoughts and beliefs and consequently reduce the symptoms of insomnia [6, 17].

Pharmacological therapies can be considered if more conservative strategies have been exhausted or are not fully effective: benzodiazepines, benzodiazepine agonists, melatonin receptor agonists and orexin receptor antagonists.

2.2. Hypersomnia

Excessive daytime sleepiness (EDS)/excessive daytime drowsiness disrupt daily performance.

Hypersomnia may be due to acute thalamus injuries, mental disorders, especially depressive symptoms, sleep deprivation or as a consequence of received treatments.

2.2.1. Diagnostic approach

The Epworth Sleepiness Scale (ESS) is a screening tool that assesses sleepiness and has eight items. ESS values equal to or greater than 10 indicate excessive daytime sleepiness (EDS), and in this case, patients should undergo polygraphy or PSG (screening for sleep apnea) [18].

All fatigued patients should be asked about sleepiness and fill in the Epworth Sleepiness Scale (ESS) as these are not always associated with sleepiness.

Magnetic resonance imaging (MRI) should be performed because of the need to identify structural lesions in the brain.

2.2.2. Management

After detecting hypersomnia, the physician should check for any medications involved and withdraw them if possible, treat acute lesions of multiple sclerosis with corticosteroids, indicate adequate sleep hygiene and assess whether specific treatment is needed to improve daily performance.

2.3. Restless leg syndrome

The four main criteria for diagnosis of RLS are: (1) unpleasant sensations in the legs; (2) worsening of the symptoms during rest; (3) relief of the symptoms by movement and (4) exacerbation of the symptoms in the evening or at night [19].

The periodic limb movement disorder (PLMD) includes repetitive periodic shaking episodes lasting between 0.5 and 5 seconds that occur during sleep every 20–40 seconds; mainly in the legs, but sometimes in the arms.

RLS and PLMD are motor disorders of sleep considered separate clinical entities, both conditions have the potential to cause disrupted sleep, share similar pathogenesis and have an increased prevalence among persons with MS. PLMD also frequently occur in the absence of RLS.

Most RLS patients (80–90%) have periodic leg movements PLM during sleep. They can cause arousals or micro-arousals leading to non-refreshing sleep, daytime sleepiness and fatigue. The prevalence of RLS in the general population ranges from 1 to 12% [20]. The prevalence of RLS in MS patients is two to five times higher than in the general population [21–24].

Differentiating RLS from other sensory and motor symptoms of MS can be difficult, as MS patients frequently suffer from spasms, dysesthesia, paraesthesia and spasticity in the legs, which worsen with immobility [25].

Predictive factors for RLS in MS patients include: older age, longer disease duration, progressive primary forms, greater disability as measured by the Expanded Disability Status Scale (EDSS), especially in the pyramidal and sensory subscales and shaking of the legs before onset of sleep [26]. Furthermore, RLS symptoms are more severe when associated with MS than when not associated with MS.

MS patients with RLS have more cervical cord lesions than those patients without RLS. These lesions possibly disrupt the ascending and descending pathways with cerebrospinal disconnection leading to these symptoms [10].

Primary RLS is a genetic form of RLS with autosomal dominant transmission [27]. Four genes have been associated with this syndrome [28] but no crossing over of those involved in MS [10].

Pathogenesis of RLS and PRLS shows dysfunction of downstream dopaminergic pathways, namely diencephalospinal and reticulospinal pathways, that project to the spinal cord. These pathways, *via* dopaminergic transmission, are responsible for the suppression of sensory inputs and motor excitability, and are susceptible to damage from diseases affecting the spinal cord. Impaired iron metabolism is also thought to contribute to the pathogenesis of RLS, as iron is a cofactor for a rate-limiting step in the synthesis of dopamine [6, 10].

Certain medications used in the management of persons with MS, such as antiemetic drugs, antipsychotic dopamine antagonists, antidepressants and antihistamines can also cause or worsen RLS [6, 10].

2.3.1. Diagnostic approach

Many descriptors can be used by patients to describe the restless sensation, including creeping, crawling, itching, burning, tightening, tingling or pain.

Symptoms of leg tightness relieved by voluntary movement suggest RLS, whereas involuntary spasms, even if a circadian component is endorsed, suggest spasticity. Rhythmic involuntary movements triggered by stretching or certain leg positions suggest clonus.

The Restless Legs Syndrome Diagnostic Index (RLS-DI) is a 10-item questionnaire. Scores range from −22 (no RLS) to +20 (definite RLS). A score of +11 yields 93.0% sensitivity and 96.1% specificity to accurately diagnose RLS [6].

Diagnosis of PLMD requires overnight PSG to assess for the presence of leg movements [6, 10].

The RLS Rating Scale is a useful tool to track treatment response and is a 10-item self-administered scale. Scores of 11–20 reflect moderate RLS.

2.3.2. Management

Iron supplementation should be implemented for a ferritin level of less than 50 ng/ml.

Reduction or discontinuation of medications and substances that can cause or worsen RLS or PLMD (dopamine antagonists, lithium, selective serotonin reuptake inhibitors, serotonin-norepinephrine reuptake inhibitors, antihistamines, tricyclic antidepressants, alcohol, tobacco and caffeine) is recommended.

Dopamine agonists (pramipexole, ropinirole and rotigotine), and the α-2-δ ligand gabapentin and anticonvulsants are first-line treatments.

Benzodiazepines and opioid agents (oxycodone and methadone) are second line treatments.

Treatment for refractory RLS, or augmentation in response to dopaminergic therapy, is also likely to be optimized by sleep specialty care [6].

2.4. Respiratory disorders during sleep

Sleep-disordered breathing is characterized by episodes of nocturnal hypopnea and apnea resulting in a reduction or a cessation of airflow in the upper airway.

Patients with sleep-disordered breathing may complain of "fatigue," decreased concentration, mood changes, erectile dysfunction, nocturia and mood changes, all these complaints are similar to those experienced in MS [29].

2.4.1. Apnea and hypopnea

Apneas and hypopneas may be caused by a collapse of the tissues and muscles in the pharynx (obstructive apnea/hypopnea) or a failure in the medullary respiratory signal (central apnea/hypopnea) [10].

Maintenance of upper airway patency during sleep requires an increase in pharyngeal tone that is primarily mediated by efferent motor output from cranial nerves X and XII to the palatal and genioglossus muscles, respectively. This process is largely influenced by afferent sensory input from pressure receptors in the upper airway, peripheral chemoreceptors in the aortic and carotid bodies, and brainstem respiratory generators. Pathophysiological processes that disrupt these tightly regulated brainstem pathways have the potential to impair nocturnal respiration. The medullary reticular formation is responsible for controlling automatic breathing during sleep [10].

Causative factors include obesity, craniofacial abnormalities, enlarged tonsils, congestive heart disease and degenerative central nervous system (CNS) disorders, to name a few [10].

Such apnea and hypopnea episodes may lead to nocturnal hypoxemia, frequent awakenings and daytime somnolence. When the apneas are associated with respiratory effort, the term obstructive apnea is used, and central apnea is used when there is a lack of respiratory effort [10].

Central sleep apnea is diagnosed when more of 50% of the events are central in patients with both central and obstructive apneas.

2.4.2. *Obstructive sleep apnea*

Obstructive sleep apnea is characterized by repeated episodes of upper airway obstruction and hypoxia during sleep [6].

The incidence of OSA in patients with MS is 2–21% and is one of the most common respiratory disorders [10].

Patients with MS who have a diagnosis of OSA and those at an elevated risk of OSA have increased fatigue and diminished quality life compared with undiagnosed or low-risk patients [6].

Sleepiness is primarily a result of acutely or chronically reduced sleep time, or poor sleep quality. Apnea severity may correlate with impaired cognition in MS [6].

2.4.2.1. *Diagnostic approach*

Questions must be asked about symptoms of snoring, pauses in breathing witnessed by a bed partner, gasping or choking upon awakening, non-restorative sleep, excessive daytime hypersomnolence or fatigue, cognitive disturbances and nighttime awakenings, any of which may arise in part from underlying OSA [6].

Dysarthria or dysphagia, obesity, increased neck circumference, crowded oropharyngeal inlet, retrognathia, or micrognathia are common physical exam findings [6].

The STOP-Bang questionnaire is a screening tool consisting of eight questions and measures that form the acronym snoring, tired, observed apnea, Blood Pressure-Body Mass Index, age, neck circumference and gender. Scores of 3 or higher indicate an elevated risk of OSA [6].

A full-night PSG is necessary to demonstrate the presence of obstructive respiratory events during sleep to confirm the diagnosis of OSA. These events may be partial (hypopneas) or complete (apneas), but must demonstrate evidence of a reduction in airflow during sleep, despite continued effort to breathe [6].

2.4.2.2. Management

Management strategies for sleep-disordered breathing should take into account the patient's primary apnea subtype, apnea severity, co-morbidities and behaviors, and other MS-specific symptoms or limitations. Guidance by a sleep medicine physician is often helpful [6]. Discontinuation of medication, such as opiates, antispasmodics or CNS depressants medications [6].

Positive airway pressure (PAP) therapy is delivered by a mechanical device and mask to splint the upper airway open during sleep. Supplemental oxygen, bi-level PAP and adaptive servo ventilation are other improvements that these devices have [6].

Oral appliances work by repositioning the mandible in the anterior and inferior position [6]. By improving nocturnal oxygen saturation and sleep quality, PAP therapy effectively reduces fatigue and can be effective in the treatment of depression. This is especially important given the link between fatigue and depression in MS [6, 18].

Disease-modifying therapy use, in particular emerged as a strong predictor of *reduced* apnea severity, raising interesting possibilities about the role of local and/or systemic inflammation in OSA [6].

2.4.3. Central sleep apnea

Central sleep apnea (CSA) is rare, and the prevalence is unclear in the general population. CSA involves repeated complete or partial reduction of airflow, caused by an intermittent lack of respiratory effort by failure in the medullary respiratory signal [10].

While the prevalence of CSA is less than that of OSA, patients with CNS disorders that affect pontine and medullary respiratory generators, including MS, may be at increased risk for this condition as well even nocturnal death (Ondine's curse) [6, 10].

CNS and brain stem-related nocturnal respiratory abnormalities such as central sleep apnea, paroxysmal hyperventilation, hypoventilation, respiratory muscle weakness and respiratory arrest have all been described and should be considered in this patient population in the evaluation of symptoms of daytime somnolence, increased fatigue and non-refreshing sleep [11].

2.4.3.1. Diagnostic approach

In patients with symptoms of daytime somnolence, increased fatigue and non-refreshing sleep, the physician must ask about nocturnal respiratory abnormalities [11] and look for evidence of reduction in airflow in the absence of respiratory effort in an overnight PSG.

In patients with both central and obstructive apneas, central sleep apnea is diagnosed when more than 50% of the events are central. The coexistence of OSA or CSA and MS has been described by several authors [2, 10, 30].

2.4.3.2. *Management*

In the cases of central sleep apnea not symptomatic or central sleep apnea during sleep-wake transition (20% of central sleep apnea cases resolve spontaneously) observation is recommended.

In other cases, PAP treatment, adaptive servo ventilation, oxygen, added dead space, carbon dioxide inhalation and overdrive atrial pacing are needed.

2.4.4. *Nocturnal urinary disorders*

Sleep disturbance is associated with outcomes such as increased risk of falls and mortality. Nocturia may both precipitate poor sleep and perpetuate insomnia (awakenings associated with nocturia may themselves be perpetuating factors) [31].

Overactive bladder (OAB) syndrome is a condition that accompanies urgency (a significant factor for sleep disruption), with or without incontinence, frequently with increased daytime frequency and nocturia [32]).

Nocturia is defined by the International Continence Society as the complaint that an individual has to wake at night one or more times to void. It reflects the relationship between the amount of urine produced while asleep, and the storage by the bladder of urine received. Nocturia is a symptom rather than a disease and causative categories have been proposed and is the most common storage symptom in the general population [32].

Nocturia can occur as part of lower urinary tract dysfunction (LUTD), notably in overactive bladder syndrome (OAB). Nocturia can also occur in association with other forms of LUTD, such as bladder outlet obstruction or chronic pelvic pain syndrome [33].

Nocturia is due to nocturnal polyuria, a decreased nocturnal bladder capacity or a mixture of the two. Various duplicating factors for nocturia have been reported, including pathological conditions such as diabetes, LUTD, cardiovascular disease, primary sleep disorders and sleep apnea [32].

Nocturia is a feature of systemic conditions affecting water and salt balance, leading to excessive production of urine at all times (global polyuria) or primarily at night (nocturnal polyuria), so that nocturia can be a systemic symptom such as cardiovascular, endocrine and renal disease can affect water and salt homeostasis, leading to an increased rate of urine production [33].

Nocturia can significantly influence quality of life, efficiency, vigor and awareness of health, primarily due to sleep disruption.

2.4.4.1. *Diagnostic approach*

Asking how many times the patient wakes up at night because of nocturia, whether urinary urgency exists and the characteristics of urination, quantity of fluid intakes, physical exercise, medication being taken, etc. is also necessary *for the diagnosis of urinary problems.*

The use of specific questionnaires such as the PSQ, ISI and ASI for the diagnosis of insomnia or the ESS for the diurnal hypersomnia helps the physician to approach the functional repercussion of the problem.

The study occasionally needs to be completed with ultrasound studies, urodynamics, MRI and urinary sediment to identify LUTD or OAB problems.

2.4.4.2. Management

Interventions targeting nocturia may potentially improve sleep quality [31].

Hygienic measures such as reduced fluid intake at the end of the evening and frequently going to the bathroom during the day can help. Adequate treatment of co-morbid conditions such as diabetes mellitus, congestive heart failure or sleep apnea requires direct intervention for improvement nocturia.

Anticholinergics, mirabegron, a-blockers, 5-a reductase inhibitors, oral phosphodiester-ase-5 inhibitors, desmopressin, diuretics, sleep-promoting agents and phytotherapy are used to treat urinary problems [33]. Half of MS patients with moderate to severe overactive bladder symptoms are treated with an anticholinergic medication [18].

Antimuscarinic drugs (Solifenacin), the most appropriate treatment for OAB, inhibited bladder stimulation may originate a decrease of drive to the brain stem, improve urination urgency and frequency and effectively reduce involuntary contractions and increase bladder capacity in patients with storage symptoms. The night time dosing of antimuscarinic drugs may improve tolerance compared to daytime dosing [32].

Antidiuretic therapy using clinician-directed dose titration has been reported to be more effective than placebo in terms of reduced nocturnal voiding frequency and duration of undisturbed sleep [33].

Nocturia severity improvement contributes to overall improvements in health-related quality of life [33].

The impact of treatment for nocturia in MS fatigue is unknown [18]. Non-pharmacological therapies such as cognitive behavioral therapy for nocturia (CBT-N) act on the abovementioned perpetuating factors. Sleep restriction entails reducing the excessive time in bed (a common occurrence in insomnia) and thereby improves sleep efficiency.

3. Effect of the quality of sleep in multiple sclerosis

Sleep disturbances have been associated with increased risk of mortality, cardiac disease, obesity and diabetes [8] and can contribute to the depression, pain and fatigue symptoms that are commonly seen in MS patients, which are often disabling [3, 9, 10].

3.1. Fatigue

Fatigue is defined as a subjective lack of physical or mental energy perceived by the patients or their caregivers which interferes with desired activities of daily living and it is the most frequent symptom in MS [18].

Between 80 and 97% [6] of patients report chronic fatigue, and more than 33% of patients rate this symptom as the most disabling [34–36].

Fatigue may occur at any stage of the disease and can even precede MS onset by several years. Fatigue affects the social and professional capabilities of patients, is a major reason for early retirement, reduced employment and is considered to be one of the main causes of impaired quality of life among MS patients, regardless of depression or disability [18].

Fatigue starts early in the morning and increases during the day. The perception of fatigue is exacerbated with environmental temperature and humidity [25], with age, [36] greater EDSS, mental or physical activity, infections and food ingestion [37].

Fatigue also deteriorates cognitive domains, such as information processing, memory and attention, [35] and it has significant socioeconomic consequences, including loss of work hours and in some instances, loss of employment, as well as family relationships and leisure time [36].

Fatigue is a symptom in MS patients and may have multi-factorial causes such as immunologic abnormalities (pro-inflammatory cytokines such as INF-α), endocrine influences (cortisol and dehydroepiandrosterone (DHEA)), axonal loss, altered patterns of cerebral activation, sleep disorders (RLS, chronic insomnia, sleep-disordered breathing and altered sleep microstructure), depression and medications used to treat MS symptoms or immunomodulatory and immunosuppressive treatments [7, 38, 39].

"Primary" fatigue is related to the pathological changes of the disease itself, and results from a spectrum where one pole is the inability to generate the force required to perform the task due to a failure of force production at the muscle level "*peripheral fatigue*"; and the other pole is the inability to sustain the required neural drive to muscle because of supraspinal, spinal and even peripheral nerve contribution "*central fatigue.*"

"Central fatigue" can be the result of both cognitive and physical exertion and can reflect either a subjective sensation (fatigue) or an objective change in performance (fatigability) [37]. Dopamine imbalance plays a major role in developing fatigue. Central fatigue is a failure of the non-motor functions of the basal ganglia.

The subjective feeling of fatigue is related to inflammation and increased levels of cytokines such as interleukin-1 (IL-1), IL-6 and TNF-alpha [40].

"Secondary" fatigue attributed to mimicking symptoms, co-morbid sleep, irritable bowel syndrome, migraine, mood disorders, depression and anxiety and medication side effects [36, 37]. Persons with secondary fatigue report greater levels of fatigue than those with isolated primary fatigue [36].

There is a great variability in MS lesions from extensive areas of destruction during MS attacks, healing processes of and neuroplasticity. The clinical manifestations of fatigue do not seem to exclusively depend on the structural damage, but rather on the balance between restorative and inflammatory/degenerative processes and the rupture of the neural network [37].

In this respect, there is evidence that supports these hypotheses, linking fatigue with structural or functional abnormalities (atrophy in the thalamus, corpus callosum, cortical gray matter regions: superior frontal and inferior parietal gyrus, parietal lobe) within various brain networks (the cortico-subcortical circuit as a substrate for MS fatigue and the involvement of a "fronto-striatal network"), greater activation of the premotor area ipsilateral to the movement with functional MRI (fMRI), decreased N-acetylaspartate-creatine ratio (NAA/Cr) as a marker of axonal dysfunction. Resting-state fMRI studies show changes in functional connectivity (FC) of the basal ganglia including reward processing and motivation. In addition to motor functions, the abovementioned aspects are involved in the pathophysiology of fatigue [18].

3.1.1. Diagnostic approach

Patients with MS report being fatigued very often, sometimes it is just the feeling of lack of energy but in others it interferes with their work or their daily life. There are tools that help quantify the degree of fatigue which are described below.

Severity Scale (FSS): is a self-administered questionnaire with nine items (questions) investigating the severity of fatigue in different situations during the previous week. Grading of each item ranges from 1 to 7, where 1 indicates strong disagreement and 7 strong agreement and the final score represents the mean value of the 9 items. A total score of less than 36 suggests that you may not be suffering from fatigue [24].

Modified Fatigue Impact Scale (MFIS): The full-length MFIS consists of 21 items (total score 0–84, 38 as a cutoff to discriminate fatigued from non-fatigued individuals) while the abbreviated version has 5 items (0–20.). The abbreviated version can be used if time is limited but the full-length version has the advantage of generating physical, cognitive and psychosocial functioning subscales. The MFIS is one of the components of the MS quality life inventory [37].

MS patients, regardless of their fatigue level, have a significantly high frequency of RLS, higher Epworth sleepiness scale (ESS) scores, and higher PSQI scores. The time in bed, wake time after sleep onset %, total arousal index, limb movement arousal index and periodic limb movement arousal index are abnormal. The sleep efficiency index and sleep continuity index are lower in fatigued MS patients than non-fatigued MS patients. The PSQI results also suggest more disrupted sleep in fatigued MS patients. For all of the reasons above, quality of sleep studies should be performed with fatigued MS patients.

Once the patient has been identified with fatigue, it is necessary to investigate whether other co-morbidities are present (depression, anxiety, sleep disturbance, diabetes, heart disease, obesity, anemia, thyroid disease and nocturnal urinary disorders), what factors influence perpetuating fatigue and what situations can be modified in their lifestyle [6].

3.1.2. Management

Interventions targeting fatigue may potentially improve sleep quality and quality of life [31].

Pharmacological interventions are also reviewed and if there is evidence that a drug is involved in fatigue, it should be suppressed or the dose decreased [18]. Disease-modifying treatments (DMTs) are generally used to reduce relapses and progression and they occasionally cause an increase in fatigue, and in these circumstances it is important to change the medication for another DMTs [40].

Hygienic measures such as energy conservation programs, specific rehabilitation interventions physical (endurance, resistance, aerobic and combined training), aquatic therapy, cooling therapies, Tai chi, stretching, mindfulness-based interventions, yoga, acupuncture, progressive muscle relaxation and sleep hygiene advice (dependent on the nature of the sleep disorder) are more effective than pharmacological interventions [41].

Adequate treatment of co-morbid conditions such as diabetes mellitus, congestive heart failure, obesity, sleep apnea and other sleep disorders, depression and anxiety with pharmacological, psychological, behavioral and educational interventions is recommended [40, 41]. Pharmacological interventions for fatigue that are effective for reducing fatigue in patients with MS include amantadine, pemoline, prokarin (1 pilot study, side effects not reported), modafinil and pemoline combined with aspirin are efficacious for reducing fatigue in patients with multiple sclerosis. Carnitine has a discreet effectiveness. In general, the risk benefit of the drugs used for fatigue makes their recommendation be evaluated in each patient, highlighting them to the amantadine [37, 41]. Aminopyridines and coenzyme Q10 have an effect on fatigue by improving nerve conduction.

Nowadays, non-invasive brain stimulation (NIBS) techniques are gaining interest in the treatment of MS fatigue [37].

Promotion of health behaviors such as quitting smoking, physical activity (a high level of physical activity was borderline significantly associated with a decrease in co-morbidity) [42] and healthy eating may prevent some co-morbidities which were slow to show improvement in fatigue after the intervention, but they are effective [36].

3.2. Cognition

Cognitive impairment is a frequent feature of MS affecting up to 65% of patients [43] at both the earlier and later stages of the disease [44] and it tends to worsen over time [45].

MS negatively affects several aspects of cognitive functions, including attention, information processing [46], learning and memory, executive function and visuospatial abilities [47], having an important impact on quality of life [48], employment status [49], daily functioning, independence [50] and participation in social activities [51, 52].

Several factors have a negative influence on cognition in MS patients, such as depression [53], fatigue and sleep disturbances. Proper sleep is important for memory consolidation [54], and sleep deprivation has been related to impaired functioning in various cognitive domains [55].

Sleep disturbance causes a decrease in sustained attention [56], interferes with information processing and executive functioning [52]. Sleep disturbed patients reported higher levels of subjective cognitive problems compared to patients with normal sleep [52].

OSA and sleep disturbance are significantly associated with diminished visual memory, verbal memory, executive function (as reflected by response inhibition), attention, processing speed and working memory [52].

Excessive daytime sleepiness can lead to poor attention, poor memory, mood disturbances and increased risk of accidents [29].

In subjects with insomnia, a functional magnetic resonance imaging (fMRI) showed hypoactivation of the medial and inferior prefrontal areas during a cognitive task, in relation to the control subjects, which returned to normal values after treatment. Insomnia or superficial sleep produces less activation of the hippocampus and less connectivity is observed in the thalamus than in the control subjects. Damage to the hippocampus and thalamus (e.g., lesions and atrophy) in MS is associated with worse cognition. In controls, both regions may be related to sleep and cognition [52].

MS patients performed worse on all cognitive tests compared to controls. MS patients had less normalized gray matter (GM) volume, normalized white matter (WM) volume, hippocampal volume and thalamic volume. The hippocampus and thalamus showed increased functional connectivity (FC) in patients compared to controls, but lower FC was observed in patients with sleep disturbances (32%) [52].

3.2.1. Diagnostic approach

Neuropsychological manifestations can even be detected in patients during early stages of the disease. The Brief Repeatable Battery-Neuropsychology (BRB-N) [57] test was developed as a short and sensitive test to identify disturbances of cognitive domains in MS patients. The BRB-N has become the most widely used neuropsychological battery for MS, [58] and it is now being applied in clinical trials to monitor cognitive changes.

Different cognitive impairment criteria have been used: <1.0 SD, <1.5 SD and <2.0 SD in one, two or three subtests of the battery, respectively [59, 60].

3.2.2. Management

Strategies to optimize sleep could improve cognitive function in patients with MS.

In the case of insomnia, relaxation techniques such as autogenic training or progressive muscle relaxation can help the patient fall asleep earlier and have a longer sleep. But they do not improve sleep, so it has no sleep recovery effect. Behavioral therapies can improve sleep, but not prolong it. A combination of relaxation techniques and behavior therapy could be the most appropriate therapy for certain sleep disorders.

The general strategies for insomnia treatment include aspects of sleep hygiene such as extensions of night time in bed and frequent naps during the day. Pharmacological treatment is usually administered with stimulants such as amphetamines, methylphenidates, pemoline and modafinil [61].

As regards sleep hygiene, it is often necessary to make some lifestyle changes such as dinner should not be too late, nor too spicy or copious, maintain a regular sleep schedule, do not spend too much time in bed other than bedtime, do not drink caffeinated beverages such as coffee, black tea or cola, or caffeine medications, 4–6 hours before bedtime, do not smoke before going to bed or during the night, try to get enough rest and darken the bedroom, ventilate the bedroom, the temperature should not exceed 18°, do not do any physically demanding sport immediately before sleep because otherwise it will stimulate too much circulation, do not drink alcohol before going to bed or avoid sleeping too much during the day.

Patients with fatigue should organize daily routine and workloads. The physician also needs to improve the efficiency of information processing and working memory in these patients with fatigue [40].

Anxiety, depression, difficulty in sleeping and fatigue may have an impact on cognitive problems. If a person with MS experiences these symptoms and has problems with memory and cognition, they need to be provided with assessment and treatment (occupational therapist and neuropsychologist).

The concept of mental toughness (MT) has recently been recognized for its psychological importance not just in coping with stress but also for its association with increased physical activity (PA), and for its impact on both stress and objective sleep quality. MT consists of four key factors such as control (of own life and emotions), commitment, challenge and confidence (in own abilities and in other people); thus covering a range of cognitive-emotional processes closely involved in coping with stress, emotions, unexpected events and social setting [62].

3.3. Depression

Patients who suffer from problematic sleep and/or fatigue (with or without anxiety) may be more likely to experience higher depressive symptoms [63].

Depression is a mental illness that causes feelings of sadness and loss of hope, changes in sleeping and eating habits, loss of interest in your usual activities and pains that have no physical explanation.

3.3.1. Diagnostic approach

A trans-diagnostic approach to symptoms may be more effective than targeting each symptom separately, such as depression treatment or pain treatment alone. Trans-diagnostic models explain how multiple co-morbid symptoms or disorders develop rather than create disorder or symptom specific models [63].

3.3.2. Management

A trans-diagnostic treatment is an intervention that targets a range of diagnoses or problems through the use of treatment strategies targeting psychological processes that are common across disorders. It may be useful to consider all five factors such as depression, pain, anxiety, sleep and fatigue in designing a treatment plan. Treatments for the constellation of biopsychosocial concerns affecting many people living with MS.

The beneficial effects on depression of CBT targeting insomnia highlight a need for a comprehensive assessment of multiple concerns such as depression, anxiety, sleep problems or fatigue when treating people with MS who report higher levels of pain [63].

3.4. Trigger for an acute multiple sclerosis exacerbation

The mechanism by which sleep disorders trigger an acute MS relapse might be multi-factorial. Normal sleeping plays an important role in maintaining the normal function of the immune system. Various studies have shown that sleep disorders are associated with elevated serum levels of pro-inflammatory cytokines and markers of oxidative stress [15].

The circadian regulation of cytokine output produces a daily rhythm in the inflammatory profile, with a pro-inflammatory state occurring at night. Disrupted sleep can interfere with this pattern leading to prolonged periods of inflammation throughout the day, thereby exacerbating symptoms. Furthermore, the circadian rhythmicity of key components of the immune system has been shown to be dysregulated in MS patients [64].

The central circadian pacemaker, located in the hypothalamic suprachiasmatic nuclei, is responsible for regulating the timing and expression of various circadian rhythms [65].

Sleep dysfunction and disruption in the circadian system alter the synchrony between these transcriptional and translational feedback loops, resulting in increased cellular permeability, which is thought to be an important underlying mechanism for initiating the inflammatory cascades causing a disease flare. In addition, the presence of pro-inflammatory cytokines has been proven to suppress the activity of circadian genes [65].

Melatonin is produced by the pineal gland that regulates circadian and seasonal rhythms. Secretion of melatonin is suppressed during daylight and enhanced during the night, promotes sleep by reducing sleep latency, decreasing wake time and increasing overall sleep quality [65].

Melatonin promotes anti-inflammatory states: it inhibits nitric oxide production, nuclear factor-κB activation and tumor necrosis factor- α, it reduces COX-2 expression and matrix metalloproteinase activity (modulating apoptosis) [65].

Circadian sleep disorders are common in MS patients and could be linked to a disruption in melatonin production, which is important in sleep-wake cycle regulation. Melatonin helps dampen the overactive immune system and low levels are associated with relapse [64].

According to studies on an animal model, sleep deprivation is associated with an accelerated autoantibody production rate and increases oxidative stress (toxic effect on oligodendrocytes causing oligodendrocyte death and myelin damage). Chronic sleep deprivation breaks down blood-brain barrier (BBB) thereby increasing permeability [15].

Sleep disorders also result in an elevated serum concentration of interleukin-6 (IL-6), which further activates polyclonal B cells and triggers an autoimmune reaction. The serum concentration of IL-6 is significantly associated with the number of relapses in female patients with relapsing-remitting multiple sclerosis (RRMS) [15]. In the study of Sahraian et al. [15], the group in relapse had worse scores of global PSIQI for the previous month than remission group (87.5% were poor quality sleepers). Age, gender, EDSS and disease duration did not associate with sleep quality in either group.

4. Co-morbidity condition

Co-morbidities have been shown to affect MS progression, time to initiation of the disease-modifying therapy (DMT), as well as treatment compliance, which may be related to the increased mortality of these patients as compared to the general population.

Co-morbidities can negatively impact sleep in MS patients, which can, in turn, lead to a worsening of symptoms, especially fatigue and pain.

Patients with sleep disorders are at risk of co-occurrence of other problems like vascular diseases, obesity and diabetes that would threaten the health of patients in the long term [17].

Circadian disruptions occur in shift workers and appear to contribute to hypertension, diabetes, breast cancer, lung cancer and elevated prostate-specific antigen. Shift work entails changes in diet, exercise and tobacco use, which can confound circadian rhythm and sleep disturbance studies [65].

4.1. Narcolepsy

Narcolepsy is classified as a chronic sleep disorder associated with sleep attacks and other features attributed to abnormalities of rapid eye movement sleep, such as hypnagogic/hypnopompic hallucinations, cataplexy, sleep paralysis and disrupted nocturnal sleep. The usual PSG features include a mean sleep latency of less than or equal to 8 minutes and two or more sleep onset rapid eye movement periods [6]. There is a high variability in the prevalence across different geographic areas, which is thought to be related to differences between the populations and current study methods [10].

Narcolepsy is estimated to affect 0.02–0.05% of the general population, the overall prevalence of narcolepsy among persons with MS is unknown [6, 10].

There are two subtypes of primary narcolepsy which are described below.

Narcolepsy type 1(immune-mediated loss of hypocretin-secreting cells in the lateral hypothalamus) [6, 10] is characterized by the presence of cataplexy (a reliable clinical marker for hypocretin deficiency) and hypocretin deficiency in CSF (<110 pg./dl).

Narcolepsy type 2: normal hypocretin levels [6, 10].

The secondary causes of narcolepsy show that MS is the fourth most common cause of narcolepsy after inherited disorders, CNS tumors and brain injury, and it has been found that 12% of the cases of secondary narcolepsy were due to MS [6, 10, 66].

In terms of genetics, 95% of narcoleptic patients and 50–60% of MS patients are positive for DR2 haplotype. The human leukocyte antigen (HLA) DQB1*0602, a known genetic risk factor for narcolepsy, also influences the presence and severity of MS. Therefore, both diseases are closely related to the same genes of the human leukocyte antigen (HLA) system, which is the basis for labeling for most autoimmune diseases. This relationship suggests that similar autoimmune factors may be at work in the development of each disorder and might be partially responsible for symptoms of fatigue and sleepiness [6, 10, 67].

The aforementioned findings merit further attention given the potential impact of sleep disorders on the health and quality of life of MS patients [10].

4.1.1. Diagnostic approach

A diagnosis of narcolepsy requires PSG and CSF hypocretin assays (only performed at a few academic institutions).

Narcolepsy cannot be established in the presence of concomitant OSA, insufficient sleep, shift work or another circadian sleep disorder [10].

In such cases, adequate treatment of concomitant sleep disorders must be confirmed prior to the multiple sleep latency testing.

The usual PSG features include a mean sleep latency of less than or equal to 8 minutes and two or more sleep onset rapid eye movement periods [6].

It is necessary to perform MRI studies to rule out secondary causes of narcolepsy [6].

4.1.2. Management

Patients with suspected narcolepsy are usually referred for diagnosis and management by sleep specialists: wake-promoting agents or stimulants may be used to increase wakefulness and vigilance.

Sodium oxybate (an endogenous metabolite of gamma-aminobutyric acid (GABA) may be used in selected cases.

REM-suppressing antidepressants may be useful for cataplexy and sleep paralysis.

In cases of secondary narcolepsy when new hypothalamic lesions are identified, a trial of high-dose steroids should be considered [6].

4.2. Overweight and obesity

Being overweight is having more body fat than is optimally healthy. The degree to which a person is overweight is generally described by the body mass index (BMI). Overweight is defined as a BMI above or equal to 25 and below 30.

Obesity is defined as a BMI over 30. The prevalence of overweight and obesity in patients with multiple sclerosis ranges from 19 to 55%. These differences are due to the distinct prevalence in the general population, differences in geographic origin, population type (military veterans or hospital users) and/or age group. It is notable that the American population has the highest numbers of obesity. Besides which, it is worth mentioning the different methodology used, including overweight with obesity in some studies [42, 68].

Spanish data (NARCOMS study) have shown that overweight people with MS had lower general and mental health scores compared to those with normal weight and found no differences in other quality of life scales of the SF-36 [69].

Depression levels were higher in the overweight versus normal weight MS Spanish patients. This finding is due to pathophysiological mechanisms common to both depression and obesity, given that chronic low-grade pro-inflammatory states can generate various abnormalities in different neural networks [69].

BMI was significantly related to levels of disability, with obese participants 1.4 times more likely to have moderate/severe disability while controlling for age, gender, time since diagnosis and number of co-morbidities. As the BMI increases, the number of co-morbidities increases with higher odds for disability and prior relapse and lower health-related quality of life [42].

Central obesity, as defined by increased waist circumference, absolute waist circumference >102 cm in men and >88 cm in women or waist-hip ratio (the circumference of the waist divided by that of the hips) of >0.9 for men and >0.85 for women, is often indicative of metabolic syndrome, and is suggested to be a more potent risk factor (cardiovascular disease, Alzheimer's diseases and type 2 diabetes) than body mass index alone.

4.2.1. Diagnostic approach

Weight, height, BMI = weight (kg)/height (m^2), waist circumference and waist-hip ratio.

4.2.2. Management

Patients who are overweight and obese are usually referred for diagnosis and management by a multidisciplinary team such as specialist nutritionist, physiotherapists, surgeons and neuropsychologists.

Gradual weight loss and gentle physical exercise and stretching are recommended. Small meals and small amounts of food, low in animal fats and fresh fruits. Bariatric surgery may be necessary in severe cases of obesity.

Co-morbidities have been shown to be associated with increased hospitalization, rate of progression to disability, decreased quality of life and increased mortality risk which is why they have to be properly treated [42].

Adverse health behavior including being overweight and obese, smoking and sedentary behavior are common in people with MS [42]. These behaviors can be modified and may significantly change the level of health. Health professionals should be focused on achieving these behavioral changes in patients with MS.

5. Influence of the treatment of multiple sclerosis in sleep

The therapeutic approach to multiple sclerosis involves pharmacological, rehabilitative, psychological, lifestyle modifying interventions, etc. These can be used independently or coordinated with each other with a holistic view. This approach involves changes in the structure of sleep, which are not always beneficial.

5.1. Treatment of relapses

Therapeutic options to treat MS relapses include oral glucocorticosteroids [70, 71] or their intravenous administration at a high dose as first line and therapeutic plasma exchange (TPE) and intravenous immunoglobulin (IVIG) as second line treatments in glucocorticosteroids unresponsive patients [72], corticotrophin injection and Acthar [73].

The action mechanisms of glucocorticosteroids in the immune system are pleiotropic, induced apoptosis of peripheral blood leucocytes and down-regulation of T-cell activity delayed for 7–10 days after a 5-day course of administration [72].

TPE is the removal of circulating antibodies, cytokines, immune complexes and complementary factors, all of which are assumed to be involved in immune-mediated neuroinflammation.

IVIG reduces or prevents the activation of inflammatory cells and alters antibody responses.

Optimal treatment of relapses increases the chance of limiting or avoiding residual deficits which have been related to the progression of disability in MS [72].

Sleep disturbance (insomnia) might be one of the side effects of corticosteroid therapy during an acute exacerbation in MS. Benzodiazepines are useful during these periods [74].

5.2. Disease-modifying therapies

Interferons are DMTs that produce major alterations of sleep, mainly by the flulike reaction, fever, headache, alteration of the mood and fatigue. It is imperative to treat these effects to improve the patient's quality of life including finding what time is best to administer the treatment. The monoclonal antibody Natalizumab could reduce fatigue [37].

5.3. Symptomatic treatment

Specific treatment of symptoms of MS manifestations occasionally interferes with sleep quality, leading to insomnia or drowsiness. The treatments the patient is receiving need to be reviewed in the event of any sleep disturbance.

Selective serotonin reuptake inhibitors, while helpful for depressive symptoms, may worsen insomnia. Stimulants and wake-promoting agents, which are commonly used for fatigue, may interfere with sleep initiation if taken during the late afternoon or early evening hours. Antihistamines, which are used as sleep aids by up to 25% of patients with MS, have the potential to worsen RLS, and thereby worsen sleep-onset insomnia.

Patients suffering from fatigue symptoms are often treated with antidepressants due to the strong association between depression and fatigue. Modafinil, amantadine and aminopyridine are known as fatigue treatment options, although the physician must monitor the real effect on sleep and adjust the administration schedules so as not to mask the effect on fatigue.

Medications used to alleviate MS-related symptoms, including over-the-counter medications, also have the potential to interfere with sleep. Given the high frequency use of these medications in this population, the physician should carefully consider screening for these medications and assessing possible effects on sleep.

5.3.1. Management

The first approach includes reviewing the list of drugs being taken by the patient and adjusting doses or suspending them if necessary to avoid interference with other situations of the patient. In this respect, the multidisciplinary approach to the patient is important.

6. Conclusions

Sleep disorders in patients with MS are frequently underdiagnosed. Clinicians caring for patients with MS should routinely screen for sleep disturbances.

All the symptoms are related, many of them share the same pathophysiology where it is not possible to identify the precipitating factor and the perpetuating factor. Sleep disturbances increase the risk of mortality, co-morbidities (cardiac disease, obesity and diabetes) and can contribute to the depression, pain, cognitive impairment and fatigue symptoms which are disabling and worsen the prognosis of multiple sclerosis.

The therapeutic approach to sleep disorders in MS involves pharmacological, rehabilitative, physical, psychological, educational and lifestyle modification interventions. These can be used independently in combination, with combined therapies being more effective.

The list of drugs being taken by the patient should always be reviewed and doses should be adjusted or suspended if necessary to avoid interference with sleeps disorders.

Conflict of interest

Montserrat González Platas and María Yaiza Perez Martín report no conflicts of interest concerning the manuscript.

Author details

Montserrat González Platas* and María Yaiza Pérez Martin

*Address all correspondence to: montserrat.gonzalezplatas@gmail.com

Neurology Service, Hospital Universitario de Canarias, La Laguna, Santa Cruz de Tenerife, Spain

References

[1] Ma S, Rui X, Qi P, Liu G, Yang J. Sleep disorders in patients with multiple sclerosis in China. Sleep Breath. 2017;**21**(1):149-154

[2] Tachibana N, Howard RS, Hirsch NP, Miller DH, Moseley IF, Fish D. Sleep problems in multiple sclerosis. European Neurology. 1994;**34**(6):320-323

[3] Merlino G, Fratticci L, Lenchig C, Valente M, Cargnelutti D, Picello M, et al. Prevalence of "poor sleep" among patients with multiple sclerosis: An independent predictor of mental and physical status. Sleep Medicine. Jan 2009;**10**(1):26-34

[4] Bamer AM, Johnson KL, Amtmann D, Kraft GH. Prevalence of sleep problems in individuals with multiple sclerosis. Multiple Sclerosis (Houndmills, Basingstoke, England: Online). Sep 2008;**14**(8):1127-1130

[5] Vitkova M, Rosenberger J, Gdovinova Z, Szilasiova J, Mikula P, Groothoff JW, et al. Poor sleep quality in patients with multiple sclerosis: Gender differences. Brain and Behavior. Nov 2016;**6**(11):e00553

[6] Braley TJ, Chervin RD. A practical approach to the diagnosis and management of sleep disorders in patients with multiple sclerosis. Therapeutic Advances in Neurological Disorders. Nov 2015;**8**(6):294-310

[7] Caminero A, Bartolomé M. Sleep disturbances in multiple sclerosis. Journal of the Neurological Sciences. Oct 15, 2011;**309**(1):86-91

[8] Kripke DF, Garfinkel L, Wingard DL, Klauber MR, Marler MR. Mortality associated with sleep duration and insomnia. Archives of General Psychiatry. Feb 2002;**59**(2):131-136

[9] Kaynak H, Altintaş A, Kaynak D, Uyanik O, Saip S, Ağaoğlu J, et al. Fatigue and sleep disturbance in multiple sclerosis. European Journal of Neurology. Official Journal of European Federation of Neurological Societies. Dec 2006;**13**(12):1333-1339

[10] González-Platas M, González-Platas J, Bermúdez-Hernández M, Pérez-Martín MY, Croissier-Elías C, Pérez-Lorensu PJ. Low prevalence of sleep disorders in demyelinating disease in a Northern Tenerife population. Journal of Clinical Sleep Medicine: JCSM: Official Publication of the American Academy of Sleep Medicine. Jun 15, 2016;**12**(6):805-811

[11] Fleming WE, Pollak CP. Sleep disorders in multiple sclerosis. Seminars in Neurology. Mar 2005;**25**(1):64-68

[12] Schutte-Rodin S, Broch L, Buysse D, Dorsey C, Sateia M. Clinical guideline for the evaluation and management of chronic insomnia in adults. Journal of Clinical Sleep Medicine: JCSM: Official Publication of the American Academy of Sleep Medicine. Oct 15, 2008;**4**(5):487-504

[13] Stanton BR, Barnes F, Silber E. Sleep and fatigue in multiple sclerosis. Multiple Sclerosis (Houndmills, Basingstoke, England: Online). Aug 2006;**12**(4):481-486

[14] Veauthier C, Gaede G, Radbruch H, Wernecke K-D, Paul F. Poor sleep in multiple sclerosis correlates with Beck depression inventory values, but not with polysomnographic data. Sleep Disorders. 2016;**2016**:8378423

[15] Sahraian MA, Rezaali S, Hosseiny M, Doosti R, Tajik A, Naser Moghadasi A. Sleep disorder as a triggering factor for relapse in multiple sclerosis. European Neurology. 2017;**77**(5–6):258-261

[16] Soldatos CR, Dikeos DG, Paparrigopoulos TJ. Athens insomnia scale: Validation of an instrument based on ICD-10 criteria. Journal of Psychosomatic Research. Jun 2000;**48**(6):555-560

[17] Abbasi S, Alimohammadi N, Pahlavanzadeh S. Effectiveness of cognitive behavioral therapy on the quality of sleep in women with multiple sclerosis: A randomized controlled trial study. International Journal of Community Based Nursing and Midwifery. Oct 2016;**4**(4):320-328

[18] Veauthier C, Hasselmann H, Gold SM, Paul F. The berlin treatment algorithm: Recommendations for tailored innovative therapeutic strategies for multiple sclerosis-related fatigue. The EPMA Journal. 2016;**7**:25

[19] Allen RP, Picchietti D, Hening WA, Trenkwalder C, Walters AS, Montplaisi J. Restless legs syndrome: Diagnostic criteria, special considerations, and epidemiology. A report from the restless legs syndrome diagnosis and epidemiology workshop at the National Institutes of Health. Sleep Medicine Mar 2003;**4**(2):101-119.

[20] Ondo WG. Restless legs syndrome. Neurologic Clinics. Aug 2009;**27**(3):779-799, vii

[21] Auger C, Montplaisir J, Duquette P. Increased frequency of restless legs syndrome in a French-Canadian population with multiple sclerosis. Neurology. Nov 22, 2005;**65**(10):1652-1653

[22] Gómez-Choco MJ, Iranzo A, Blanco Y, Graus F, Santamaria J, Saiz A. Prevalence of restless legs syndrome and REM sleep behavior disorder in multiple sclerosis. Multiple Sclerosis (Houndmills, Basingstoke, England: Online). Jul 2007;**13**(6):805-808

[23] Manconi M, Ferini-Strambi L, Filippi M, Bonanni E, Iudice A, Murri L, et al. Multicenter case-control study on restless legs syndrome in multiple sclerosis: The REMS study. Sleep. Jul 1, 2008;**31**(7):944-952

[24] Deriu M, Cossu G, Molari A, Murgia D, Mereu A, Ferrigno P, et al. Restless legs syndrome in multiple sclerosis: A case-control study. Movement Disorders Official Journal of Movement Disorders Society. Apr 15, 2009;**24**(5):697-701

[25] Crayton H, Heyman RA, Rossman HS. A multimodal approach to managing the symptoms of multiple sclerosis. Neurology. Dec 14, 2004;**63**(11 Suppl 5):S12-S18

[26] Manconi M, Rocca MA, Ferini-Strambi L, Tortorella P, Agosta F, Comi G, et al. Restless legs syndrome is a common finding in multiple sclerosis and correlates with cervical cord damage. Multiple Sclerosis (Houndmills, Basingstoke, England: Online). Jan 2008;**14**(1):86-93

[27] Bonati MT, Ferini-Strambi L, Aridon P, Oldani A, Zucconi M, Casari G. Autosomal dominant restless legs syndrome maps on chromosome 14q. Brain. Jan 6, 2003;**126**(6):1485-92

[28] Trenkwalder C, Paulus W. Restless legs syndrome: Pathophysiology, clinical presentation and management. Nature Reviews Neurology. Jun 2010;**6**(6):337-346

[29] Caples SM, Gami AS, Somers VK. Obstructive sleep apnea. Annals of Internal Medicine. Feb 1, 2005;**142**(3):187-197

[30] Ferini-Strambi L, Filippi M, Martinelli V, Oldani A, Rovaris M, Zucconi M, et al. Nocturnal sleep study in multiple sclerosis: Correlations with clinical and brain magnetic resonance imaging findings. Journal of the Neurological Sciences. Sep 1994;**125**(2):194-197

[31] Fung CH, Vaughan CP, Markland AD, Huang AJ, Mitchell MN, Bliwise DL, et al. Nocturia is associated with poor sleep quality among older women in the study of osteoporotic fractures. J Am Geriatr Soc. 2017;**65**(11):2502-2509

[32] Kwon T, Oh TH, Choi S, Cho WY, Min K, Lee JZ, et al. Influence of daytime or nighttime dosing with solifenacin for overactive bladder with nocturia: Impact on nocturia and sleep quality. Journal of Korean Medical Science. Sep 2017;**32**(9):1491-1495

[33] Sakalis VI, Karavitakis M, Bedretdinova D, Bach T, Bosch JLHR, Gacci M, et al. Medical treatment of nocturia in men with lower urinary tract symptoms: Systematic review by the European Association of Urology Guidelines panel for male lower urinary tract symptoms. European Urology. Nov 2017;**72**(5):757-769

[34] Krupp L. Fatigue is intrinsic to multiple sclerosis (MS) and is the most commonly reported symptom of the disease. Multiple Sclerosis (Houndmills, Basingstoke, England: Online). Aug 2006;**12**(4):367-368

[35] Bakshi R. Fatigue associated with multiple sclerosis: Diagnosis, impact and management. Multiple Sclerosis (Houndmills, Basingstoke, England: Online). Jun 2003;**9**(3):219-227

[36] Fiest KM, Fisk JD, Patten SB, Tremlett H, Wolfson C, Warren S, et al. Fatigue and comorbidities in multiple sclerosis. International Journal of MS Care. Apr 2016;**18**(2):96-104

[37] Chalah MA, Riachi N, Ahdab R, Créange A, Lefaucheur J-P, Ayache SS. Fatigue in multiple sclerosis: Neural correlates and the role of non-invasive brain stimulation. Frontiers in Cellular Neuroscience. 2015;**9**:460

[38] Veauthier C. Younger age, female sex, and high number of awakenings and arousals predict fatigue in patients with sleep disorders: A retrospective polysomnographic observational study. Neuropsychiatric Disease and Treatment. 2013;**9**:1483-1494

[39] Pokryszko-Dragan A, Bilińska M, Gruszka E, Biel Ł, Kamińska K, Konieczna K. Sleep disturbances in patients with multiple sclerosis. Neurological Sciences: Official Journal of the Italian Neurological Society and of the Italian Society of Clinical Neurophysiology. Aug 2013;**34**(8):1291-1296

[40] Dettmers C, DeLuca J. Editorial: Fatigue in multiple sclerosis. Frontiers in Neurology. 2015;**6**:266

[41] Miller P, Soundy A. The pharmacological and non-pharmacological interventions for the management of fatigue related multiple sclerosis. Journal of the Neurological Sciences. Oct 15, 2017;**381**:41-54

[42] Marck CH, Neate SL, Taylor KL, Weiland TJ, Jelinek GA. Prevalence of comorbidities, overweight and obesity in an international sample of people with multiple sclerosis and associations with modifiable lifestyle factors. PLoS One. 2016;**11**(2):e0148573

[43] Amato MP, Zipoli V, Portaccio E. Multiple sclerosis-related cognitive changes: a review of cross-sectional and longitudinal studies. Journal of the Neurological Sciences. Jun 15, 2006;**245**(1–2):41-46

[44] Piras MR, Magnano I, Canu EDG, Paulus KS, Satta WM, Soddu A, et al. Longitudinal study of cognitive dysfunction in multiple sclerosis: Neuropsychological, neuroradiological, and neurophysiological findings. Journal of Neurology, Neurosurgery, and Psychiatry. Jul 2003;**74**(7):878-885

[45] Reuter F, Zaaraoui W, Crespy L, Faivre A, Rico A, Malikova I, et al. Cognitive impairment at the onset of multiple sclerosis: Relationship to lesion location. Multiple Sclerosis (Houndmills, Basingstoke, England: Online). Jun 2011;**17**(6):755-758

[46] Beatty WW, Monson N. Problem solving by patients with multiple sclerosis: Comparison of performance on the Wisconsin and California card sorting tests. Journal of the International Neuropsychological Society. Mar 1996;**2**(2):134-140

[47] Calabrese P. Neuropsychology of multiple sclerosis – An overview. Journal of Neurology. Feb 2006;**253**(Suppl 1):I10-I15

[48] Putzki N, Fischer J, Gottwald K, Reifschneider G, Ries S, Siever A, et al. Quality of life in 1000 patients with early relapsing-remitting multiple sclerosis. European Journal of Neurology. Jun 2009;**16**(6):713-720

[49] Schiavolin S, Leonardi M, Giovannetti AM, Antozzi C, Brambilla L, Confalonieri P, et al. Factors related to difficulties with employment in patients with multiple sclerosis: A review of 2002–2011 literature. International Journal of Rehabilitation Research. (Internationale Zeitschrift Fur Rehabilitationsforschung. Revue Internationale De Recherches De Readaptation). Jun 2013;**36** (2):105-111

[50] Engel C, Greim B, Zettl UK. Diagnostics of cognitive dysfunctions in multiple sclerosis. Journal of Neurology. May 2007;**254**(Suppl 2):II30-II34

[51] Rao SM, Leo GJ, Ellington L, Nauertz T, Bernardin L, Unverzagt F. Cognitive dysfunction in multiple sclerosis. II. Impact on employment and social functioning. Neurology. May 1991;**41**(5):692-696

[52] van Geest Q, Westerik B, van der Werf YD, Geurts JJG, Hulst HE. The role of sleep on cognition and functional connectivity in patients with multiple sclerosis. Journal of Neurology Jan 2017;**264**(1):72-80

[53] Arnett PA, Rao SM, Bernardin L, Grafman J, Yetkin FZ, Lobeck L. Relationship between frontal lobe lesions and Wisconsin card sorting test performance in patients with multiple sclerosis. Neurology. Mar 1994;**44**(3 Pt 1):420-425

[54] Walker MP. The role of sleep in cognition and emotion. Annals of the New York Academy of Sciences. Mar 2009;**1156**:168-197

[55] Lo JC, Groeger JA, Santhi N, Arbon EL, Lazar AS, Hasan S, et al. Effects of partial and acute total sleep deprivation on performance across cognitive domains, individuals and circadian phase. PLoS One. 2012;**7**(9):e45987

[56] Lehmann P, Eling P, Kastrup A, Grothues O, Hildebrandt H. Self-reported sleep problems, but not fatigue, lead to decline in sustained attention in MS patients. Multiple Sclerosis (Houndmills, Basingstoke, England: Online). Apr 2013;**19**(4):490-497

[57] Rao SM, Leo GJ, Bernardin L, Unverzagt F. Cognitive dysfunction in multiple sclerosis. I. Frequency, patterns, and prediction. Neurology. May 1991;**41**(5):685-691

[58] Huijbregts SCJ, Kalkers NF, de Sonneville LMJ, de Groot V, Reuling IEW, Polman CH. Differences in cognitive impairment of relapsing remitting, secondary, and primary progressive MS. Neurology. Jul 27, 2004;**63**(2):335-339

[59] Sepulcre J, Vanotti S, Hernández R, Sandoval G, Cáceres F, Garcea O, et al. Cognitive impairment in patients with multiple sclerosis using the brief repeatable battery-neuropsychology test. Multiple Sclerosis (Houndmills, Basingstoke, England: Online). Apr 2006;**12**(2):187-195

[60] Pérez-Martín MY, Eguia-Del Río P, González-Platas M, Jiménez-Sosa A. Cognitive status in patients with multiple sclerosis in Lanzarote. Neuropsychiatric Disease and Treatment. 2016;**12**:1553-1559

[61] Happe S. Excessive daytime sleepiness and sleep disturbances in patients with neurological diseases: Epidemiology and management. Drugs. 2003;**63**(24):2725-2737

[62] Sadeghi Bahmani D, Gerber M, Kalak N, Lemola S, Clough PJ, Calabrese P, et al. Mental toughness, sleep disturbances, and physical activity in patients with multiple sclerosis compared to healthy adolescents and young adults. Neuropsychiatric Disease and Treatment. 2016;**12**:1571-1579

[63] Amtmann D, Askew RL, Kim J, Chung H, Ehde DM, Bombardier CH, et al. Pain affects depression through anxiety, fatigue, and sleep in multiple sclerosis. Rehabilitation Psychology. Feb 2015;**60**(1):81-90

[64] Mills EA, Mirza A, Mao-Draayer Y. Emerging approaches for validating and managing multiple sclerosis relapse. Frontiers in Neurology. 2017;**8**:116

[65] Parekh PJ, Oldfield Iv EC, Challapallisri V, Ware JC, Johnson DA. Sleep disorders and inflammatory disease activity: Chicken or the egg? American Journal of Gastroenterology. Apr 2015;**110**(4):484-488

[66] Nishino S, Kanbayashi T. Symptomatic narcolepsy, cataplexy and hypersomnia, and their implications in the hypothalamic hypocretin/orexin system. Sleep Medicine Reviews. Aug 2005;**9**(4):269-310

[67] Iseki K, Mezaki T, Oka Y, Terada K, Tomimoto H, Miki Y, et al. Hypersomnia in MS. Neurology. Dec 24, 2002;**59**(12):2006-2007

[68] Marrie R, Horwitz R, Cutter G, Tyry T, Campagnolo D, Vollmer T. High frequency of adverse health behaviors in multiple sclerosis. Multiple Sclerosis (Houndmills, Basingstoke, England: Online). Jan 2009;**15**(1):105-113

[69] Cambil-Martín J, Galiano-Castillo N, Muñoz-Hellín E, Díaz-Rodríguez L, Laguarta-Val S, Fernández-de-Las-Peñas C, et al. Influence of body mass index on psychological and functional outcomes in patients with multiple sclerosis: A cross-sectional study. Nutritional Neuroscience 2016;**19**(2):79-85

[70] Grau-López L, Teniente-Serra A, Tintoré M, Rovira A, Ramió-Torrenta L, Brieva L, et al. Similar biological effect of high-dose oral versus intravenous methylprednisolone in multiple sclerosis relapses. Multiple Sclerosis (Houndmills, Basingstoke, England: Online). Apr 2015;**21**(5):646-650

[71] Ramo-Tello C, Grau-López L, Tintoré M, Rovira A, Ramió i Torrenta L, Brieva L, et al. A randomized clinical trial of oral versus intravenous methylprednisolone for relapse of MS. Multiple Sclerosis (Houndmills, Basingstoke, England: Online). May 2014;**20**(6):717-725

[72] Ehler J, Blechinger S, Rommer PS, Koball S, Mitzner S, Hartung H-P, et al. Treatment of the first acute relapse following therapeutic plasma exchange in formerly glucocorticosteroid-unresponsive multiple sclerosis patients-a multicenter study to evaluate glucocorticosteroid responsiveness. Intl J Mol Sci. 2017;**18**(8):1749

[73] Gold LS, Suh K, Schepman PB, Damal K, Hansen RN. Healthcare costs and resource utilization in patients with multiple sclerosis relapses treated with H.P. Acthar Gel®. Advances in Therapy. 2016;**33**:1279-1292

[74] Perrin Ross A, Williamson A, Smrtka J, Flemming Tracy T, Saunders C, Easterling C, et al. Assessing relapse in multiple sclerosis questionnaire: Results of a pilot study. Multiple Sclerosis International. 2013;**2013**:470476

6

Brain Reorganization in Late Adulthood: Rapid Left-to-Right Switch of Handedness Through Memory-Drawing Training

Lora T. Likova

Abstract

The neural correlates of hand preference are still debatable, and the very few studies on the mechanisms of enforced change of handedness from left to right are all restricted to early childhood. We were able to address the question of retraining handedness in late adulthood for the first time, well outside the accepted critical period for brain plasticity, through a unique training utilizing the complex motor task of blind memory-guided drawing, in a totally blind, congenitally left-handed man. Ten hours of this Cognitive-Kinesthetic Drawing Training, which the author initially developed to drive neuroplasticity in blindness rehabilitation, was sufficient to generate a profound switch in the cortical lateralization of motor control. This study provides new insights into the neuroplasticity of motor control architecture. The results are of high relevance to the long-standing debate about the sources of hemispheric asymmetry. The unprecedented effect on handedness of the rapid Cognitive-Kinesthetic Drawing Training implies a powerful potential of this training for further rehabilitation domains, such as the rehabilitation of stroke or trauma affecting hand control.

Keywords: neuroplasticity, drawing, training, learning, memory, neurorehabilitation, lateralization, left-handed, handedness, Cognitive-Kinesthetic training

1. Introduction

The neural correlates of hand preference are still debatable, and the very few studies on the mechanisms of enforced change of handedness are all restricted to handedness switching from left to right in early childhood [1]. The question of *retraining* handedness in *late adulthood,* well outside the accepted critical period for brain plasticity, has not been previously studied. The author was able to address this question for the first time by driving neuroplasticity through a unique training on the complex motor task of blind memory-guided drawing, in a congenitally left-handed man who had become totally blind 10 years before. The unprecedented effect on handedness of the rapid Cognitive-Kinesthetic Drawing Training—which the author initially developed for blindness rehabilitation [2–7], implies a powerful potential of this training for further rehabilitation domains, such as the rehabilitation of stroke or trauma affecting hand control.

Left-handers are often excluded from neuroscience study cohorts in order to focus on a more uniform population. However, left-handed individuals represent a substantial portion of the human population, and therefore, it is important to account for this aspect of neural coding in order to better understand brain functioning [8]. Most studies have found that, in both right- and left-handers, movements of the preferred hand activate mainly the contralateral hemisphere [9–18], whereas movements of the non-preferred hand tend to result in a more balanced pattern of activation in the two hemispheres, indicating greater involvement of ipsilateral cortex [1, 12]. For example, it has been found that right-handers had greater activation in the left premotor area for either hand [13], indicating a general dominance of the left hemisphere in motor function, whereas left-handers showed a symmetrical of activation in the premotor cortex contralateral to the moving hand (either left or right). A parallel pattern of such a contralaterality for either hand in the right-handed, but not in the left-handed, was found in another brain region—the sensorimotor cortex [19]. It should be noted, however, that there are still many discrepancies in the literature, which are often attributed to differences in experimental design, including the type of motor task.

Does forceful switching from left-to-right handedness in adulthood change the patterns of cortication activation in left-handers or not? How much of the observed inter-hemispheric patterns are entirely genetically predetermined or can be affected by experience, such as training? There are only a few studies addressing these questions, with divergent results (e.g., [1, 16, 20–24]).

2. The Cognitive-Kinesthetic Drawing Training

The Cognitive-Kinesthetic Drawing Training is a noninvasive approach to blindness rehabilitation that the author has developed based on a novel conceptual paradigm [3–6]. It utilizes a special protocol of *memory-guided drawing*. My previous studies show that this training affects a widely distributed brain network, including both lower-level regions, such as the primary visual cortex (even in the blind), and higher level regions as the hippocampus or a swath of temporal cortex regions [6]. It also enhances top-down connectivity from the hippocampus and other memory-related regions such as the perirhinal cortex [25–26] to early visual areas.

The results from my previous study [6] also revealed the remarkable learning dynamics of functional reorganization in the hippocampal complex and the temporal-lobe object processing hierarchy over a two-month-long consolidation period. In particular, the hippocampal pattern of profound *learning-based transformations* was strongly reflected in the primary visual cortex (V1), with the memory retrieval function showing massive growth as a result of the Cognitive-Kinesthetic memory training and consolidation, while the initially strong hippocampal response during tactile exploration and encoding became almost nonexistent. Furthermore, the inferior temporal cortex manifested a striking *alternating patch structure* [6] (**Figure 1**, bottom panel) reminiscent of the face and object patches reported along the temporal lobe [27]. However, in my study, the differentiation was a function of the *temporal evolution of learning* changes, that is, it was reflecting the effect of training *over time (*instead being a function of face/object category). This cascade of alternating discrete regions also underwent a radical *sequence of transformations* as a

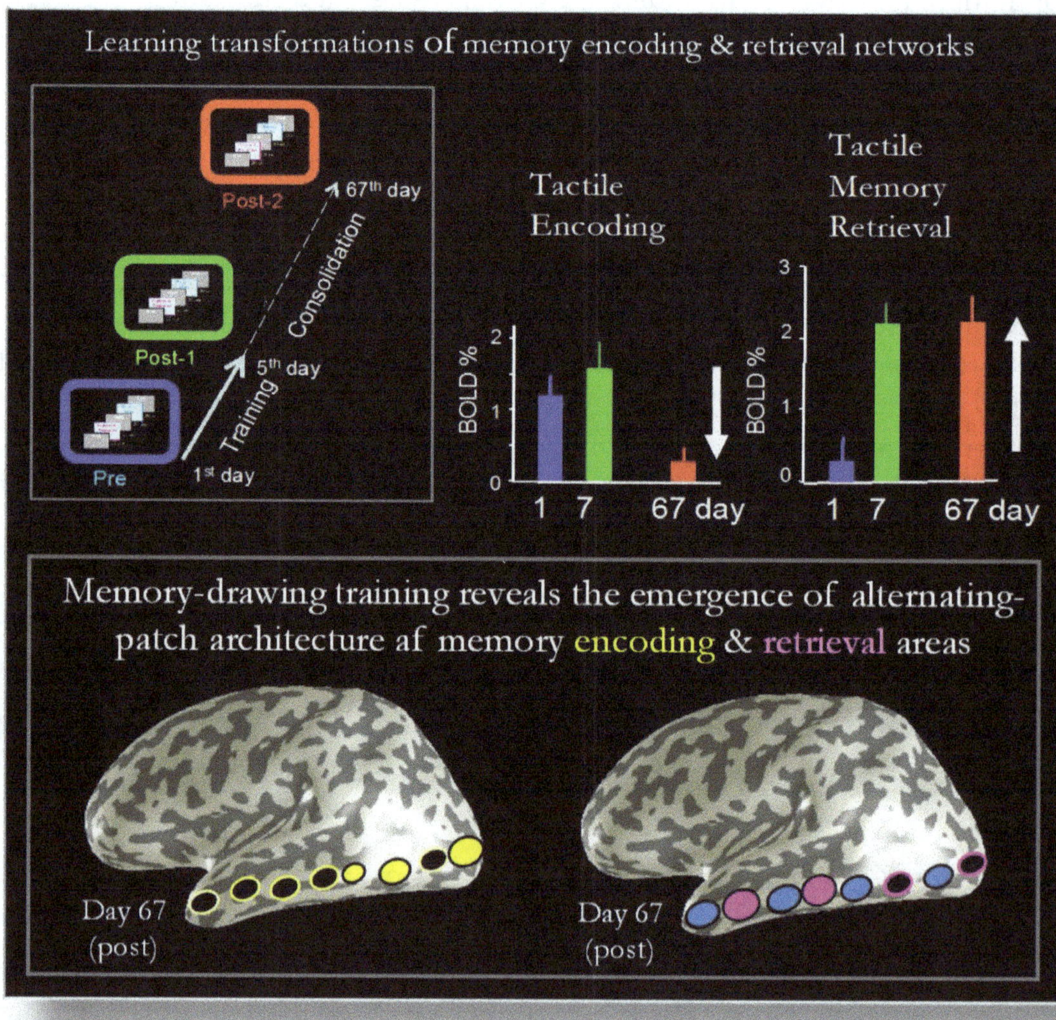

Figure 1. Learning evolution along IT driven by the Cognitive-Kinesthetic memory-drawing training. **Upper panel:** Left: Experimental design, including 3 fMRI assessments: i) a pre-training (*pre/blue*), ii) an immediate after training (*post1/green*), and iii) two months after consolidation period with no training (*post2/red*) assessments. Right: Example of the dramatic reorganization of BOLD responses in an IT region for the *tactile encoding,* and the *tactile memory retrieval tasks* from Day1 (pre-training), to day 7 (immediately post-training) to day 67 (2 months after training). **Bottom panel:** Alternating-patch structure of dissociated, largely non-overlapping encoding and retrieval regions after consolidation (day 67; after training). Left: Memory-encoding task. Yellow—areas still active after consolidation; black—areas not activated anymore. Right: Memory-retrieval task: Purple—areas that become active; blue—suppressed areas; black—areas not involved anymore (after Likova [6]).

function of the *stage of learning*, toward a *complete functional specialization* in terms of either *encoding* or *retrieval* after consolidation. Several distinct patterns of this learning evolution *within* each of the patches (see, e.g., in **Figure 1**, top panel) implied a complex reorganization of the object processing sub-networks throughout both the *training* and the following *consolidation* period.

3. Generalization of drawing-learning effects

While there have been many cross-sectional comparisons of blind and sighted capabilities, the only research focused on *interventions* to enhance basic spatial-cognition abilities in people with blindness has been that based on my Cognitive-Kinesthetic drawing training. This intervention has been shown to improve *spatial memory* and *memory-guided spatiomotor coordination* to a dramatic extent. Although it is typically assumed that drawing is dependent on vision, previous work indicates that individuals with congenital blindness are able to learn to draw over some unspecified time period that often may take years [28–30]. My studies have shown, however, that everyone—blind, sighted, or visually impaired—can learn this skill in only a few hours through an appropriate training, such as the Cognitive-Kinesthetic methodology [3–4, 31–33].

I have further hypothesized that the improvements from the Cognitive-Kinesthetic training would *transfer*, or—*generalize,* to a wide range of *untrained* basic spatial-cognition abilities that extend well beyond the drawing task *per se* [6]. "Basic" abilities were conceptualized as those that are foundational to other tasks, such as the ability to perceive, and remember object features, textures, spatial configurations, and patterns, together with abilities for spatial analysis and new concept learning. My rationale for this *transfer of learning*, or *Generalization of Learning*, hypothesis derived from the fact that the act of drawing complex images from memory "orchestrates" multiple spatial-cognition abilities [2–3, 31–33]. A recent study confirmed my Generalization of Learning Hypothesis [34] by showing significant improvements in a large standardized battery of untrained cognitive tests [35–36] for the blind and low vision following the 10 hours of Cognitive-Kinesthetic training in a cohort of congenitally blind and severe low-vision participants.

4. Switching of handedness as a form of learning effect?

In the earlier cited studies, the Cognitive-Kinesthetic Drawing Training was designed and applied as a noninvasive intervention for a rapid enhancement of *spatial memory, spatial cognition* in general, and precise *memory-guided motor control* in both the blind and the sighted. The memory drawing protocol in the form developed for this training, fully engages the whole *perception-cognition-action loop* [3–4], which was a key element of my *conceptual framework* underlying the training. (Note here the expansion of the traditional "perception-action" loop to include the central component of "cognition" (**Figure 2**), as I believe it is critical to its generalization to the gamut of spatial-cognition abilities.)

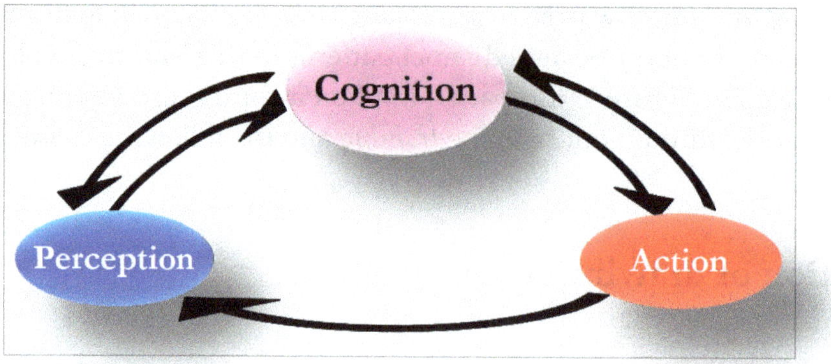

Figure 2. Perception-Cognition-Action Loop. Note the inclusion of the *cognition* module as a central mediator into the traditional perception-action loop [4].

In this chapter, we ask whether the learning effect of this training could extend to the ***action*** component of the processing *loop* involved. Specifically, can it drive reorganization of motor-architecture for *switching handedness*?

5. Methods and procedures

5.1. Participant and the Cognitive-Kinesthetic Training

The participant was a 57-year-old male who had full vision until age of 47, when his vision began declining in one eye and then the other, and he was diagnosed with Leber's hereditary optic neuropathy. Within a year, he was blind, seeing only some light in the far periphery. He had been left-handed since birth. The participant gave informed consent for the experimental protocol, which was approved by the Smith-Kettlewell Institutional Review Board as in full conformance with the Declaration of Helsinki.

After only a total of 10 hours of the Cognitive-Kinesthetic Drawing Training (2 hours/day for 5 days [3]), this left-handed blind participant learned to develop detailed and robust *memory representations* of *haptically* explored (with the ***preferred/left*** hand) raised-line depictions of complex images, such as human faces and objects, in order to draw them with his ***non-preferred/right*** hand. Thus, in order to generate the structured motor output of the drawing, he had to learn how to use these enhanced haptic memory representations to *replace* his *lost "eye-hand coordination"* by a *"memory-hand coordination"* mechanism now that he was blind.

In the process, this blind participant learned to *draw freely* with his *non-preferred/right* hand, guided *solely* by the haptic memory acquired with the other hand. This man had never been able to draw well even with his preferred/left hand while still sighted, so he and his family were greatly surprised by this successful outcome.

> *I never could draw very well ... That's why it's very interesting to me that I would've been the person that did not have drawing skills before, and to be able to do something like this now .., wow, it is exciting - you have thought me drawing better than I could when I could see ... and - to do this with my right hand ...!.*

In an additional session, he subsequently practiced drawing the *already* memorized images with his preferred/left hand.

5.2. Experimental design

A key component of the study was measuring whole-brain functional MRI (fMRI) activation before and after applying the Cognitive-Kinesthetic Drawing Training, allowing us to determine the neuroplastic changes in a *causal* framework (**Figure 3**).

As in previous studies with the Likova Cognitive-Kinesthetic training method, fMRI was run *before* and *after* the training for a battery of *raised-line* models of faces and objects as the drawing targets in a three-task block fMRI design [3–4]. The three tasks were as follows: *Haptic Exploration* (*HE*) involving perceptual exploration and encoding in memory of the raised-line model to be drawn; *Memory Draw* (*MD*)—the task to draw this model freehand, guided solely by the encoded haptic memory; *Scribble* (*S*) was a negative memory-control and motor-control task for the hand movements alone. Each task duration was 20 s, with a 20-s baseline condition (*Rest*, *R*) intervening between tasks. Importantly, as opposed to the usual null periods, the participant not only rested motionless but was also instructed and practiced to clear any memory or imagery from awareness (*"blank-mind"*). The start of each task or rest interval was prompted by an auditory cue. The whole task sequence with interleaved rest intervals (*R, HE, R, MD, R, S, R*) was repeated 12 times in each 1.5-hour fMRI session using a new face or object image for each repeat. The *HE* task was always performed with the preferred/left hand. The *MD* and *S* tasks were performed with the non-preferred/right, and additionally, with the preferred/left hand in separate scans.

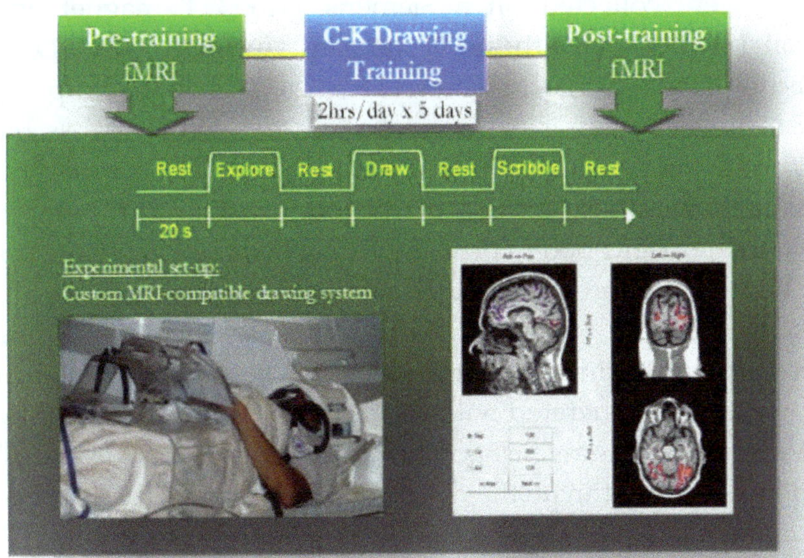

Figure 3. Experimental design. The rapid Cognitive-Kinesthetic drawing training (2 hours/day × 5 days) was preceded and followed by fMRI scans. In the scanner, three tasks were performed in a block paradigm: *Haptic Exploration, Memory Draw,* and *Scribble.* Each task and interleaved rest period were 20 s in duration. An innovative MRI-compatible lectern (lower left) provided for tactile stimulus presentation and both nonvisual and visual drawing. Functional brain activation is color coded in red (lower right).

5.3. Innovative experimental platform

The overall experimental platform integrated a number of innovations, such as, a *multisensory magnetic resonance (MR)-Compatible Tablet system*, and a novel type of parametric brain mapping—*Categorical-Change Maps* [37] that we developed especially for the purpose of assessing *brain plasticity changes* as a result of a causal intervention, and the *Cognitive-Kinesthetic Training*.

The custom MR-Compatible Tablet system (**Figure 3**) allows for participant-controlled tactile-stimulus presentation for haptic exploration and drawing in the scanner. This system consists of a plexiglass lectern extending across the participant's lap, topped with a dual-slot height-adjustable surface [3]. In the left slot was the raised-line drawing stimulus to be haptically explored during the *HE* task, and in the right slot was an MR-compatible electronic drawing tablet (EMS Medical Systems, Bologna, Italy) to be used during the *MD* and *S* tasks. Between scans, the participant was instructed how to remove the topmost raised-line drawing stimulus (which was just explored and drawn) from the left slot and place it by their side, exposing the next stimulus in the prescribed sequence. Participants used a plastic stylus to draw and scribble, with the movement of the stylus across the drawing tablet being recorded and presented in real time to the experimenters on a display in the control room. Auditory cues were presented through MR-compatible headphones (Resonance Technologies, Salem, MA). Our custom MR-compatible tablet system allowed participants to draw comfortably on the plastic lectern across their torso/lap without moving their head. Additionally, during scanning, the participant's head was stabilized in the head coil with firm but comfortable padding around all sides to minimize movement.

5.4. Brain imaging data acquisition and preprocessing

Functional MRI data were collected on a Siemens Trio 3 T magnet equipped with a 12-channel head coil (Siemens Healthcare, Erlangen, Germany). BOLD responses were obtained using an echo-planar (EPI) acquisition (TR = 2 s, TE = 28 ms, flip angle = 80°, voxel size = 3.0 × 3.0 × 3.5 mm) consisting of 35 axial slices extending across the whole brain. Preprocessing was conducted using FSL (FMRIB Analysis Group, Oxford, UK) and included slice-time correction and two-phase motion correction, consisting of both within-scan and between-scan six-parameter rigid-body corrections. To facilitate segmentation and registration, a whole-brain high-resolution T1-weighted anatomical scan was also obtained for each participant (voxel size = 0.8 × 0.8 × 0.8 mm). White matter segmentation in this T1 scan was conducted using FreeSurfer (Martinos Center for Biomedical Imaging, Massachusetts General Hospital) and gray matter was generated with the mrGray function in the mrVISTA software package (Stanford Vision and Imaging Science and Technology, Palo Alto, USA). The Stanford package mrVISTA allows us to estimate the neural activation amplitudes for each task within respective regions of interest (ROIs) using a standard general linear model (GLM) procedure for each task regressor applied to the average signal across all voxels within each ROI.

5.5. Categorical-Change parametric mapping: a novel concept and methodology for the assessment of brain plasticity changes

In studies on brain plasticity, it is critical to be able to fully assess functional brain *changes* due to either an intervention, a natural development, or other causes, such as loss of vision.

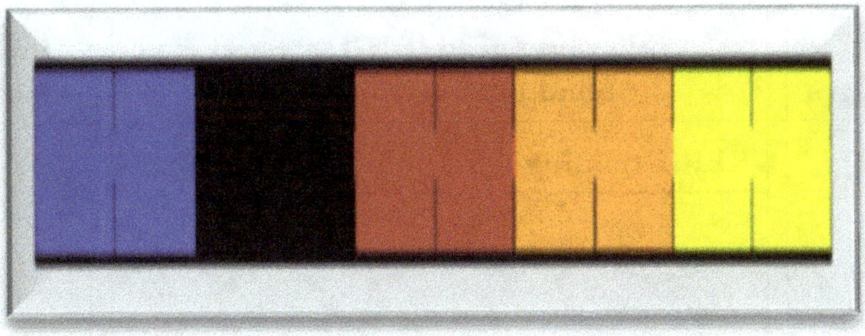

Figure 4. Color coding for Categorical-Change mapping in the case of *positive baseline* activation. *Orange*: No significant change; *Red*: Reduced but still positive activation; *Yellow*: Increased positive activation; *Black*: Lost activation; *Blue*: BOLD signal inverted from positive into negative.

We have conceptualized a system of ***brain-change categories*** and developed a novel type of voxel-wise parametric mapping that can provide the needed *multifaceted assessment of neuroplasticity* [37], and thus, bridge a major gap in this field. This is based on (1) assessing the activation (in each voxel of the brain) during an initial state (e.g., *before* training; *baseline*) and (2) the change in activation (e.g., *after* training) ***relative*** to that baseline.

In the current study, we employed a subset of the categorical-change mapping to visualize **at once** *all five possible categories* of post-training change (or lack thereof) of any ***positive baseline*** activation prior to the state change or intervention.

The color coding for novel type of maps is shown in **Figure 4**. If an activated region did not undergo any significant change relative to the initial state, it is visualized in orange; if its positive activation was increased—in yellow; if it was reduced but still positive—in red; if the activation was lost—in black; while if the sign of the BOLD signal was inverted from positive into negative reflecting a changed in the nature of processing, it is shown in blue.

Note that we have developed the categorical-change mapping to assess the ***full spectrum of possible changes***, relative to a given pre-intervention state. In other words, this mapping tool can also be applied to brain regions that in the ***baseline*** state have ***negative*** BOLD signal, or have ***no activation*** at all. These two options are beyond the scope of the present analysis, however.

6. Results

6.1. Drawing qualities

A total of only 10 hours of the Cognitive-Kinesthetic Drawing, spread out over 5 days, led to dramatic motor control changes in this *congenitally left-handed* blind participant, who was able for the first time to obtain a highly precise control of his *non-preferred right* hand.

The scope and quality of this unexpected new ability of the *non-preferred* hand is illustrated in **Figure 5**. The *central panel* shows a comparison of his pre-training versus post-training drawing

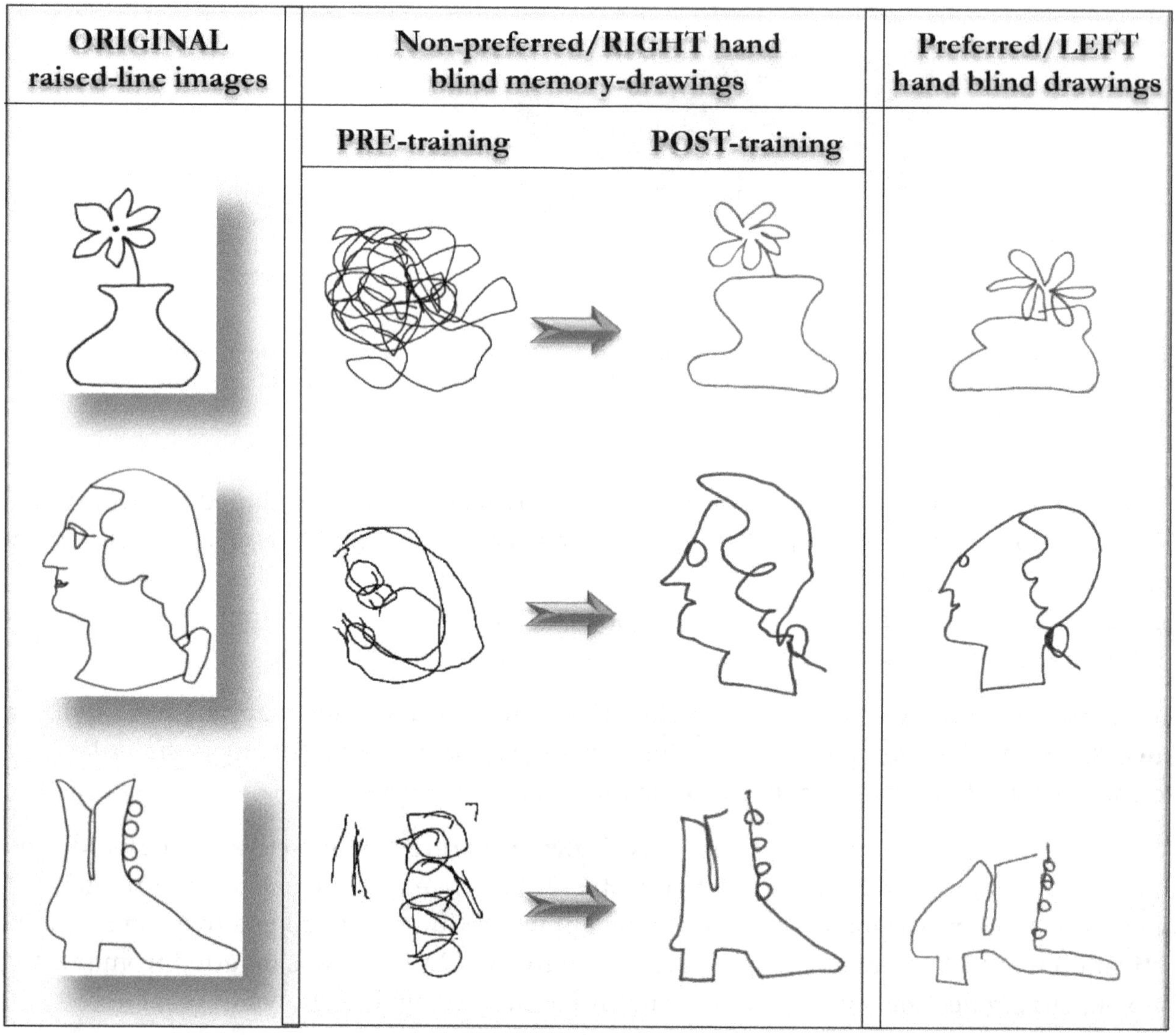

Figure 5. Examples of drawings made by the left-handed blind participant, who underwent the Cognitive-Kinesthetic drawing training. **Left panel:** Raised-line originals used in the haptic exploration and memorization phase. The exploration was always done with the preferred/left hand. **Middle panel:** Drawing from memory with the ***non-preferred/right*** hand, showing the dramatic improvement *from pre-training to post-training,* despite the fact that this hand has never been used before for drawing, writing, or any other habitual motor activity. **Right panel:** Drawings with the ***preferred/left*** hand. These drawings are guided by the same memory that was guiding the other hand; the memory per se, however, was based always on the haptic exploration of the originals with the preferred/left hand. Note that the two hands seem to express two different personalities.

done with the right (non-preferred) hand. Note, these are performed entirely *non-visually,* guided solely by the *memory from the haptic* exploration of the raised-line originals shown in the *left panel.* Note that the exploration was always done with the *preferred/left* hand.

After completing the training of the non-preferred/right hand, the participant had a session of practicing drawing with his all-life preferred (but untrained on the blind memory drawing) left hand. He was then asked to use the untrained left hand to draw the same images guided by the *already* acquired memory (**Figure 3**, *right panel*). Because the left hand had been the dominant one for almost six decades, and moreover, as the haptic exploration and memorization phase

(*HE*) was always done with this hand, the expectation would be for these to provide definitive advantages for *left*-handed drawing.

Conversely, in the main study (drawing with the non-preferred/right hand), the fact that the image information was gathered through exploration with the opposite (left) hand, sets the expectation that the *right*-hand drawing would be at a disadvantage. However, this seems to be the case only *before* the training. Note the rapidly achieved dramatic improvement ***from pre-training to post-training*** for the right hand (**Figure 3**, *middle panel*) despite this disadvantage, and despite the fact that his right hand had never been used before for drawing, writing, or any other habitual motor activity. It is thus surprising, that the *post-training* reproductions with the right hand resembled the originals better than those done with the whole-life-preferred left hand (**Figure 5**, *right panel*). Note again that both phases of the process—*haptic memory encoding* and *retrieval for memory drawing*—were done without the involvement of any vision in this blind participant.

Although the drawing quality and similarity are evident to the human eye, we further assessed the drawing quality by *bi-dimensional regression analysis* [38]. First, for each original image, landmarks were set at unique points that could be easily identified by the naked eye in the original figures and the resulting drawings. Second, bi-dimensional analysis was run for the correspondence between landmarks on the original images and those available on their reproduction by drawing. The specific measure for analyzing the quality of drawings was the fit of an affine bi-dimensional regression (expressed as Fisher-Z values of the respective Rs). The number of landmarks depended on the complexity for each template image.

The bi-dimensional regression scores indicated an improvement averaging about a factor of six *from pre- to post-training* accuracy with the trained hand. Consistent with the perceptual evaluation done earlier, the *post-training* bi-dimensional regression values were significantly higher overall for the non-preferred (but Cognitive-Kinesthetically trained) right hand versus the preferred but untrained left hand, even though the left hand was the one used in acquiring the spatial memory that guided each of the hands along the drawing trajectories.

Interestingly, although the line stability, and image completeness produced by the preferred/left hand were very good, the accuracy of reproduction with this preferred but untrained hand was lower by about a factor of two relative to the strong improvement with the training of the non-preferred/right hand. What was even more surprising was that, stylistically, it could be said that the two hands seemed to express two different personalities.

6.2. Brain plasticity driven by the Cognitive-Kinesthetic Drawing Training

6.2.1. Baseline A: the activation in the brain network engaged by the left hand in memory drawing as baseline

The fMRI recordings run *before* and *after* the training provided a measure of the neuroplastic functional changes underlying the behavioral improvements. To assess not simply *what* has been changed, but ***how*** was it changed and what specific *categories of change* had occurred in the cortex, we used our novel approach of Categorical-Change parametric brain mapping described earlier.

Using the categorical-change parametric mapping, **Figure 6** shows the types of changes that happened in the cortical network activated during memory drawing with the preferred/left hand (*baseline*), when the non-preferred/right hand instead performed the same memory drawing task either *before* training (*top panel*) or *after* training (*bottom panel*).

6.2.1.1. Pre-training (top panel)

The architecture of the *baseline network* (used as a mask) indicates that the movements of the *preferred/left* hand activated predominantly its *contralateral*/right hemisphere, as expected.

As also expected, the categorical-change mapping shows that *before* training, the drawing movements of the *non-preferred/right* hand resulted in a more ***balanced inter-hemispheric*** pattern of activation, indicating preservation of the greater involvement of the ipsilateral (right) hemisphere, consistent with previous studies on switching handedness (see Introduction). This result demonstrates that in its attempt to perform such a complex and precision-demanding motor task *before* training, the non-preferred/right hand continued to depend on the functional architecture of the preferred/left hand. Third, the figure shows that all motor, premotor, and sensorimotor regions in *both* hemispheres that were engaged by the preferred left hand were engaged to an even higher degree by the non-preferred hand.

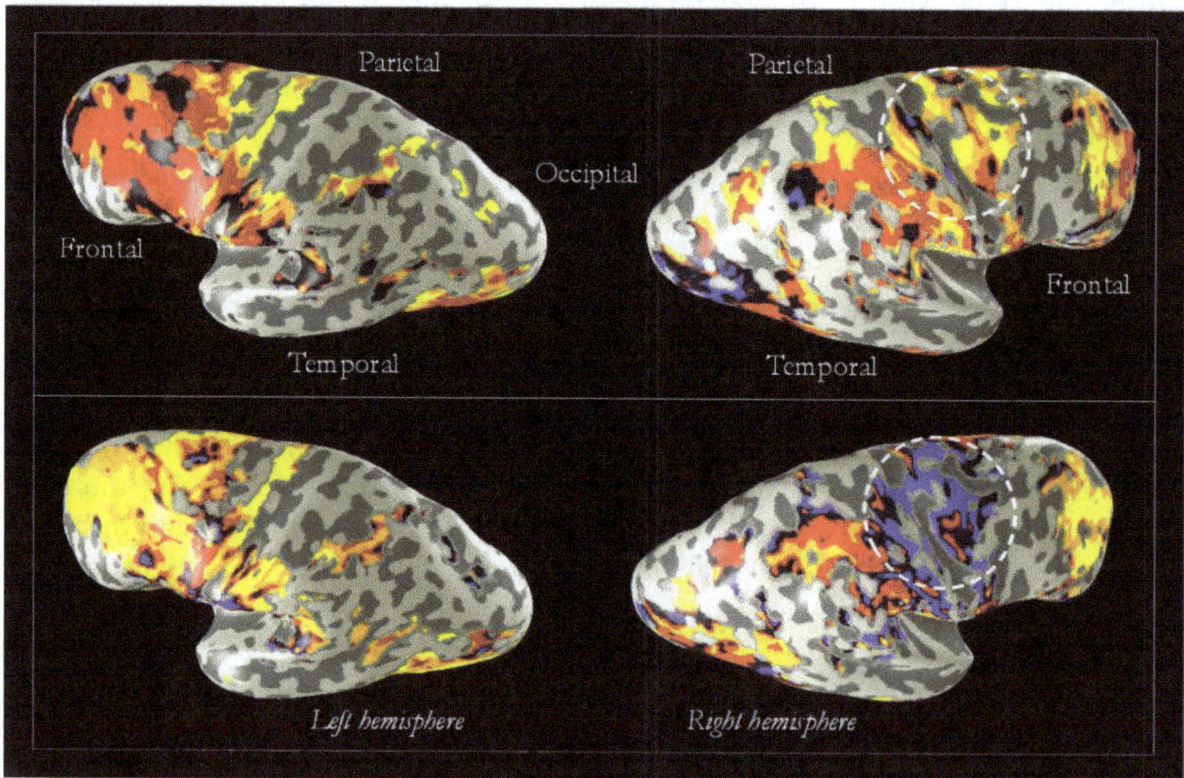

Figure 6. Categorical changes in cortical activation relative to that for memory-guided drawing with the untrained left hand *(baseline)*. The *positive* activation in the brain network engaged by memory drawing with the *left hand* was used as the ***baseline*** for the comparisons in both panels. The differences from that *baseline* for the non-preferred/right-hand activation *before training* are shown in the top panel; *after training*, they are shown in the bottom panel. The voxel-wise changes are presented on inflated views of the lateral surfaces of the left and right hemispheres. Color coding as in **Figure 4**: *Orange*—No change relative to baseline; *Yellow*—Increased positive signal; *Red*—Decreased positive signal; *Black*—Reduction to no significant signal; *Blue*—Negative signal.

6.2.1.2. Post-training (bottom panel)

Remarkably, after the Cognitive-Kinesthetic training, we observed a dramatic reorganization of motor architecture of the *non-preferred/right* hand toward a strongly expressed *contralateral* (left hemisphere) dominance. This previously unobserved reorganization is also clearly confirmed by the categorical-change map analysis in Section 6.2.2. below, where the *pre-training right-hand* network was used as baseline.

6.2.2. Baseline B: the activation in the brain network engaged by the non-preferred/right in memory drawing before training as a baseline

In this section, the network activated by the non-preffered/right hand during MD was used as the basline in the analysis. Consistent with findings from Section 6.2.1. above (see **Figure 6**), the categorical-maps shown in **Figure 7** confirm both the *bilateral* pattern of (positive) activation of the *non-preferred* hand *before* training (used as the baseline mask) and the ***transformation*** of this *bilaterality* into a *strong contralaterality* as a result of training. Another striking finding from the categorical comparison in **Figure 7** was the *massive suppression* (blue) of the BOLD responses in the motor and premotor cortex of the *ipsilateral*/right hemisphere. Furthermore, contrary to what may be expected, this happened in conjunction not with an increase but with an almost *unchanged (orange) or even reduced (red)* activation in these motor control regions of the *contralateral*/left hemisphere relative to pre-training. In other words, the increased contralaterality (left hemisphere greater than right) was *not* caused by increased contralateral/left activation but by an *ipsilateral suppression,* in spite of the fact that this right hemisphere has been the dominant one for the *entire life* of this participant.

It is noteworthy that drawing, particularly if it is solely guided by memory as in the Cognitive-Kinesthetic training applied here, is a highly complex task *orchestrating* a wide

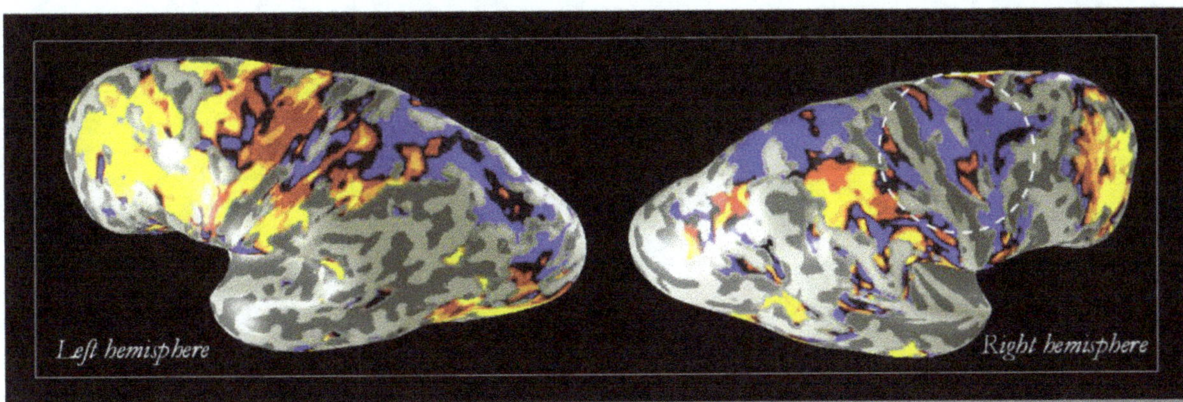

Figure 7. Rapid switch of handedness. To establish the categories of ***training-induced*** changes in the cortical network controlling the ***non-preferred/right*** hand during *MemoryDraw*, our categorical-change mapping was used with the *pre-training* activation pattern of the ***right*** hand as a ***baseline*** in a comparison with its activation ***after*** the right hand underwent the 10 hours of ***training***. The ***training-induced*** categorical changes in the ***functional architecture of the non-preferred right*** are shown on the lateral surfaces of the left and right hemisphere. Color coding as in **Figure 4**: *Orange* — No change relative to baseline; *Yellow* — Increased positive signal; *Red* — Decreased positive signal; *Black* — Reduction to no significant signal; *Blue* — Negative signal

range of perceptual, cognitive, and precise motor functions, thus engaging widely *distributed networks* throughout the brain; their detailed analysis, however, is beyond the scope of this chapter.

6.3. Patterns of hemispheric asymmetry

To quantitatively assess and compare the hemispheric patterns of activation across conditions, we applied the approach used in [1] of comparing the number of voxels, or—volume, activated in each condition. We, however, significantly expanded this approach by taking both positive and negative voxel activations and considering them separately. The voxel numbers were calculated for the conjunction of the motor, premotor, supplementary motor, and somatosensory cortices. The respective FreeSurfer ROIs were used to define the respective cortical regions for quantitative analysis.

Figure 8 shows that both the preferred/left hand (*left panel*) and the non-preferred/right hand pre-training (*middle panel*) conformed to pre-existing models: (1) the activation for the left hand was *predominantly contralateral* (right > left; see *left panel*), whereas (2) a more *balanced, bilateral* pattern of activation was observed for the drawing movements of the *right hand (middle panel)*, indicating a greater ipsilateral involvement.

The *right panel* of **Figure 8**, on the other hand, reveals a radical reorganization in the motor control architecture of the right (non-preferred) hand as a result of the Cognitive-Kinesthetic drawing training. The bilateral pattern of (strongly positive) activation *before* training (*middle panel*) rapidly changed into a strongly contralateral (left hemispheric) pattern *after* training (*right panel*).

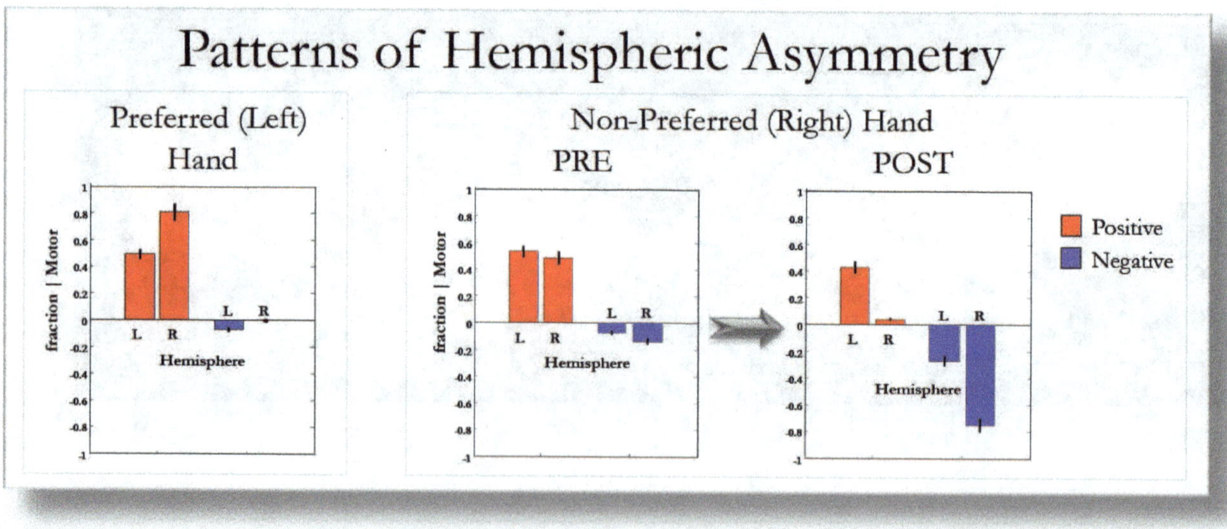

Figure 8. Cognitive-Kinesthetic training effects on the pattern of inter-hemispheric interactions. Three distinct patterns of inter-hemispheric interaction were observed. The distributions of positive (*red*) and negative (*blue*) voxels per hemisphere (*L, left; R, right*) in the conjunction of the motor, premotor, supramotor, and somatosensory cortices during memory-guided drawing is shown for the preferred/left hand (*left panel*), the non-preferred/right hand *pre*-training (*middle panel*), and the non-preferred/right hand *post*-training (*right panel*).

7. General discussion

It is generally accepted that, in both *left- and right-handed* subjects, the preferred hand is controlled mainly by the hemisphere *contralateral* to that hand, whereas the *non-preferred* hand is controlled by *both hemispheres*. In relation to *left-to-right switches* in handedness, the switched individuals have been found to share features of both left-handers and right-handers regarding their motor control architectures. ([1], see Introduction).

Before training, the results for both the *preferred*/left and the *non-preferred*/right hand conformed to these preexisting models: the *preferred*/left hand produced predominantly *contralateral* activation, whereas the *non-preferred*/right hand produced a more balanced *bilateral* activation, indicating control by both hemispheres.

After training, however, the bilateral pattern expected in switchers was not observed any more. Instead, the non-preferred/right hand underwent a strong training-based reorganization of its motor control architecture, so as its bilateral activation pattern radically changed post-training into a contralateral one. Remarkably, this *contralaterality* (left hemisphere > right hemisphere) was caused not by increased contralateral (left) activation but by a massive suppression in the ipsilateral (right) hemisphere; it is particularly surprising that this happened despite the fact that the right hemisphere has been the dominant one since birth.

These findings show for the first time that the dominance of the preferred hemisphere can be rapidly overturned, and that this can happen even in late adulthood after decades of established dominance. Note that, until now, despite long-standing efforts across many disciplines to achieve a fully-fledged hand switching in left-handers, the best that has been achieved has been to engage the contralateral left hemisphere without being able to overturn the ipsilateral right hemisphere control [1, 12]. The fact that the Cognitive-Kinesthetic Drawing Training was able to transform the bilateral into a definitive contralateral pattern, and to do so effectively and efficiently, implies a serious deficiency in the current knowledge on motor control plasticity, and the need for enhanced investigation into this process. Moreover, the power of this memory-driven motor training to rapidly drive motor-control plasticity, in addition to the previously shown effects on memory and spatial cognition, for example [2–5, 39–41], suggests strong involvement of cognitive mechanisms in this process, as codified earlier by the introduction of the "perception-cognition-action loop" concept.

The resulting neural reorganization in this congenitally left-handed individual was correlated with similarly remarkable enhancement in the memory-drawing performance of the non-preferred hand, which post-training resembled the original much better than pre-training, and moreover, significantly better than the experienced preferred hand. This was particularly unexpected because the left hand had several additional advantages. First, the *haptic exploration* of the originals was *always* done with the *left* hand, thus providing a direct perception and encoding of this hand's movements along the lines of that image. In contrast, the non-preferred right hand *never* received any direct encoding of the trajectory but for planning and execution of the drawing trajectory it had to use the memory image developed through the other hand. Second, the nature of the left-hand exploration phase represents a strong form of *dual* memory encoding for that hand. There was no difficulty or delay, however, to successfully use thus acquired memory for guiding drawing with the right hand. It should be noted that, in the drawing phase, the hand under training receives multifaceted, Cognitive-Kinesthetic feedback, which affects the initial haptic memory, corrects and sharpens it, thus adding another layer of enhancement and embodiment to the overall encoding.

An important practical implication of these findings is that the effects of the Cognitive-Kinesthetic Training can generalize over the full "perception-cognition-action loop" involved throughout the process, which suggests its usefulness not only in the domains of spatial cognition and memory rehabilitation but also in motor control rehabilitation as well.

8. Conclusions

This study is the first to show results that contradict the models of the nondominant hand always being controlled by both hemispheres, as had been previously thought. It is particularly remarkable that this brief memory-guided drawing training was able to switch lifelong handedness, overturning almost six decades of dominance of the right hemisphere by inducing profound suppression in the previously dominant hemisphere. In terms of handedness research as a whole, the study suggests a critical role for functional mechanisms, such as inter-hemispheric competition, as opposed to an inherent structural predetermination in hand dominance. The results are consequently of high relevance to the long-standing debate about the sources of hemispheric asymmetry. The unprecedented effect on handedness of the rapid Cognitive-Kinesthetic Drawing Training also implies the powerful potential of this training for further rehabilitation domains, such as the rehabilitation of stroke or trauma affecting hand control.

Acknowledgements

This research was supported by the National Eye Institute at the National Institute of Health (RO1EY024056) and National Science Foundation (NSF/SL-CN: 1640914) awarded to Lora Likova. The author would like to thank Christopher W. Tyler for helpful discussions on the manuscript, Kristyo Mineff for assisting with the drawing training, Spero Nicholas for helping with the functional Magnetic Resonance Imaging (fMRI) data collection, and preprocessing.

Author details

Lora T. Likova

Address all correspondence to: lora@ski.org

Smith-Kettlewell Eye Research Institute, San Francisco, CA, USA

References

[1] Grabowska A, Malgorzata G, Binder M, Forsberg L, Rymarczyk K, Urbanik A. Switching handedness: fMRI study of hand motor control in right-handers, left-handers and converted left-handers. Acta Neurobiologiae Experimentalis. 2012;**2012**(72):439-451

[2] Likova LT. Drawing in the blind and the sighted as a probe of cortical reorganization. In: Proceedings of the IS&T/SPIE Electronic Imaging. International Society for Optics and Photonics; 2010. pp. 752708-752720

[3] Likova LT. Drawing enhances cross-modal memory plasticity in the human brain: A case study in a totally blind adult. Frontiers in Human Neuroscience. 2012;**6**(44):1-15

[4] Likova LT. A cross-modal perspective on the relationships between imagery and working memory. Frontiers in Psychology. 2013;**3**(561):1-14

[5] Likova LT. Learning-based cross-modal plasticity in the human brain: Insights from visual deprivation fMRI. In: Papageorgiou TD, Christopoulos GI, Smirnakis SM, editors. Advanced Brain Neuroimaging Topics in Health and Disease-Methods and Applications. InTech. 2014. In press. pp. 327-358. Ch 13

[6] Likova LT. Temporal evolution of brain reorganization under cross-modal training: Insights into the functional architecture of encoding and retrieval networks. In: IS&T/SPIE Electronic Imaging. International Society for Optics and Photonics; 2015. pp. 939417-939432

[7] Likova LT. Addressing long-standing controversies in conceptual knowledge representation in the temporal pole: A cross-modal paradigm. Imaging Science & Technology. 2017;**2600954**:268-272

[8] Willems RM, Van der Haegen L, Fisher SE, Francks C. On the other hand: Including left-handers in cognitive neuroscience and neurogenetics. Nature, Reviews Neuroscience. 2014;**15**:193-201. DOI: 10.1038/nrn3679

[9] Kim S-G, Ashe J, Hendrich K, Ellermann JM, Merkle H, Ugurbil K, Georgopoulos AP. F unctional magnetic resonance imaging of motor cortex: Hemispheric asymmetry and handedness. Science. 1993;**261**:615-617

[10] Grabowska A, Herman A, Nowicka A, Szatkowska I, Szeląg E. Individual differences in the functional asymmetry of the human brain. Acta Neurobiologiae Experimentalis (Wars). 1994;**54**:155-162

[11] Volkman J, Schnitzler A, Witte OW, Freund H-J. Handedness and asymmetry of hand representation in human motor cortex. Journal of Neurophysiology. 1998;**79**:2149-2154

[12] Solodkin A, Hlustik P, Noll DC, Small SL. Lateralization of motor circuits and handedness during finger movements. European Journal of Neurology. 2001;**8**:425-434

[13] Hlustik P, Solodkin A, Gullapalli RP, Noll DC, Small SL. Functional lateralization of the human premotor cortex during sequential movements. Brain and Cognition. 2002;**49**: 54-62

[14] Verstynen T, Diedrichsen J, Albert N, Aparicio P, Ivry RB. Ipsilateral motor cortex activity during unimanual hand movements relates to task complexity. Journal of Neurophysiology. 2005;**93**:1209-1222

[15] Hervé PY, Mazoyer B, Crivello F, Perchey G, Tzourio-Mazoyer N. Finger tapping, handedness and grey matter amount in the Rolando's genu area. NeuroImage. 2005;**25**:1133-1145

[16] Klöppel S, Mangin JF, Vongerichten A, Frackowiak RS, Siebner HR. Nurture versus nature: Long-term impact of forced right-handedness on structure of pericentral cortex and basal ganglia. The Journal of Neuroscience. 2010;**30**:3271-3275

[17] Wu X, Chen K, Liu Y, Long Z, Wen X, Jin Z, Yao L. Ipsilateral brain deactivation specific to the nondominant hand during simple finger movements. Neuroreport. 2008;**19**:483-486

[18] Rocca MA, Falini A, Comi G, Scotti G, Filippi M. The mirror-neuron system and handedness: A "right" world? Human Brain Mapping. 2008;**29**:1243-1254

[19] Singh LN, Higano S, Takahashi S, Kurihara N, Furuta S, Tamura H, Shimanuki Y, Mugikura S, Fujii T, Yamadori A, Sakamoto M, Yamada S. Comparison of ipsilateral activation between right and left handers: A functional MR imaging study. Neuroreport. 1998;**9**:1861-1866

[20] Carter-Saltzman L. Biological and sociocultural effects on handedness: Comparison between biological and adoptive families. Science. 1980;**209**:1263-1265

[21] Siebner HR, Limmer C, Peinemann A, Drzezga A, Bloem BR, Schwaiger M, Conrad B. Long-term consequences of switching handedness: A positron emission tomography study on handwriting in "converted" lefthanders. The Journal of Neuroscience. 2002;**22**:2816-2825

[22] Annett M. Handedness and Brain Asymmetry. The Right Shift Theory. USA, Canada: Psychology Press, Taylor and Francis Inc.; 2002

[23] Draganski B, Gaser C, Busch V, Schuierer G, Bogdahn U, May A. Neuroplasticity: Changes in grey matter induced by training. Nature. 2004;**427**:311-312

[24] Pascual-Leone A, Amedi A, Fregni F, Merabet LB. The plastic human brain cortex. Annual Review of Neuroscience. 2005;**28**:377-401

[25] Cacciamani L, Likova L. Memory-Guided Drawing Training Increases Granger Causal Influences from the Perirhinal Cortex to V1 in the Blind. Neurobiology of Learning and Memory. Elsevier; 2017;**141**:101-107. DOI: 10.1016/j.nlm.2017.03.013

[26] Likova L, Cacciamani L, Nicholas S, Mineff K. Top-down working memory reorganization of the primary visual cortex: Granger causality analysis. Journal of Vision. 2017; **17**(10):594-594

[27] Tsao DY, Moeller S, Freiwald WA. Comparing face patch systems in macaques and humans. Proceedings of the National Academy of Sciences of the USA. 2008;**105**(49):19514-19519

[28] Kennedy JM. Drawing & the Blind: Pictures to Touch. New Haven: Yale University Press; 1993

[29] Kennedy JM, Juricevic I. Foreshortening, convergence and drawings from a blind adult. Perception. 2006;**35**:847-851

[30] Ponchilla PE. Non-visual sports and arts: Fertile substrates for the growth of knowledge about brain plasticity in people who are blind or have low vision. In: Rieser JJ, editor. Blindness and Brain Plasticity in Navigation and Object Perception. London: Lawrence Erlbaum Associates; 2008

[31] Piaget J, Inhelder B. The Child's Concept of Space. Chicago: Routledge & Paul; 1956

[32] Eliot J, Smith IM. An International Directory of Spatial Tests. Windsor Berkshire: NFER-Nelson; 1983

[33] Del Giudice E, Grossi D, Angelini R, Crisanti AF, Latte F, Fragassi NA, Trojano L. Spatial cognition in children. I. Development of drawing-related (visuospatial and constructional) abilities in preschool and early school years. Brain and Development. 2000;**22**(6):362-367

[34] Likova L, Cacciamani L. Transfer of learning in the blind: Enhancement of spatial-cognitive abilities through drawing. Journal of Visual Impairment & Blindness. (In press)

[35] Dial JG, Chan F, Mezger C, Parker HJ. Comprehensive vocational evaluation system for visually impaired and blind persons. Journal of Visual Impairment & Blindness. 1991;**85**:153-156

[36] Dial J, Mezger C, Gray S, Massey T, Chan F, Hull J. Manual: Comprehensive Vocational Evaluation System. Dallas: McCarron-Dial Systems; 1990

[37] Likova L, Tyler C, Mineff K, Nicholas S. Categorical change mapping: A new approach to investigating neuroplasticity (under submission)

[38] Carbon CC. Bidimensional regression modeling using R. Journal of Statistical Software. 2013;**52** Code Snippet 1. http://www.jstatsoft.org/

[39] Cacciamani L, Likova LT. Memory-guided drawing training increases granger causal influences from the perirhinal cortex to V1 in the blind. Neurobiology of Learning and Memory. 2017;**141**:101-107. DOI: 10.1016/j.nlm.2017.03.013. PMC5589194

[40] Cacciamani LC, Likova LT. Tactile object familiarity in the blind brain reveals the supramodal perceptual-mnemonic nature of the perirhinal cortex. Frontiers in Human Neuroscience. 2016;**10**:92. DOI: 10.3389/fnhum.2016.00092. PMC4828456

[41] Likova LT, Cacciamani L. Transfer of learning in the blind: Enhancement of spatial-cognitive abilities through drawing. Journal of Visual Impairment and Blindness. 2018 (in press)

7

Model Systems to Define Remyelination Therapies

Robert H. Miller, Molly Karl, Reshmi Tognatta,
Ahdeah Pajoohesh-Ganji and Mohammad Abu-Rub

Abstract

Demyelinating diseases of the central nervous system (CNS), such as multiple sclerosis (MS), are characterized by multiple focal *demyelinating* lesions, resulting in various functional deficits. The pathology of MS is defined by local loss of myelin sheaths in the brain and spinal cord associated with infiltration of peripheral immune cells. Classically, MS starts with a series of relapses and remissions, followed several years later by a more progressive form of the disease and a steady functional decline. Although the mechanism of disease initiation is poorly understood, disease progression is associated with immune system activation toward CNS antigens including myelin proteins. Animal models of MS have been critical in the development of MS therapies, with experimental allergic encephalitis (EAE) being the most common. This model has been instrumental in defining the role of T cells in disease progression and in the development of targeted therapies. Understanding the biology of myelin repair has, however, largely come from other model systems including local targeted demyelination in vivo, slice preparations, and in vitro. This has led to the identification of a diverse array of potential new targets to modulate disease progression. Development of these new avenues is the target of intensive ongoing research.

Keywords: remyelination, therapeutics, animal model, multiple sclerosis, oligodendrocytes, astrocytes, experimental allergic encephalitis (EAE)

1. Introduction

Myelin is the fatty insulation that surrounds axons, enhances axonal conduction rates, and protects axons from damage in the nervous system. In the central nervous system (CNS), the majority of myelin is a product of oligodendrocytes, and a single oligodendrocyte may myelinate multiple segments of different axons. During development, oligodendrocytes are generated from precursors (OPCs—oligodendrocyte precursor cells) that arise in specific locations of the brain and spinal cord as a result of local inductive cues (discussed in more detail later). While oligodendrocytes and myelin are found throughout the CNS, the amount of myelin in white matter is substantially greater than that in gray matter. Indeed, the primary reason that white matter appears white is due to its high concentration of lipid-rich myelin. Because myelin plays a central role in modulating neuronal activity, its loss is frequently associated with functional deficits. Myelin loss or demyelination occurs in various different pathological conditions including developmental disorders such as the leukodystrophies, adult-onset insults such as stroke, and classical demyelinating diseases such as multiple sclerosis (MS) and related disorders. MS, the most common CNS demyelinating disease, was originally described over 100 years ago, and initial descriptions of the disease highlighted an illness of increasing functional deficits. Our understanding of the disease course and its progression has advanced over time, and it is now clear that MS is a more complex disorder in terms of clinical presentation and underlying pathogenesis [1–6].

In classic cases, MS initially presents as a sudden-onset neurological deficit that resolves over a period of time. Subsequent attacks (relapses) are followed by periods of remission; however, over time, remission fails to result in a return to normal functionality and deficits slowly accumulate. Following this relapsing-remitting phase (relapsing-remitting MS), the disease enters a more chronic phase in which deficits accumulate in a progressive manner (progressive MS) (**Figure 1**). Not all patients follow this disease trajectory. In a distinct subset of patients, the

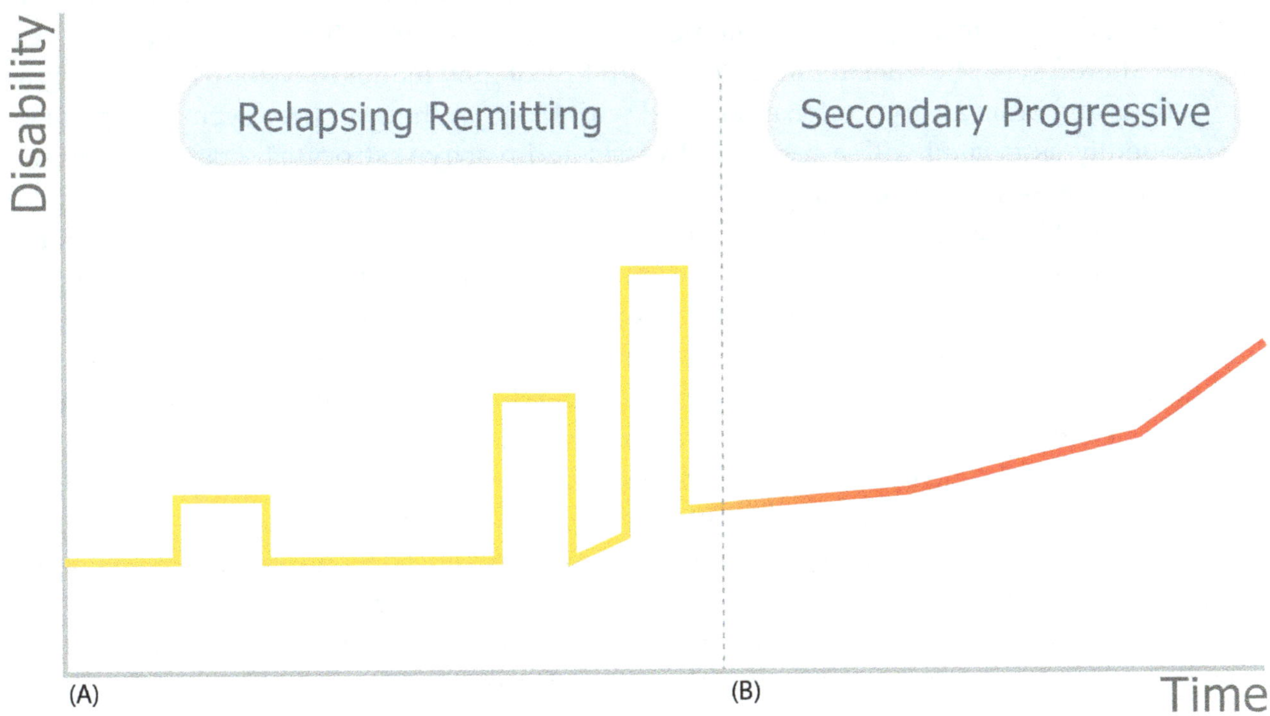

Figure 1. Graph showing typical disease activity in relapsing remitting MS, characterized by defined clinical attacks followed by full functional recovery (A) or incomplete recovery between attacks with residual deficits (B), eventually leading to worsening disability (C).

disease presents initially as progressive functional impairment without obvious remissions—a condition known as primary progressive MS. Alternatively, some patients never progress beyond the relapsing remitting phase, and others only experience a single attack. In MS and numerous MS-related conditions, myelin loss is localized and multiple areas of demyelination or plaques may be present in a single patient. Each of the plaques appears to progress or resolve independently during the progression of the disease.

The variability in presentation and progression makes the accurate diagnosis of MS complicated [6]. This is further compounded by the lack of biomarkers that unambiguously identify MS, and consequently, a diagnosis of MS is dependent on several factors in an overall presentation rather than a single definitive test. Identifying factors include medical history and clinical examination, magnetic resonance imaging (MRI) imaging, and the presence of oligoclonal bands in CSF. While MRI and other imaging modalities are highly effective at identifying lesions in CNS white matter, they are not able to specifically characterize MS-associated demyelinated lesions, and other conditions such as inflammation may generate similar MRI findings. Recent advances in imaging modalities have enhanced the specificity of these approaches for demyelination, and it seems likely that more specific approaches will be implemented in the clinic in the near future. One such approach is using PET imaging to detect areas of myelin loss [7]. The development of selective tracers of myelin that can be visualized in a noninvasive manner is promising; however, the widespread application of this approach is likely to be limited by the short half-life of the probes and the necessity of a local cyclotron for their production.

While generally considered to be a disease of white matter, and myelin in particular, there is now strong data indicating that MS plaques also occur in gray matter, including synapses, and that altered synaptic transmission along with loss of gray matter may contribute to cognitive deficits and brain atrophy often associated with MS [8]. Wherever they occur, MS plaques are frequently associated with a core blood vessel and reactive astrocytes. The close association of blood vessels with MS plaques is indicative of the role of the immune system in the pathogenesis of MS, which is universally recognized as an autoimmune disease. Considerable evidence indicates that T cells that recognize myelin antigens enter the CNS and attack myelin and oligodendrocytes. This inflammatory insult recruits other cells including cells of the innate immune system such as macrophages and microglia that contribute to CNS damage. The majority of existing MS therapies are directed toward either suppressing the immune response or blocking the entry of T cells and other cells of the peripheral immune system into the CNS. While such approaches have been quite effective at modulating the severity and interval of relapses in relapsing remitting MS, it has become clear that they fail to block overall progression of the disease and brain atrophy, and neurodegeneration is only slightly improved. Such observations have led to a concerted effort to identify therapies for MS that are targeted toward promoting myelin repair or inhibiting damage within the CNS but have been somewhat hampered by the lack of understanding of the causes of MS.

The chronic nature of MS and the likelihood that the disease has been ongoing for an extended interval prior to becoming symptomatic make it extremely difficult to identify the initial pathogenic signal. One attractive hypothesis is that a potential trigger for MS is a response to a prior infection or other environmental signal [9]. This notion is supported by the findings that MS patients have elevated immunological responses to various pathogens, which may account for some aspects of the epidemiology of MS. A wide range of pathogens including spirochetes, chlamydia, and a range of viruses have been linked to MS [1]. It seems likely that the role of such pathogens is to enhance susceptibility to MS rather than directly induce disease. One of the strongest links in MS is viral infection [10], and a number of different viruses have been implicated including Epstein-Barr, human herpes virus 6, and human endogenous retroviruses [10–12]. Precisely how the viral infection contributes to MS development has not been clarified, but it may reflect the initial stimulation of immune cells to viral antigens or the induction of oligodendrocyte death as a result of viral infection.

One aspect of MS that has been extensively studied is its genetic linkage [13], and instead of a gain or loss of function of one individual gene, there are a range of genetic associations linked to MS. In particular, MHC class 11 molecules such as HLA-DR and HLA-DQ alleles are considered risk factors for the disease [14]. Given the immunological nature of the disease, the association with immunomodulatory genes is expected; however, the mechanisms by which these genetic changes increase disease susceptibility are still unclear. For example, certain MHC molecules can promote the development of an autoimmune response following a sub-acute challenge from a structurally similar antigen. The contribution of genetic or epigenetic changes in cells of the oligodendrocyte lineage or myelin that contribute to MS susceptibility remains to be clarified.

To understand the biology of MS requires a clear understanding of the cellular and molecular mechanisms that mediate myelination and myelin maintenance, and much of our understanding of the control of myelination comes from studies in development. Oligodendrocytes, the myelinating cells of the CNS [15–18], are generated from precursor cells (OPC or oligodendrocyte precursor cells) that arise in distinct location of the embryonic CNS in response to selective inductive cues and subsequently disperse throughout the CNS [17, 19–21]. The early commitment of neural stem cells to the oligodendrocyte lineage depends on environmental cues that include sonic hedgehog and the subsequent induction of transcriptional signaling pathways that promote the appearance of OPCs, their proliferation, and subsequent migration. One of the major mitogens and potential growth factors that support the expansion of the oligodendrocyte lineage is platelet-derived growth factor alpha (PDGFα). The receptor PDGFαR is expressed predominantly by OPCs in vivo and allows for the unambiguous identification of OPCs in the setting of demyelination and repair. In the spinal cord, OPCs originate at the ventral midline during embryonic development and subsequently disperse widely through gray and white matter. This migration is guided by a number of different signals including Netrin 1 and Wnts and appears to track with the vasculature. Prior to myelination, OPCs differentiate to oligodendrocytes, a process that includes the cessation of proliferation and the induction of additional transcription factors including Myrf that are essential for oligodendrocyte maturation. The differentiation of oligodendrocytes is clearly environmentally regulated. For example, myelin debris has been shown to inhibit the differentiation of oligodendrocytes and may be an important factor in the control of remyelination where delayed myelin clearance may inhibit repair [22, 23]. Once oligodendrocytes mature, there is a defined time window during which they extend multiple processes to contact adjacent axons and initiate myelination. Less is known about the molecular interactions that orchestrate the initiation of myelination. Several parameters such as axonal size and electrical activity have been implicated as important in the early stages of myelination. In addition, several factors have been suggested to inhibit the onset of myelination, and these include LINGO-1 and the expression of PSA-NCAM on axonal surfaces. Following differentiation and maturation, oligodendrocytes begin to generate myelin sheaths. An individual oligodendrocyte initially generates an excess number of myelin sheaths, some of which grow and are stabilized, while others shrink and are subsequently lost. What regulates the growth and retraction of myelin sheaths is not well understood, but recent studies suggest that it may be regulated by axonal activity.

Myelin is a specialized plasma membrane that provides a fatty insulation around axons and allows the rapid conduction of electrical impulses by increasing conduction velocity, reducing the threshold for firing, and providing axonal protection [24]. Myelin sheaths are discontinuous and are linked by Nodes of Ranvier (**Figure 2**) that have a characteristic morphology and are areas of high concentration of ion channels that support electrical impulse propagation. Nodes of Ranvier appear to be particularly sensitive to damage, and their disruption results in perturbation of axonal conduction. The region between two nodes is known as the internode, and it is made up of a number of specific proteins [25], including the major proteins myelin basic protein (MBP) and proteolipid protein (PLP) as well as other minor proteins such as myelin-associated glycoprotein (MAG), myelin oligodendrocyte protein (MOG), 2′3′ cyclic nucleotide 3′phosphdiesterase (CNP), and myelin-associated oligodendrocyte basic protein (MOBP) [26].

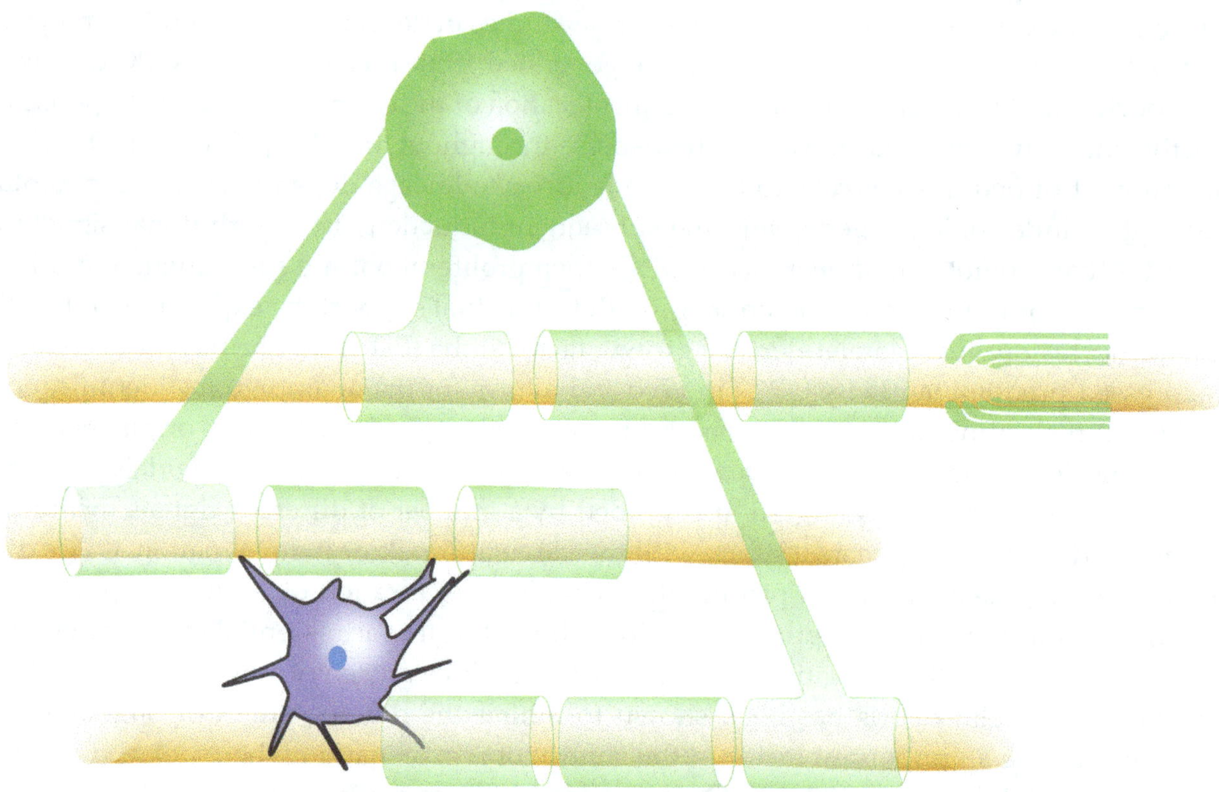

Figure 2. CNS myelin. Schematic representation of an oligodendrocyte ensheathing several axons in the CNS. Segments of myelin sheaths are separated by Nodes of Ranvier, which are contacted by astrocyte foot processes.

Each of these myelin components is presumably important for normal myelin function. For example, MBP mutant animals such as *shiverer* fail to form compact myelin and have limited life span [27], while animals lacking PLP develop normally but manifest axonal pathology later in life [28, 29].

The normal development of myelin is also dependent on additional CNS cell types: axonal processes are targets for myelination, and astrocytes are important in the development and survival of cells of the oligodendrocyte lineage [30]. Astrocytes are a heterogeneous cell population that have been proposed to perform multiple functions that support development and maintenance of the brain and spinal cord. During development, astrocytes guide the migration of neurons from their germinal zones to their final destination [31] and act as substrates for long-distance axonal growth to their targets. In the adult, astrocytes are important for the removal of neurotransmitters, control of the ionic environment, and maintenance of the blood-brain barrier as well as either supporting or inhibiting regeneration through the formation of glial scars [32–34] that are comprised of astrocyte processes and extracellular matrix. A similar glial scar is formed around chronic demyelinating lesions and has been suggested to block myelin repair [35], although recent studies indicate that the astrocyte response is beneficial in certain animal models.

Histological studies provide an evidence of neuronal damage in MS, including axonal loss in areas of demyelination [29, 36] or even frank brain atrophy due to widespread loss of neuronal cell bodies and their axons [37]. It is unclear whether the axonal loss is secondary to myelin loss or independent of it via direct antigenic targeting. The role of astrocytes in MS disease pathogenesis is less well defined. For example, in areas of demyelination, a reactive astrocytic response is commonly characterized by elevated expression of glial fibrillary acidic protein (GFAP) that may be either protective or pathogenic [38]. Disruption of the blood-brain barrier is also important in the formation of demyelinating lesions in MS, and astrocytes have been proposed to play an important role in the maintenance of the blood-brain barrier in the adult CNS. The best evidence for an astrocytic role in demyelination comes from the studies of the MS variant known as neuromyelitis optica (NMO) that preferentially presents in the optic nerve and spinal cord. In a significant subset of NMO patients, demyelination is thought to result from the binding of pathogenic antibodies against aquaporin 4, a molecule expressed on the end feet of astrocytes around blood vessels. Antibody binding results in astrocyte death and subsequent demyelination, although the molecular linkages in this cascade are unknown.

The cellular complexity and heterogeneity of MS-like diseases represent a significant challenge in developing effective animal models that accurately mimic disease progression, and this has led to the generation of a number of different models, each of which highlights distinct components of the disease [39]. Some of the most powerful and best-studied models of MS are those that utilize selective stimulation of the peripheral immune system as the major driver of CNS pathogenesis, and these are discussed in more detail later.

2. Animal models of demyelinating diseases: strengths and weaknesses

2.1. Immunological models for CNS demyelination

Multiple sclerosis is characterized by the engagement of the immune system, and this has been primarily modeled through approaches collectively known as experimental allergic encephalitis (EAE) [40, 41]. In general, EAE is an inflammation-mediated demyelinating disease that is induced in host animals through immunization with CNS tissue resulting in a host of functional deficits that correlate with immune cell infiltration into the CNS. The functional deficit is then scored on a 1–5 scale: 1 presents with a flaccid tail, 2 with hindlimb weakness, 3 with hindlimb paralysis, 4 with forelimb and hindlimb paralysis, and 5 death. In most studies, the scale is expanded to between 2.5 and 3.5, allowing for better definition of functional changes.

Initial development of EAE involved injection of spinal cord homogenates into rabbits resulting in hindlimb paralysis and other functional deficits. Subsequently, immunization of monkeys with spinal cord homogenate derived from rabbit CNS [42] showed the pathological accumulation of cells around blood vessels of the brain and spinal cord. Variability in individual animal responses limited initial studies; however, this has largely been resolved through the use of immune stimulants such as complete Freund's adjuvant (CFA) combined with pertussis toxin. This model has been refined through identification of effective protein antigens. These antigens are predominantly myelin-associated proteins including myelin basic protein (MBP), myelin-oligodendrocyte glycoprotein (MOG), and proteolipid protein (PLP) [41]. Minor myelin components are also capable of generating disease suggesting that most myelin components can act as effective priming antigens. The identification of specific myelin protein peptides that provoke a reproducible and consistent disease following immunization into genetically defined host populations has resulted in several major models of EAE that are now commonly used. These include the induction of EAE in the *SJL* mouse genotype following immunization with the $PLP_{139\text{-}151}$ peptide, which generates a relapsing remitting disease mimicking some characteristics of relapsing remitting MS. An alternative model utilizes C57/Bl6 mice immunized with the MOG $peptide_{35\text{-}55}$. This model is often used to recapitulate more advanced stages of MS because it generates a more chronic disease course. Other less common models include the induction of EAE in PL/J mice following immunization with MBP or MOBP and immunization of Biozzi ABH mice with MOG protein that models selective aspects of MS.

Several major themes have emerged from studies on the mechanisms of disease in murine EAE. One common finding is a primary role for T cells in disease development. Adoptive transfer clearly demonstrated that T cells specific for MBP antigen were capable of transferring disease to naïve hosts [43]. The functional deficits in this model were transient, resolving within 1–2 weeks, and were not characterized by extensive demyelination suggesting the pathology in MS reflects multiple pathogenic processes. One strong candidate that contributes to EAE and MS pathology is B cells [44]. B cells play multiple roles in immune-mediated pathology in the CNS. On the one hand, they facilitate activation and expansion of T cell populations within the CNS and enhance the recruitment of other immune cells into the CNS.

On the other hand, B cells produce antibodies directed against the different myelin antigens. For example, some MS lesions are characterized by an overexpression of anti-myelin antibodies, with MOG as a potential antigenic target [45]. Understanding the roles of B cells in the underlying pathogenesis of MS and other neuro-inflammatory diseases now seems to be at the forefront of research development after demonstrating that two B-cell inhibitors, Rituximab and Ocrelizumab, were shown to be highly effective in some MS patients, including those with primary progressive MS [46–48].

The role of the innate immune system in demyelinating pathologies is also an area of current focus. Microglial cells are also known to undergo reactive changes, whereby they aid in myelin clearance, but also could potentially participate in antigen presentation along with dendritic cells. One hypothesis is that pathological mechanisms vary by the stage of disease. Relapsing remitting disease, for example, may be largely driven by influx from the peripheral adaptive immune cells, whereas secondary and primary progressive forms of the disease are largely driven by the innate immune system.

Myelin components are not the only antigenic targets in MS. For example, axon-specific proteins, such as the neurofilament triplet, and node of Ranvier components, such as Contactin/TAG-1 and S100, have also been associated with EAE and MS [49]. It is unclear, however, whether the aforementioned proteins are primary disease targets or their involvement is secondary to myelin loss. It is likely, however, that as the disease progresses, the ongoing destruction of neural tissue expands the pathological basis of the disease resulting in more widespread damage and worsening functional deficits.

EAE models have been invaluable in elucidating critical aspects of MS biology and other demyelinating CNS diseases and have been reviewed in detail [40, 41]. One of the major advantages is that EAE utilizes well-defined antigenic targets and can be adaptable to numerous genetic animal models. This has allowed the identification of several well-defined networks resulting in T cell activation and trafficking, as well as shed light into the role of T cell subsets in disease progression. What is important is that these disease models still serve as primary tools not only for disease modeling but also for validating and identifying new therapeutic targets.

Another aspect of MS pathology that has started to gain ground is the effect on long-term synaptic plasticity, which is the physiological mechanism responsible for learning and memory and also is a key determinant of clinical recovery after cortical injury. It has now become clear that MS is frequently associated with cognitive and behavioral changes, which have been detected in the early stages of the disease, and are certainly more common than previously thought [50]. These changes are likely the result of synaptic impairment or altered synaptic plasticity. Among the different brain regions, the hippocampus is the most vulnerable. Despite its obvious importance, very few studies have been directed at understanding the hippocampal synaptic plasticity after EAE and not all are in agreement with what effect EAE has on hippocampal long-term synaptic plasticity. There is, however, sufficient evidence to indicate that activated microglia are responsible, and that changes in synaptic plasticity are rather dynamic, effectively mirroring the stages of the disease and severity of inflammation. Along those lines, it has also been suggested that enhanced cortical plasticity is predictive of functional recovery after a relapse [51].

An important variant of immune-mediated models of demyelination is the generation of local rather than systemic lesions [52]. This has been achieved by sensitizing host animals with subthreshold levels of encephalogenic peptides and subsequently delivering a local injection of a pro-inflammatory cytokine to stimulate local demyelination. For example, injection of $_{1-125}$MOG peptide and incomplete Freund's adjuvant into Lewis rats results in an immune response but no overt clinical symptoms. Subsequent local injection of tumor necrosis factor alpha (TNF-α) or interferon-gamma (INF-γ) results in localized infiltration of immune cells, local demyelination, and axonal damage. Such studies revealed a rapid local functional deficit reflecting immune-mediated damage. This was followed by some functional recovery, although axonal damage remained. There are several strengths to this model including the ability to assess long-term consequences of a localized immune response and the capability to develop novel therapies to modulate initial immunological insult and promote long-term functional recovery. Such a model has several weaknesses including the localized nature of the insult and the method of induction of inflammatory stimuli. Local injection of cytokines results in damage to the blood-brain barrier and the stimulation of a robust astroglial response making mechanistic interpretation of the outcome of these studies difficult. There are a number of important differences between MS and EAE. EAE is generated through injection of selected antigens, while the trigger for MS is unclear. To date, there has been no description of a spontaneously occurring form of MS in animals. Second, the inclusion of unrelated antigens when inducing EAE has led to developing disease mechanisms and therapies that have otherwise failed clinical trials

Many of the current therapies used in the treatment of MS have emerged from studies of EAE, and it is not surprising that they are targeted toward regulation of immune cell responses. Such recent treatments include Fingolimod (FTY720) directed against the sphingosine-1-phosphate receptor that regulates T and B cell responses appears to directly stimulate remyelination in the CNS [53, 54], and Natalizumab directed toward adhesion molecules on lymphocytes blocks the entrance of those cells in the parenchyma of the CNS [55]. Such therapies, while modulating relapse activity, have generated unexpected side effects in the setting of clinical applications that have in certain cases limited their utilization. Furthermore, long-term studies suggest that while such therapies are effective at modulating inflammatory responses, they are less effective at controlling the disease activity or promoting recovery in the CNS. Current studies are becoming increasingly focused on developing approaches to promote myelin repair in the CNS, and EAE is not particularly suited to identification of repair mechanism.

2.2. Demyelination induced by gliotoxins

One of the major drawbacks of the aforementioned immune-mediated models of demyelination is that both pathological and repair processes occur simultaneously, which complicates the interpretation of potential repair strategies. To define the pathways mediating myelin repair, a variety of alternative models are available, and these include both focal and systemic glial toxin treatments. These models, while they do not recapitulate the complex etiology and pathogenesis of MS, have two major strengths. First, the onset of the insult can be tightly regulated in time and space; second, the epochs of demyelination and remyelination are largely separate, allowing for the characterization of molecular cues regulating each aspect of lesion generation and repair.

The most common model utilizes the generation of focal areas of demyelination induced by direct injection of chemicals that selectively ablate oligodendrocytes and their myelin. Many different demyelinating agents have been used, although the most common include lysolecithin, ethidium bromide, and antibodies against the major sphingolipid component of myelin, galactocerebroside.

Lysolecithin (L-α-Lysophosphatidylcholine or LPC) when injected into white matter as a 1% solution induces focal demyelination [56, 57]. Common locations for LPC-induced lesions include spinal cord white matter, the midline of the corpus callosum, and caudal cerebellar peduncle. Injection of LPC results in a rapid loss of myelin and oligodendrocytes. Compared to other models, LPC lacks absolute cellular specificity, and there is a reduction in astrocytes and some axonal loss in the lesion. One powerful feature of LPC lesions is their ability to recover. In general, demyelination occurs rapidly, and the lesion area is largely devoid of myelin 2–3 days after lesion generation. Oligodendrocyte precursor cells repopulate the lesion sites around 5 days and subsequently proliferate and differentiate into oligodendrocytes, with remyelination taking place between 7 and 14 days in rodents on average. The latter varies with the lesion site and animal age. By 30 days post-lesion, remyelination is essentially complete (**Figure 3**). These observations have led to the identification of several distinct molecular mechanisms, such as Notch and Wnt pathways, retinoid X receptor gamma signaling, growth factors such as hepatocyte growth factor and neuregulin, hormones including progesterone, cell cycle proteins such as cyclin-dependent kinases, chemokine receptors such as CXCR2, the NOGO receptor LINGO-1, and death receptor 6 (DR6) signaling. In white matter tracts containing large-caliber axons, the remyelinated axons have thinner myelin sheaths than the originals (**Figure 3**).

An alternative glial toxin, ethidium bromide results in cell loss due to its DNA-intercalating properties; therefore, all nucleated cells are affected in this model. Ethidium bromide is injected directly into white matter tracts, and the lesions tend to be larger than LPC lesions and have been utilized to assay the effects of age, sex, growth factors, and the role of microglia/macrophage activation on remyelination. As expected, ethidium bromide injections cause a more widespread loss of astrocytes, oligodendrocytes, and OPCs while sparing axons. This is followed by the influx of macrophages in and around the lesion and the development of reactive astrocytosis, which aims to seal off the lesion site [58]. In contrast to LPC-induced lesions, a significant amount of remyelination in ethidium bromide-induced lesions in the spinal cord is accomplished by Schwann cells. It was initially assumed that such Schwann cells were derived from peripheral nerves or spinal nerve roots adjacent to the lesion; however, fate mapping studies suggest that OPCs generate Schwann cells in the absence of astrocytes [59] raising the possibility that astrocyte regulate the fate of OPCs. Given the more widespread loss of neural cells, ethidium bromide lesions are less commonly used for the identification of remyelinating therapies.

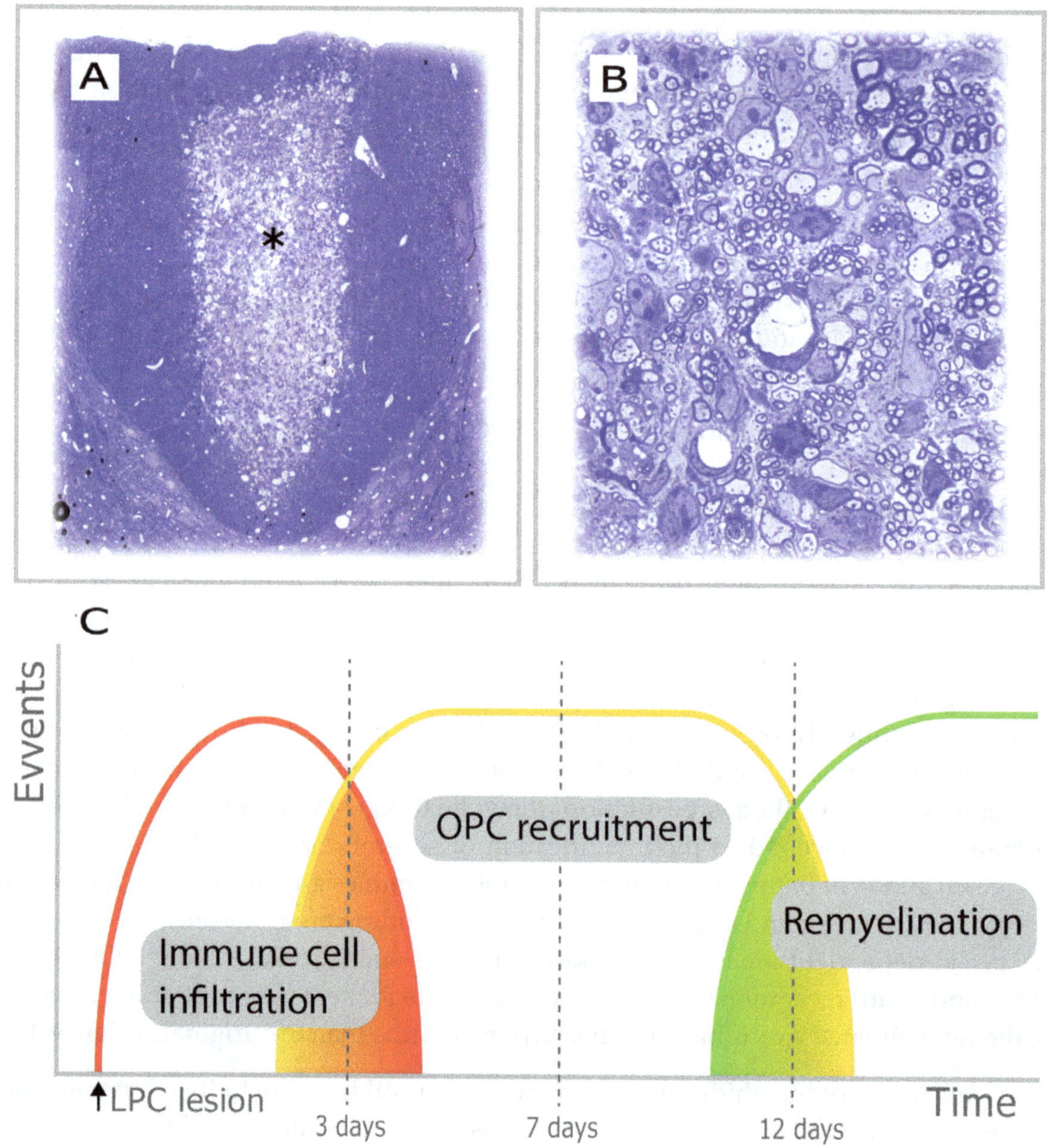

Figure 3. A) Representative image of dorsal spinal column cross section, stained with Toluidine blue, showing an LPC-induced demyelinating lesions denoted by the asterisk. B) Representative high magnification image of an LPC lesion during remyelination. C) Graph depicting typical disease progression in a characteristic LPC lesion; including immune cell infiltra-tion around 3 days, followed by OPC recruitment peaking at 7 days, and then the onset of remyleination at apporximately 12 days post injection.

To provide enhanced cellular specificity, cell type-specific surface antibodies have been used to target the complement cascade and induce selective cell lysis [60]. This model has been effective using antibodies to galactocerebroside (GalC), the major myelin sphingolipid to eliminate mature oligodendrocytes. Initial studies demonstrated that a single intraspinal injection of complement proteins plus anti-GalC resulted in demyelination and partial loss of oligodendrocytes. Analysis of the mechanism of myelin repair suggested that it was the result of recruitment of OPCs and not Schwann cells or mature oligodendrocytes [61].

A major strength of the local toxin models is that they provide a localized region of reproducible synchronized demyelination allowing for analysis of remyelination in the absence of concurrent demyelination. The timing of remyelination differs between the models, although all undergo spontaneous repair. Another advantage of using these models is their adaptability; lesions can be generated in animals of any age, at any accessible location, and from different genetic backgrounds. The disadvantage is that the mechanism of cell death is non-physiologic, and so whether this truly models naturally occurring lesion development, disease progression, and clinical phenotype is unclear. One particular aspect where these models have proven beneficial is the development of myelin-promoting therapies, as opposed to those modulating immune responses. For example, using an LPC-induced demyelination model, LINGO-1 was identified as a potential therapeutic target, whereby anti-LINGO-1 antibodies promoted OPC differentiation and subsequent remyelination [62, 63].

LINGO-1 knockout mice show precocious myelination, suggesting that LINGO-1 antagonists might be useful to accelerate myelin repair. Using both the LPC and cuprizone models (see below) of demyelination, anti-LINGO-1 antibody treatments significantly increase the speed of remyelination, suggesting a new therapeutic option for MS patients. The anti-LINGO-1 Li81 antibody is the first MS therapy directly targeting remyelination and is currently in MS clinical trials.

A second commonly used approach for glial toxin-induced demyelination is systemic oral delivery of toxins that preferentially target oligodendrocytes. Systemic delivery of a glial toxin in a noninvasive manner has a number of advantages. For example, it overcomes the complexity associated with direct injections into the CNS and provides a larger demyelinating area allowing for easier molecular analysis. The most frequently utilized systemic toxin is cuprizone.

Ingestion of the copper chelator cuprizone (biscyclohexanone oxaldihydrazone) results in demyelination of specific brain regions, which is thought to reflect mitochondrial stress and an innate immune response [64]. Cuprizone-induced demyelination results from loss of oligodendrocytes rather than direct insults to myelin sheaths, and mice aged 6–9 weeks given 0.2–0.3% cuprizone treatment of for 5–6 weeks develop acute demyelination of the corpus callosum and other rostral white matter regions. Interestingly, the spinal cord is less susceptible, which could be in part due to a differential sensitivity by spinal oligodendrocytes to cuprizone, and/or nonuniform penetration in different CNS tissues. Oligodendrocyte apoptosis is also associated with extensive reactive astrogliosis and microglial activation. Acute demyelination is followed by spontaneous remyelination that occurs following removal of cuprizone from the diet. When cuprizone treatment is prolonged to 12 weeks or longer, remyelination is very sparse, resulting in a model of chronic demyelination.

The extended time course of disease induction and repair makes the cuprizone model useful for studying the biological processes related to both demyelination and remyelination in the CNS. The cuprizone model has been extensively used to examine the potential of various compounds to stimulate myelin repair [65, 66]. Because the time course of cuprizone treatment is so long, demyelination is progressive and remyelination begins while demyelination is still taking place. Combining cuprizone with rapamycin, which blocks mTor signaling, decreases the efficiency of remyelination, making it easier to analyze and quantify repair processes. The cuprizone model is easier to use compared to other models in that the toxin is included in regular mouse chow that is fed to the animals each day. There are, however, a number of concerns with this model. First, cuprizone is generally limited to mice, and there is a clear genetic linkage to the susceptibility for cuprizone toxicity. Likewise, there are differences in susceptibility between gender and age that are poorly understood [67]; however, proof-of-principle studies demonstrate that signals known from in vitro studies to stimulate oligodendrocyte differentiation such as thyroid hormone (T3) promote remyelination in the cuprizone model, making it useful for therapeutic discovery.

2.3. Cell death models of demyelination

A number of studies have begun to suggest that demyelination may be a primary result of oligodendrocyte death, with activation of the immune system as a secondary event. Whether in the complex setting of disease damage to oligodendrocytes is direct or indirect likely depends on the immediate pathological conditions. An alternative cellular target that may trigger oligodendrocyte damage and demyelination is myelinated axons. Axonal damage and loss are frequently seen in MS lesions [36] and models of immune-mediated demyelination, although it is unclear whether axonal degeneration follows myelin loss or whether demyelination is a consequence of axonal degeneration. To distinguish between these possibilities, animal models in which oligodendrocytes are directly targeted for cell death are being developed to assess whether the loss of oligodendrocytes results in demyelination, how effectively and rapidly remyelination occurs, and whether localized demyelination results in axonal damage. Information from such studies will help define new mechanisms of CNS pathology and novel targets for therapeutic intervention. Currently, there are three major ways for selectively inducing oligodendrocyte cell death in the adult vertebrate CNS.

One approach to drive selective death of neural cells involves the selective expression of a toxic molecule targeted to specific cell types [68]. For example, extensive loss of oligodendrocytes has been achieved through the targeted expression of the alpha subunit of the diphtheria toxin (DT). Diphtheria toxin (DT) is composed of two subunits (alpha and beta), each having different functions. The beta subunit interacts with cell receptors to facilitate the entry of the toxin into the cell, whereas the alpha subunit is the cytotoxic component that acts intracellularly.

The cytotoxicity of DT results from inhibition of protein translation and cell death. In the absence of its beta subunit, DT is unable to penetrate cells, limiting the nonspecific induction of cell death in neighboring cells. Targeting the expression of the DT to oligodendrocytes is achieved using Cre/LoxP technology using a major myelin protein promoter, and its activation is through tamoxifen-induced removal of transcriptional stop sequences resulting in death of oligodendrocytes. One interesting finding from these studies is that extensive loss of oligodendrocyte cell bodies is not correlated with rapid myelin loss. After a post-treatment delay of approximately 3 weeks, the mice displayed progressive motor deficits associated with significant myelin degradation and vacuolization. A second unexpected outcome of these studies was that the widespread loss of oligodendrocytes did not trigger a rapid immune response.

While remyelination was extensive, and the animals appeared to recover completely with longer survival times, recovery was compromised and there was an infiltration of T cells into the CNS. Adoptive transplantation of these T cells into naïve hosts was sufficient to transfer disease. It is likely that the initial insult served to prime the immune system, which eventually led to an autoimmune response and subsequent CNS demyelination [69].

The DT model also differs from MS in a number of key ways. As discussed above, MS is a spontaneous disease, and the lesions develop in a variable manner in both time and space. MS is also not toxin-induced, although there might be a role for pathogens in initial disease stages. The cell death model, on the other hand, depends on the use of a toxin that effectively terminates protein translation, causing cell ablation, and subsequent recruitment of phagocytic cells. Another key difference between the two is that the clearance of myelin in MS following oligodendrocyte loss is rather rapid and is driven by both resident and peripheral immune cells. In contrast, myelin clearance is clearly delayed in the DT model, which would indicate that it is either inhibited or nonexistent. A major concern for the DT model is the complete nature of oligodendrocyte loss, which differs significantly from the focal loss of oligodendrocytes in MS.

In a related model, the specificity of the toxic insult is targeted through receptor expression in a null background [70]. For example, expression of the DT receptor (DTR) under the control of an oligodendrocyte-specific promoter results in cell type sensitivity to diphtheria toxin. Exposure to DT results in the induction of cell death by inhibiting protein synthesis. The clinical phenotype includes ataxia, limb paralysis, and tail spasticity that appear around 10 days post-injection and progressively develop. Perturbations in somatosensory evoked potentials together with histological markers of neurodegeneration, and abnormal Nodes of Ranvier indicate dysfunctional neural networks. The pathology differs between the models; while the DT mice display severe demyelination, the DTR mice show little demyelination. This may reflect that in the DTR model, there is a more extensive engagement of axonal damage leading to death before demyelination develops.

A potential strength of the DTR model is that it may provide a model system to examine the mechanisms and develop targeted therapies against axonal damage in demyelinating diseases since axonopathy is a frequent pathological finding in MS.

During CNS development, many cell types including oligodendrocytes are produced in excess and the additional cells are eliminated through apoptosis-mediated cell death. Cell type-specific induction of apoptosis through activation of an inducible caspase 9 construct driven off a selective promoter has been used to specifically eliminate lymphocytes and oligodendrocytes [71]. Induction of oligodendrocyte apoptosis in the adult CNS results in rapid demyelination and local activation of microglia in the absence of T cell infiltration [72, 73]. During development, activation of oligodendrocyte apoptosis in the first postnatal week inhibits myelination, which subsequently recovers but has increased susceptibility to adult insults [72]. The role of oligodendrocyte apoptosis in early stages of MS is not well defined; however, apoptotic oligodendrocytes have been reported in the early lesions [74], suggesting this may contribute to MS plaque formation. Similarly, activated microglia but an absence of peripheral immune cells has been described in some early lesions.

Overall, while models of selective oligodendrocyte death have provided important insights into the response of the neural cells and the pathway of myelin loss, they have not yet been used to identify new pathways of pathology or illuminate new targets for therapeutic interventions. Whether they will provide a useful platform for the development of therapies for distinct subsets of MS awaits further refinement and analysis.

2.4. In vitro discovery platforms for therapeutic development

Over the past decade, there has been significant development of new platforms for remyelination drug discovery. These include the use of isolated purified cell preparations, rodent IPS cells that provide an unlimited supply of cells, human cell line-derived neural cells, human IPS cells, and in silico model systems. Each of these platforms has its own advantages and disadvantages. In general, such in vitro approaches have been relatively powerful in identifying pathways that regulate myelin formation from mature oligodendrocytes but have been less effective at identifying signaling pathways that regulate the proliferation and survival of oligodendrocytes and their precursors.

With the development of culture models for CNS neural cells and the ability to unambiguously identify distinct cell populations, the ability to identify molecular signaling that promoted the development of oligodendrocytes was feasible. Early studies utilized mixed cultures derived from either white matter such as the optic nerve, mixed gray and white matter such as the spinal cord or predominantly grey matter such as cerebral cortex. Addition of selected growth factors or other signaling molecules that resulted in an increase in mature oligodendrocytes was considered potential therapy. There are two major concerns with this approach. First, the cellular target(s) of the added molecules is unclear, since the culture contains not only cells of the oligodendrocyte lineage but also astrocytes, neurons, and innate immune cells of the CNS, any of which might mediate the response. The second concern is that increased numbers of mature oligodendrocyte may result from either enhanced progenitor proliferation, reduced cell death, or increased cell differentiation, and distinguishing between these mechanisms has proven challenging. To refine the cellular target(s) of potential therapeutics, purified cell cultures have been utilized. Purification of rodent or murine OPCs either through differential antibody binding (panning) or FACS sorting allows for assessment of the direct response of the cell population to therapeutic exposure. Such approaches have been used recently to identify signaling mechanisms that promote the appearance of mature oligodendrocytes [75–78]. One concept that has gained significant support in recent years is the notion that the rate-limiting step in remyelination is the differentiation and maturation of oligodendrocytes to myelinating cells. Several more refined approaches have been developed to identify factors that directly regulate oligodendrocyte maturation. These include the use of purified OPCs initially derived from human material. The emergence of IPS technology combined with identification of molecular environments that promote the survival of human cells has facilitated the identification of several small molecules that mediate oligodendrocyte maturation such as retinoic receptors, benztropine and miconazole. In the majority of such screens, the readout has been enhanced by expression of myelin proteins such as MBP. While this has proven useful, the ultimate goal of remyelinating therapies is the generation of new myelin. Recent studies have used a biophysical approach to identify signals that promote the formation of myelin on artificial substrates. When grown in the presence of inert fibers of the appropriate dimensions, oligodendrocytes will begin to enwrap them as if they were immature axons. Molecules that enhance that process are considered strong candidate to promote remyelination in the CNS, and molecules including Clemastine an anti-histamine drug have been identified in similar assays.

While the reductionist approaches provide important insights into isolated cellular responses of the oligodendrocyte lineage, they lack any physiological setting. As a result, it is unclear whether signals that modulate oligodendrocyte maturation in isolation will promote myelin repair in the developing or diseased CNS. One model to address this concern is the use of slice cultures. Slices of the CNS grown on the air/medium interface develop robust myelination. The most successful slices are those derived from cerebellum and coronal sections through the corpus callosum. Treatment of such slices with LPC results in rapid demyelination and allows for analysis of drug-induced repair in an efficient and physiological environment. In most studies, multiple different models are used to determine the efficacy individual compounds to promote remyelination.

3. Conclusions and comments

There is a broad range of animal models that address distinct aspects of multiple sclerosis and other demyelinating diseases. Each of the models has specific strengths and weaknesses in furthering our understanding of the pathogenic processes that mediate demyelination and in identifying new opportunities for the effective promotion of myelin repair. EAE models have led to the development of many therapeutic targets aimed at halting disease progression. More recently, other models such as those targeting oligodendrocyte cell death have been instrumental in fine-tuning our understanding of the pathology of demyelination/remyelination in MS and other similar diseases. Each of the model systems discussed in this review deserves particular credit, as it has helped solve a different piece of the puzzle. For example, while EAE models have unraveled many of the immunological bases of the CNS demyelination, particularly the role of T cells in MS, the use of glial toxins such as LPC or ethidium bromide has emerged as extremely useful in reshaping our understanding of the environmental and cell-based mechanisms of remyelination, and the models of oligodendrocyte death provide insights into factors driving the pathology. It seems likely that new models will be forthcoming that more effectively address the role of cells other than those of the immune and oligodendrocyte lineage. Understanding the role of microglia and astrocytes, as well as further clarity around the mechanism of vascular components in disease progression, will allow new therapeutic avenues to be developed in future studies.

Acknowledgements

This work was supported by NIH grant NS 30800 to R.H. Miller.

Author details

Robert H. Miller[1*], Molly Karl[1], Reshmi Tognatta[2], Ahdeah Pajoohesh-Ganji[1] and Mohammad Abu-Rub[1]

*Address all correspondence to: rhm3@gwu.edu

1 School of Medicine and Health Sciences, George Washington University, Washington, DC, USA

2 Gladstone Institute, San Francisco, CA, USA

References

[1] Joy JE, Johnston Jr RB. Multiple Sclerosis: Current Status and Strategies for the Future. Washington DC: National Academy Press; 2001

[2] Lassmann H, Bruck W, Lucchinetti C. Heterogeneity of multiple sclerosis pathogenesis: Implications for diagnosis and therapy. Trends in Molecular Medicine. 2001;**7**(3):115-121

[3] Lublin FD, Reingold SC. Defining the clinical course of multiple sclerosis: Results of an international survey. National Multiple Sclerosis Society (USA) Advisory Committee on Clinical Trials of New Agents in Multiple Sclerosis. Neurology. 1996;**46**(4):907-911

[4] Lucchinetti C, Bruck W, Parisi J, Scheithauer B, Rodriguez M, Lassmann H. Heterogeneity of multiple sclerosis lesions: implications for the pathogenesis of demyelination. Annals of Neurology. 2000;**47**(6):707-717

[5] Moore GRW. Neuropathology and Pathophysiology of the Multiple Sclerosis Lesion. Philadelphia: F.A. Davis Company; 1998

[6] Poser CM, Paty DW, Scheinberg L, McDonald WI, Davis FA, Ebers GC, Johnson KP, Sibley WA, Silberberg DH, Tourtellotte WW. New diagnostic criteria for multiple sclerosis: Guidelines for research protocols. Annals of Neurology. 1983;**13**(3):227-231

[7] Wang Y, Wu C, Caprariello AV, Somoza E, Zhu W, Wang C, Miller RH. In vivo quantification of myelin changes in the vertebrate nervous system. The Journal of Neuroscience. 2009;**29**(46):14663-14669

[8] Grothe M, Lotze M, Langner S, Dressel A. The role of global and regional gray matter volume decrease in multiple sclerosis. Journal of Neurology. 2016;**263**(6):1137-1145

[9] Correale J, Gaitan MI. Multiple sclerosis and environmental factors: the role of vitamin D, parasites, and Epstein-Barr virus infection. Acta Neurologica Scandinavica. 2015;**132**(199):46-55

[10] Kakalacheva K, Munz C, Lunemann JD. Viral triggers of multiple sclerosis. Biochimica et Biophysica Acta. 2011;**1812**(2):132-140

[11] Das Sarma J. A mechanism of virus-induced demyelination. Interdisciplinary Perspectives on Infectious Diseases. 2010;**2010**:109239

[12] Tselis A. Evidence for viral etiology of multiple sclerosis. Seminars in Neurology. 2011;**31**(3):307-316

[13] Oksenberg JR, Seboun E, Hauser SL. Genetics of demyelinating diseases. Brain Pathology. 1996;**6**(3):289-302

[14] Gourraud PA, Harbo HF, Hauser SL, Baranzini SE. The genetics of multiple sclerosis: an up-to-date review. Immunological Reviews. 2012;**248**(1):87-103

[15] Bunge MP, Bunge RP, Pappas GD. Electron microscopic demonstrations of connections between glia and myelin sheaths in the developing mammalian central nervous system. The Journal of Cell Biology. 1962;**12**:448-453

[16] Bunge RP. Glial cells and the central myelin sheath. Physiological Reviews. 1968;**48**: 197-251

[17] Miller RH. Regulation of oligodendrocyte development in the vertebrate CNS. Progress in Neurobiology. 2002;**67**:451-467

[18] Raine CS. Morphological aspects of myelin and myelination. In: Morell P, editor. Myelin. New York and London: Plenum Press; 1977. pp. 1-49

[19] Ono K, Yasui Y, Rutishauser U, Miller RH. Focal ventricular origin and migration of oligodendrocyte precursors into the chick optic nerve. Neuron. 1997;**19**:1-20

[20] Pringle NP, Richardson WD. A singularity of PDGF alpha-receptor expression in the dorsoventral axis of the neural tube may define the origin of the oligodendrocyte lineage. Development. 1993;**117**(2):525-533

[21] Rowitch D. Glial specification in the vertebrate neural tube. Nature Reviews Neuroscience. 2004;**5**:409-419

[22] Kotter MR, Li WW, Zhao C, Franklin RJ. Myelin impairs CNS remyelination by inhibiting oligodendrocyte precursor cell differentiation. The Journal of Neuroscience. 2006;**26**(1):328-332

[23] Robinson S, Miller RH. Contact with central nervous system myelin inhibits oligodendrocyte progenitor maturation. Developmental Biology. 1999;**216**(1):359-368

[24] Morell P, Roberson M, Meissner G, Toews AD. Myelin: From electrical insulator to ion channels. In: Dynamic Interactions of Myelin Proteins. New York: Wiley-Liss, Inc.; 1990. pp. 1-24

[25] Norton WT, Poduslo SE. Myelination in rat brain: Method of myelin isolation. Journal of Neurochemistry. 1973;**21**:749-757

[26] Campagnoni AT. Molecular biology of myelin proteins from the central nervous system. Journal of Neurochemistry. 1988;**51**:1-14

[27] Nave K-A. Neurological mouse mutants: A molecular-genetic analysis of myelin proteins. In: Kettnmann NH, Ransom B, editors. Neuroglia. New York: Oxford University Press; 1995. pp. 571-587

[28] Griffiths I, Klugmann M, Anderson T, Yool D, Thomson C, Schwab MH, Schneider A, Zimmermann F, McCulloch M, Nadon N, Nave KA. Axonal swellings and degeneration in mice lacking the major proteolipid of myelin. Science. 1998;**280**(5369):1610-1613

[29] Rosenbluth J, Nave KA, Mierzwa A, Schiff R. Subtle myelin defects in PLP-null mice. Glia. 2006;**54**(3):172-182

[30] Montgomery DL. Astrocytes: form, functions, and roles in disease. Veterinary Pathology. 1994;**31**(2):145-167

[31] Rakic P. Neuron-glia relationship during granule cell migration in developing cerebellar cortex. A Golgi and electronmicroscopic study in *Macacus rhesus*. The Journal of Comparative Neurology. 1971;**141**(3):283-312

[32] Fitch MT, Doller C, Combs CK, Landreth GE, Silver J. Cellular and molecular mechanisms of glial scarring and progressive cavitation: in vivo and in vitro analysis of inflammation-induced secondary injury after CNS trauma. The Journal of Neuroscience. 1999;**19**(19):8182-8198

[33] Fitch MT, Silver J. CNS injury, glial scars, and inflammation: Inhibitory extracellular matrices and regeneration failure. Experimental Neurology. 2008;**209**(2):294-301

[34] Silver J, Miller JH. Regeneration beyond the glial scar. Nature Reviews. Neuroscience. 2004;**5**(2):146-156

[35] Fuller ML, DeChant AK, Rothstein B, Caprariello A, Wang R, Hall AK, Miller RH. Bone morphogenetic proteins promote gliosis in demyelinating spinal cord lesions. Annals of Neurology. 2007;**62**(3):288-300

[36] Trapp BD, Peterson J, Ransohoff RM, Rudick R, Mork S, Bo L. Axonal transection in the lesions of multiple sclerosis. The New England Journal of Medicine. 1998;**338**(5):278-285

[37] Waxman SG. Demyelinating diseases--new pathological insights, new therapeutic targets. The New England Journal of Medicine. 1998;**338**(5):323-325

[38] Sofroniew MV. Reactive astrocytes in neural repair and protection. The Neuroscientist. 2005;**11**(5):400-407

[39] Didonna A. Preclinical models of multiple sclerosis: Advantages and limitations towards better therapies. Current Medicinal Chemistry. 2016;**23**(14):1442-1459

[40] Gold R, Linington C, Lassmann H. Understanding pathogenesis and therapy of multiple sclerosis via animal models: 70 years of merits and culprits in experimental autoimmune encephalomyelitis research. Brain. 2006;**129**(Pt 8):1953-1971

[41] Mix E, Meyer-Rienecker H, Hartung HP, Zettl UK. Animal models of multiple sclerosis – Potentials and limitations. Progress in Neurobiology. 2010;**92**(3):386-404

[42] Rivers TM, Sprunt DH, Berry GP. Observations on attempts to produce acute disseminated encephalomyelitis in monkeys. The Journal of Experimental Medicine. 1933;**58**(1):39-53

[43] Ben-Nun A, Wekerle H, Cohen IR. The rapid isolation of clonable antigen-specific T lymphocyte lines capable of mediating autoimmune encephalomyelitis. European Journal of Immunology. 1981;**11**(3):195-199

[44] Franciotta D, Salvetti M, Lolli F, Serafini B, Aloisi F. B cells and multiple sclerosis. Lancet Neurology. 2008;**7**(9):852-858

[45] Haase CG, Guggenmos J, Brehm U, Andersson M, Olsson T, Reindl M, Schneidewind JM, Zettl UK, Heidenreich F, Berger T, Wekerle H, Hohlfeld R, Linington C. The fine specificity of the myelin oligodendrocyte glycoprotein autoantibody response in patients with multiple sclerosis and normal healthy controls. Journal of Neuroimmunology. 2001;**114**(1-2):220-225

[46] Hauser SL, Waubant E, Arnold DL, Vollmer T, Antel J, Fox RJ, Bar-Or A, Panzara M, Sarkar N, Agarwal S, Langer-Gould A, Smith CH, H.T. Group. B-cell depletion with rituximab in relapsing-remitting multiple sclerosis. The New England Journal of Medicine. 2008;**358**(7):676-688

[47] Kappos L, Li D, Calabresi PA, O'Connor P, Bar-Or A, Barkhof F, Yin M, Leppert D, Glanzman R, Tinbergen J, Hauser SL. Ocrelizumab in relapsing-remitting multiple sclerosis: A phase 2, randomised, placebo-controlled, multicentre trial. Lancet. 2011;**378**(9805):1779-1787

[48] Montalban X, Hauser SL, Kappos L, Arnold DL, Bar-Or A, Comi G, de Seze J, Giovannoni G, Hartung HP, Hemmer B, Lublin F, Rammohan KW, Selmaj K, Traboulsee A, Sauter A, Masterman D, Fontoura P, Belachew S, Garren H, Mairon N, Chin P, Wolinsky JS, Investigators OC. Ocrelizumab versus placebo in primary progressive multiple sclerosis. The New England Journal of Medicine. 2017;**376**(3):209-220

[49] Charles P, Tait S, Faivre-Sarrailh C, Barbin G, Gunn-Moore F, Denisenko-Nehrbass N, Guennoc AM, Girault JA, Brophy PJ, Lubetzki C. Neurofascin is a glial receptor for the paranodin/Caspr-contactin axonal complex at the axoglial junction. Current Biology. 2002;**12**(3):217-220

[50] Chiaravalloti ND, DeLuca J. Cognitive impairment in multiple sclerosis. Lancet Neurology. 2008;**7**(12):1139-1151

[51] Mori F, Kusayanagi H, Nicoletti CG, Weiss S, Marciani MG, Centonze D. Cortical plasticity predicts recovery from relapse in multiple sclerosis. Multiple Sclerosis. 2014;**20**(4):451-457

[52] Merkler D, Ernsting T, Kerschensteiner M, Bruck W, Stadelmann C. A new focal EAE model of cortical demyelination: Multiple sclerosis-like lesions with rapid resolution of inflammation and extensive remyelination. Brain. 2006;**129**(Pt 8):1972-1983

[53] Balatoni B, Storch MK, Swoboda EM, Schonborn V, Koziel A, Lambrou GN, Hiestand PC, Weissert R, Foster CA. FTY720 sustains and restores neuronal function in the DA rat model of MOG-induced experimental autoimmune encephalomyelitis. Brain Research Bulletin. 2007;**74**(5):307-316

[54] Miron VE, Ludwin SK, Darlington PJ, Jarjour AA, Soliven B, Kennedy TE, Antel JP. Fingolimod (FTY720) enhances remyelination following demyelination of organotypic cerebellar slices. The American Journal of Pathology. 2010;**176**(6):2682-2694

[55] Rose JW, Foley J, Carlson N. Monoclonal antibody treatments for multiple sclerosis. Current Neurology and Neuroscience Reports. 2008;**8**(5):419-426

[56] Gregson NA. Lysolipids and membrane damage: lysolecithin and its interaction with myelin. Biochemical Society Transactions. 1989;**17**(2):280-283

[57] Hall SM. The effect of injections of lysophosphatidyl choline into white matter of the adult mouse spinal cord. Journal of Cell Science. 1972;**10**(2):535-546

[58] Blakemore WF. Ethidium bromide induced demyelination in the spinal cord of the cat. Neuropathology and Applied Neurobiology. 1982;**8**(5):365-375

[59] Zawadzka M, Rivers LE, Fancy SP, Zhao C, Tripathi R, Jamen F, Young K, Goncharevich A, Pohl H, Rizzi M, Rowitch DH, Kessaris N, Suter U, Richardson WD, Franklin RJ. CNS-resident glial progenitor/stem cells produce Schwann cells as well as oligodendrocytes during repair of CNS demyelination. Cell Stem Cell. 2010;**6**(6):578-590

[60] Piddlesden SJ, Lassmann H, Zimprich F, Morgan BP, Linington C. The demyelinating potential of antibodies to myelin oligodendrocyte glycoprotein is related to their ability to fix complement. The American Journal of Pathology. 1993;**143**(2):555-564

[61] Woodruff RH, Franklin RJ. Demyelination and remyelination of the caudal cerebellar peduncle of adult rats following stereotaxic injections of lysolecithin, ethidium bromide, and complement/anti-galactocerebroside: A comparative study. Glia. 1999;**25**(3):216-228

[62] Mi S, Miller RH, Lee X, Scott ML, Shulag-Morskaya S, Shao Z, Chang A, Thill G, Levesque M, Zhang M, Hession C, Sah D, Trapp BD, He Z, Jung V, McCoy JM, Pepinsky RB, LINGO-1 negatively regulates myelination by oligodendrocytes. Nature Neuroscience. 2005;**8**:745-751

[63] Mi S, Miller RH, Tang W, Lee X, Hu B, Wu W, Zhang Y, Shields CB, Zhang Y, Miklasz S, Shea D, Mason J, Franklin RJ, Ji B, Shao Z, Chedotal A, Bernard F, Roulois A, Xu J, Jung V, Pepinsky B. Promotion of central nervous system remyelination by induced differentiation of oligodendrocyte precursor cells. Annals of Neurology. 2009;**65**(3):304-315

[64] Liu L, Belkadi A, Darnall L, Hu T, Drescher C, Cotleur AC, Padovani-Claudio D, He T, Choi K, Lane TE, Miller RH, Ransohoff RM. CXCR2-positive neutrophils are essential for cuprizone-induced demyelination: relevance to multiple sclerosis. Nature Neuroscience. 2010;**13**(3):319-326

[65] Koutsoudaki PN, Hildebrandt H, Gudi V, Skripuletz T, Skuljec J, Stangel M. Remyelination after cuprizone induced demyelination is accelerated in mice deficient in the polysialic acid synthesizing enzyme St8siaIV. Neuroscience. 2010;**171**(1):235-244

[66] Moharregh-Khiabani D, Blank A, Skripuletz T, Miller E, Kotsiari A, Gudi V, Stangel M. Effects of fumaric acids on cuprizone induced central nervous system de- and remyelination in the mouse. PLoS One. 2010;**5**(7):e11769

[67] Kipp M, Clarner T, Dang J, Copray S, Beyer C. The cuprizone animal model: new insights into an old story. Acta Neuropathologica. 2009;**118**(6):723-736

[68] Traka M, Arasi K, Avila RL, Podojil JR, Christakos A, Miller SD, Soliven B, Popko B. A genetic mouse model of adult-onset, pervasive central nervous system demyelination with robust remyelination. Brain. 2010;**133**(10):3017-3029

[69] Traka M, Podojil JR, McCarthy DP, Miller SD, Popko B. Oligodendrocyte death results in immune-mediated CNS demyelination. Nature Neuroscience. 2016;**19**(1):65-74

[70] Oluich LJ, Stratton JA, Xing YL, Ng SW, Cate HS, Sah P, Windels F, Kilpatrick TJ, Merson TD. Targeted ablation of oligodendrocytes induces axonal pathology independent of overt demyelination. The Journal of Neuroscience. 2012;**32**(24):8317-8330

[71] Straathof KC, Pule MA, Yotnda P, Dotti G, Vanin EF, Brenner MK, Heslop HE, Spencer DM, Rooney CM. An inducible caspase 9 safety switch for T-cell therapy. Blood. 2005;**105**(11):4247-4254

[72] Caprariello AV, Batt CE, Zippe I, Romito-DiGiacomo RR, Karl M, Miller RH. Apoptosis of oligodendrocytes during early development delays myelination and impairs subsequent responses to demyelination. The Journal of Neuroscience. 2015;**35**(41):14031-14041

[73] Caprariello AV, Mangla S, Miller RH, Selkirk SM. Apoptosis of oligodendrocytes in the central nervous system results in rapid focal demyelination. Annals of Neurology. 2012;**72**(3):395-405

[74] Barnett MH, Prineas JW. Relapsing and remitting multiple sclerosis: pathology of the newly forming lesion. Annals of Neurology. 2004;**55**(4):458-468

[75] Deshmukh VA, Tardif V, Lyssiotis CA, Green CC, Kerman B, Kim HJ, Padmanabhan K, Swoboda JG, Ahmad I, Kondo T, Gage FH, Theofilopoulos AN, Lawson BR, Schultz PG, Lairson LL. A regenerative approach to the treatment of multiple sclerosis. Nature. 2013;**502**(7471):327-332

[76] Mei F, Fancy SPJ, Shen YA, Niu J, Zhao C, Presley B, Miao E, Lee S, Mayoral SR, Redmond SA, Etxeberria A, Xiao L, Franklin RJM, Green A, Hauser SL, Chan JR. Micropillar arrays as a high-throughput screening platform for therapeutics in multiple sclerosis. Nature Medicine. 2014;**20**(8):954-960

[77] Najm FJ, Lager AM, Zaremba A, Wyatt K, Caprariello AV, Factor DC, Karl RT, Maeda T, Miller RH, Tesar PJ. Transcription factor-mediated reprogramming of fibroblasts to expandable, myelinogenic oligodendrocyte progenitor cells. Nature Biotechnology. 2013;**31**(5):426-433

[78] Najm FJ, Madhavan M, Zaremba A, Shick E, Karl RT, Factor DC, Miller TE, Nevin ZS, Kantor C, Sargent A, Quick KL, Schlatzer DM, Tang H, Papoian R, Brimacombe KR, Shen M, Boxer MB, Jadhav A, Robinson AP, Podojil JR, Miller SD, Miller RH, Tesar PJ. Drug-based modulation of endogenous stem cells promotes functional remyelination in vivo. Nature. 2015;**522**(7555):216-220

8

Docosahexaenoic Acid Promotes Recovery of Motor Function by Neuroprotection and Neuroplasticity Mechanisms

John V. Priestley and Adina T. Michael-Titus

Abstract

The omega-3 polyunsaturated fatty acid, docosahexaenoic acid (DHA), has been shown to promote recovery of motor function after spinal cord injury. This is likely to be at least partly due to neuroprotective effects of DHA. However, recent studies have shown that DHA also supports neuroplasticity after injury, such as promoting sprouting of spared corticospinal tract (CST) axons. In this chapter, we review the published studies showing that DHA promotes recovery of motor function in rodent models of spinal cord injury (SCI), and consider the available data on the underlying mechanisms. This includes effects on inflammation and on neuronal and oligodendrocyte survival at the injury site, and effects on spared CST axons and serotonergic axons. Current data support the hypothe-sis that DHA promotes recovery of motor function by both neuroprotection and neuroplasticity mechanisms. The significance of this, and the implications of combin-ing DHA with rehabilitation strategies, will be discussed.

Keywords: thoracic spinal cord injury, cervical spinal cord injury, central pattern generator, V2a interneurons, DHA

1. Introduction

1.1. Polyunsaturated fatty acids and their role in neurology

Polyunsaturated fatty acids (PUFA) of the omega-3 and omega-6 series are lipids with major structural and signalling roles. The long-chain omega-3 PUFA docosahexaenoic acid (DHA) is present in significant concentrations in the central nervous system (CNS), where its synthesis from the dietary precursor alpha-linolenic acid (LNA) occurs through desaturation, elongation and β-oxidation reactions. Its intermediate precursors are eicosapentaenoic acid (EPA) and docosapentaenoic acid (DPA). In humans, the conversion of LNA into DHA is below 5% [1, 2]. Therefore, an adequate dietary supply of DHA is required, especially because due to modern food manufacturing, there has been a significant decrease in the omega-3 intake and the omega-3 to omega-6 PUFA dietary ratio in the Western diet [3]. These changes have been linked to an increase in the incidence and the prevalence of diseases such as cancer, cardiovascular disease, rheumatoid arthritis, osteoporosis and asthma [4]. After absorption, the omega-3 PUFA can cross cellular membranes through specialized fatty acid transporters and interact with fatty acid-binding proteins (FABP). These proteins are a family of lipid chaperones involved in the extracellular and intracellular transport of fatty acids [5]. FABP bind long-chain fatty acids, with different ligand selectivity and binding affinity profiles. Changes in FABP levels have been reported following injury. For example, B-FABP is found in the brain and has very high affinity for DHA; it is detected in plasma as a high specificity and sensitivity biomarker of brain injury [6]. More recently, Figueroa et al. [7] reported increases in tissue levels of FABP-5 after spinal cord injury.

The principal omega-3 PUFA in the brain is DHA, representing 10–20% of the total fatty acid composition. Retinal tissue is also highly enriched in DHA. This fatty acid is a component of phospholipids, in particular phosphatidylethanolamine and phosphatidylserine; it is concentrated in cytoplasmic and synaptosomal membranes, growth cones, microsomal and mitochondrial membranes, and is also a component of myelin [8]. DHA-enriched phospholipids are present in the inner leaflet of the cytoplasmic membrane, and DHA chains are very flexible and transition rapidly between conformational states. This creates a unique microenvironment for the functioning of many proteins embedded in membranes, such as neurotransmitter receptors [9]. After release from membrane phospholipids by phospholipases, long-chain omega-3 PUFA such as DHA can be metabolized and produce a wide range of metabolites, designated with the generic term of "docosanoids", which include protectins, D-series resolvins and maresins. These DHA metabolites have intrinsic biological effects, which are mediated through specific receptors [10, 11]. Therefore, some of the effects induced by DHA may be due not to a direct action of the fatty acid but to specific metabolites which are derived from it, and which could attain significant levels, especially under conditions of chronic DHA supplementation [12].

DHA has an essential role in normal neurodevelopment, in particular for vision and cognition [13]. Supplementation with DHA has been shown to improve various aspects of learning and memory in children [14]. More than two decades ago, Martinez and collaborators [15] carried out seminal studies in children with peroxysomal disorders, which lead to a major DHA deficit, and showed that supplementation with DHA can lead to significant improvement in neurological function, and this is accompanied by improved myelination of the immature brain. At around the same time, studies initiated by Lazdunski and collaborators were providing evidence that omega-3 PUFA had significant neuroprotective potential under conditions which lead to CNS injury, such as seizures and ischaemia [16]. DHA has been increasingly linked to a variety of conditions, such as Alzheimer's disease and Parkinson's disease, and also schizophrenia, depression and attention deficit-hyperactivity disorder [17–19], and this has consolidated the idea that dietary supplementation with DHA could have therapeutic value across a spectrum of major disorders in neurology and psychiatry.

1.2. Pathways controlling movement in the rat and possible strategies for promoting recovery of movement following spinal cord injury (SCI)

Locomotion in rodents is controlled by a central pattern generator (CPG) which generates the basic rhythm of limb flexion and extension and which, for the hindlimbs, is located in the lower thoracic and upper lumbar spinal cord. In recent years, great progress has been made in dissecting the organization of the CPG, by identifying subtypes of neurons based on their developmental expression of specific transcription factors (summarized in [20, 21]). Genetic ablation of specific transcription factors can then be used to probe the functional roles of different neuronal subtypes (see e.g. [22, 23]). **Figure 1** illustrates one possible model of the

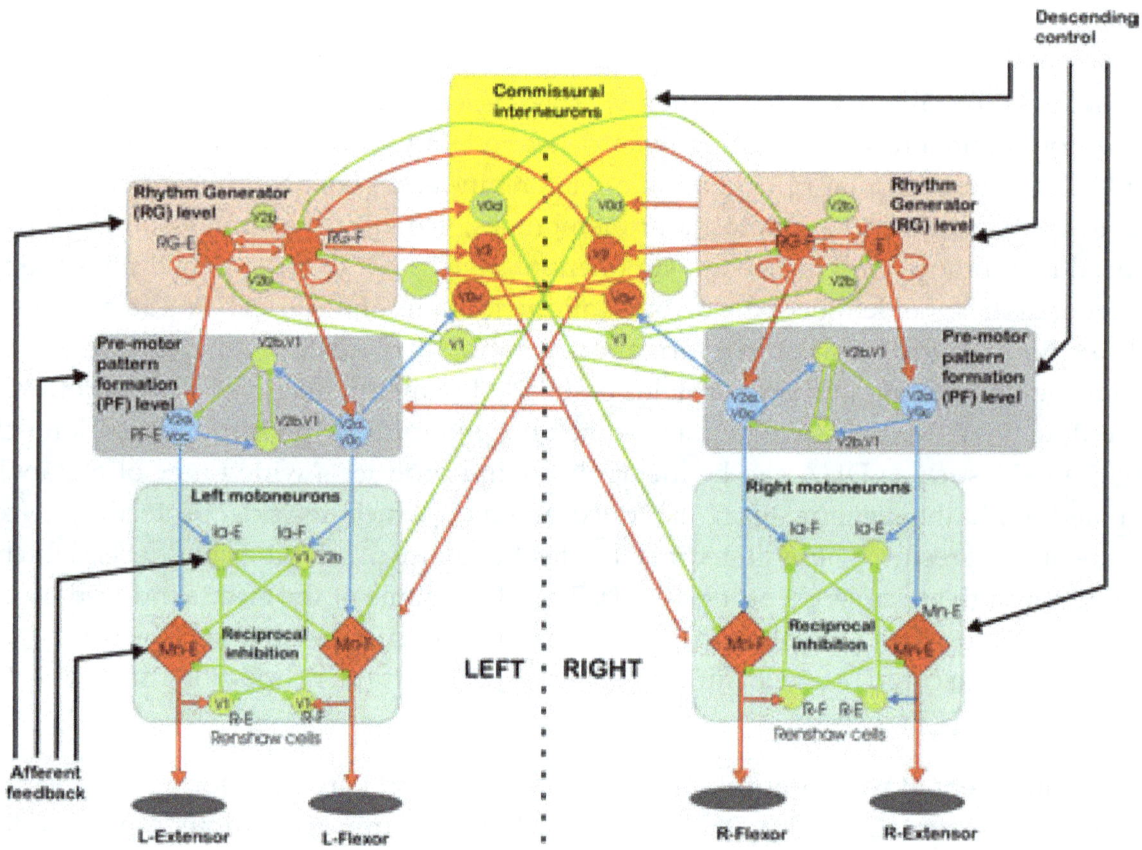

Figure 1. Schematic model of the rodent CPG controlling hind limb movement. Excitatory neurons are shown in red, and inhibitory neurons are shown in green. Rhythm generator (RG), pattern formation (PF) and motoneurons (Mn) are present for both flexion and extension on both sides of the spinal cord. V0d, V0v, V0c, V1, V2a, V2b and V3 are different types of interneurons which in some cases correspond to existing well-characterized neuronal types (e.g. V1 neurons include Renshaw cells). V2a neurons are shown in blue and have direct projections to motoneurons, plus projections to V2b/V1 PF inhibitory interneurons and to V0v excitatory commissural interneurons. Afferent feedback and descending control occur bilaterally, but for simplicity have only been shown ipsilaterally. The diagram is based on diagrams contained in Harris-Warrick [20] and Rybak and colleagues [21].

CPG based on studies reported in [22, 23]. Flexor and extensor motoneurons are thought to have separate rhythm generators (RG) which provide input to a pattern formation (PF) network that controls flexor/extensor alternation. The RG network also connects to commissural interneurons which coordinate left/right hindlimb movement. As an example of the complexity of the system, we have highlighted the V2a class of excitatory interneuron in **Figure 1**. V2a neurons can be identified by their expression of the homeodomain protein Chx10 and receive input from the RG centres. They project to three different targets, namely (1) motoneurons, (2) V2b inhibitory interneurons that are part of the PF centre, and (3) V0v commissural interneurons [21]. They therefore can influence locomotion by direct monosynaptic inputs to motoneurons and by regulating the flexor/extensor and left/right coordinating centres. However, V2a interneurons are not only present in the lumbar CPG, they also occur in the cervical spinal cord and play a key role in skilled forelimb movement, by conveying an internal copy of the premotor signals. This is possible because of their dual innervation of cervical motoneurons and precerebellar interneurons [22].

The CPG can generate alternating hindlimb movements independently, but in the intact animal, the CPG is modulated by afferent feedback and by descending control. The effects of SCI depend on the spinal level of the injury. Rats subject to complete transection above the level of the lumbar locomotor centres show some spontaneous recovery of hindlimb movement [24], and this can be increased by a variety of treatments, including weight supported treadmill training [24], delivery of growth factors [25, 26] and implantation of various exogenous cells [27–29]. At least some of this recovery of function appears to be related to regeneration or sprouting of descending bulbospinal [30, 31] and corticospinal [25] pathways. In contrast, the lasting paraplegia that results from a SCI at lumbar level is thought to result from loss of spinal interneurons, possibly including components of the CPG [32]. An efficacious treatment for SCI might need to preserve and/or restore descending control pathways and repair damage to intrinsic networks such as the CPG.

2. The effects of PUFA treatment on recovery of movement following experimental SCI

2.1. Thoracic hemisection SCI

DHA promotes recovery of quadrupedal locomotion in rats and mice following thoracic hemisection [33], compression [34–36] and contusion [37] SCI, when acutely administered post-injury. Recovery is further improved if an acute injection of DHA is followed by a DHA-supplemented diet (**Figure 2**). The DHA treatment results in increased neuronal and oligodendrocyte survival [34] and decreased macrophage and microglial activation [36, 38] at the injury site. However, since the motoneuron pools that contribute to locomotion are not at thoracic level, it is likely that the effects on locomotion are due to preservation of descending axons passing through the injury site rather than preservation of thoracic neurons themselves. Analysis of axon numbers at the SCI site using generic axonal markers such as neurofilament and myelin basic protein (MBP) reveals that DHA preserves axons in white matter tracts [39] but, with the exception of serotonin (5-hydroxytryptamine, 5-HT), the origin and role of those axons have not been much explored. As outlined above, corticospinal and bulbospinal projections play an important role in motor control but mainly innervate motoneurons indirectly, via interneurons, and so are difficult to analyse (however, see Section 4 on pyramidotomy below). In contrast, 5-HT axons are derived from the medullary raphe nuclei, innervate many motoneurons monosynaptically and play key roles in modulating motoneuron excitability [40]. DHA treatment preserves the number of 5-HT axons at the level of a thoracic compression injury [39], including axons that appear to contact motoneurons (see **Figure 3**). It is therefore likely that at least some of the motor recovery is due to increased preservation of 5-HT axons that pass through the injury site and innervate motoneurons at lumbar level. 5-HT axons have a great capacity to sprout and make new connections [41]. Another possibility is therefore that some 5-HT axons are spared by the SCI but that DHA promotes sprouting and restoration of synaptic circuits by these axons. These possibilities have not been examined directly following thoracic SCI, but the effects of DHA on 5-HT axons have been studied in much more detail following cervical injury.

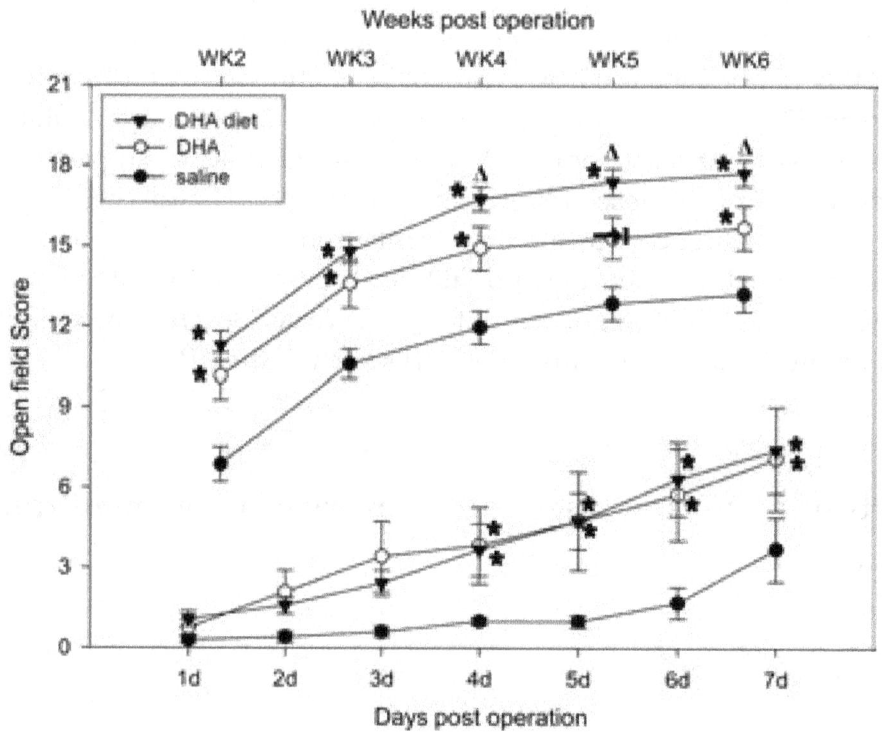

Figure 2. Locomotor performance of thoracic compression SCI rats injected with saline or DHA and of animals injected with DHA and then fed on a DHA-enriched diet. Results for days 1–7 are shown in the bottom half of the graph, plotted against the bottom X-axis. Results for 2–6 weeks are shown in the top half of the graph, plotted against the top X-axis. Both DHA- and saline-treated animals showed similar low levels of locomotor function 1 day after surgery, as assessed on the BBB open field task. During the first week, DHA-treated animals had improved motor function recovery compared with saline-treated animals (days 5, 6 and 7; $^*p < 0.05$). Between week 2 and week 6, DHA-treated animals continued to perform better than saline-treated animals ($^*p < 0.05$). In addition, from the 4th week onwards, animals injected with DHA followed by maintenance on the DHA-enriched diet, performed better than animals only injected with DHA (weeks 4, 5 and 6; $^{\Delta}p < 0.05$). Error bars represent SEMs. Reproduced from [34] with permission.

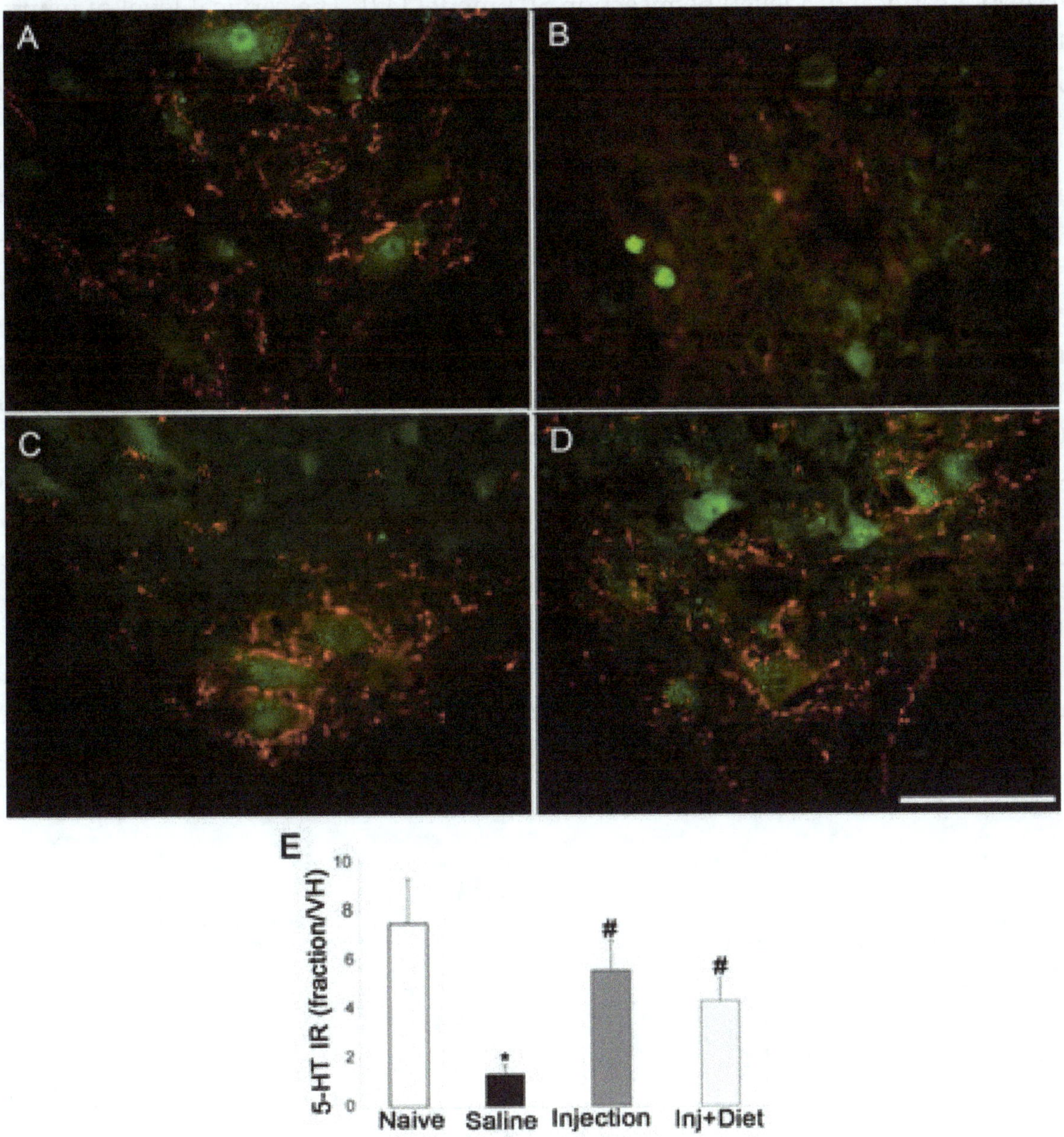

Figure 3. Immunofluorescence micrographs showing thin, 5-HT immunoreactive (IR) axons (red) that innervate NeuN labelled neurons (green) in the ventral horn (VH). In naïve animals (A), a dense network of beaded 5-HT-positive fibres can be seen surrounding large NeuN neurons. At 6 weeks post-thoracic compression injury, a marked loss of 5-HT-positive fibres was seen in saline-treated animals (B) compared with the groups receiving DHA injection alone (C), or in combination with a DHA-enriched diet (D). Quantitative analysis (E) at 6 weeks post-injury revealed a significant loss of 5-HT IR in the VH of saline-treated animals following injury. A significant amelioration in the loss of 5-HT IR was observed in the VH in both DHA-treatment groups (significantly different from *naïve or #saline-treated animals at $p < 0.05$; scale bar = 100 μm). Reproduced from [39] with permission.

2.2. Experimental cervical SCI

The majority of experimental studies have focused on thoracic injury, but the most common clinical injury is at cervical level (57% of SCI). Recently, we have therefore examined the effects of DHA in a cervical (C5 level) hemisection SCI model [42]. The cervical level of injury also has the advantage of allowing us to examine the effects of DHA treatment on a skilled motor task, namely retrieval of food using the forepaws. Rats are trained to retrieve food by extending a forelimb through a gap in a perspex box and grasping food pellets which are on a staircase [43]. Following SCI at C5 level, rats lose the ability to recover the food pellets, but recover partial function if treated acutely with DHA (**Figure 4**). Following cervical hemisection, 5-HT axons show a remarkable degree of plasticity. Rostral to the hemisection, there is an increase in 5-HT immunoreactivity which is maintained up to 3 weeks. Caudal to the hemisection, there is a transient loss of 5-HT immunoreactivity at 1 week, but levels are restored by 3 weeks (**Figure 5B**). DHA treatment results in an even greater number of 5-HT immunoreactive axons caudal to the injury (**Figure 5B**), and increased density of 5-HT axons contacting motoneurons (**Figure 5C–E**). However, 5-HT axons are not the only ones to sprout in response to DHA treatment. Corticospinal tract (CST) axons on the intact side of the spinal cord were identified by anterograde labelling with the tracer biotinylated dextran amine (BDA). Following hemisection, a small number of these axons sprout across the midline to innervate the denervated side of the spinal cord. However, after DHA treatment, this number doubles [42]. It is therefore possible that the recovery of skilled movement is due to sprouting of 5-HT and CST axons and formation of novel circuits. However, since the increase in axons occurs at the same level as the hemisection, it is possible that the increase in 5-HT and CST axons is due to neuroprotection rather than neuroplasticity. We have therefore examined the effect of DHA treatment in a third model of SCI, namely unilateral pyramidotomy in the mouse [42].

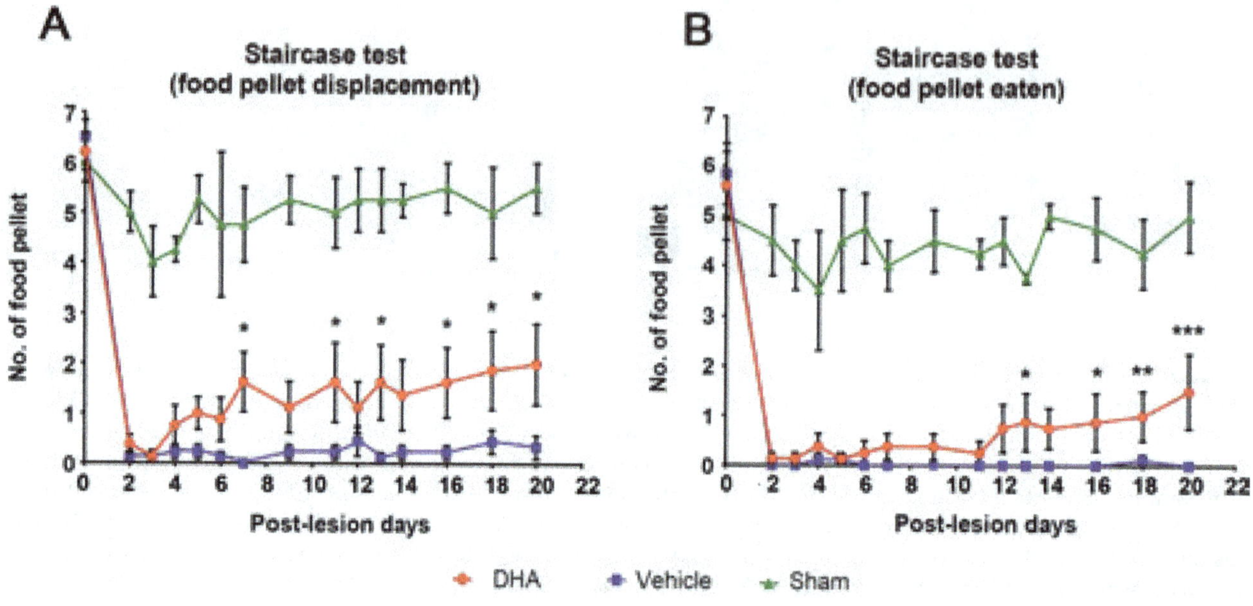

Figure 4. DHA enhances functional recovery following cervical lateral hemisection in the rat. A, B, In the Montoya staircase test, all injured animals lost the ability to displace (gross motor function) or eat (fine motor function) the food pellet after cervical lateral hemisection 2 d after injury. The animals treated with vehicle did not recover any food retrieval ability (blue squares), but DHA-treated animals gradually recovered food retrieval ability (red circles) from around 2 weeks onwards, compared with uninjured sham operated animals (green triangles). *$p < 0.05$, **$p < 0.01$, ***$p < 0.001$, compared to vehicle-treated animals. Results represent mean ± SEM. Reproduced from [42] with permission.

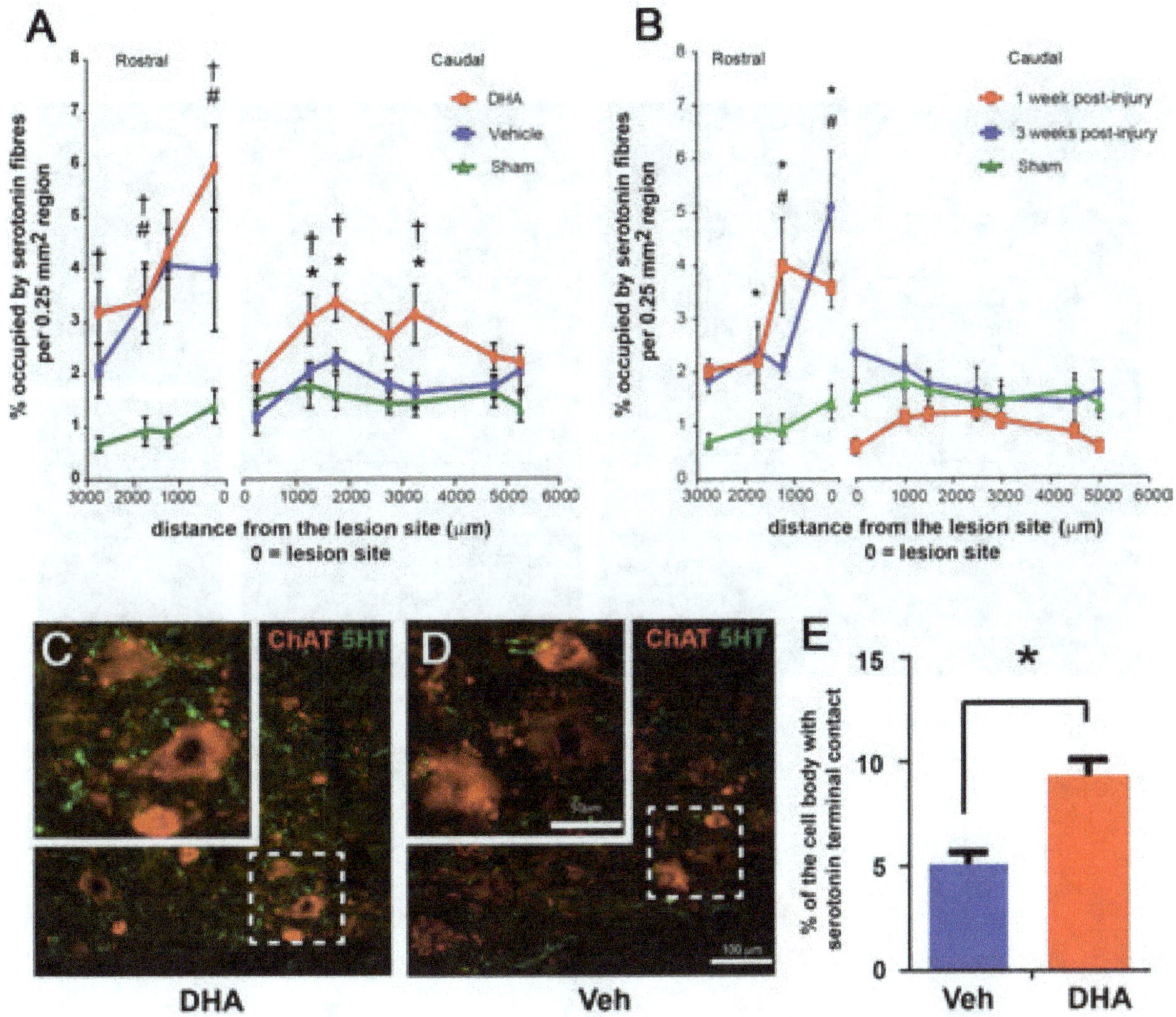

Figure 5. DHA enhances 5-HT (serotonin) fibre regrowth following cervical lateral hemisection in the rat. (*A*) Serotonin fibres in the rostral part of the lesion site were significantly increased in both treatment groups at 3 weeks post-injury, but only the DHA-treated group (red circles), not the vehicle group (blue squares), had significantly increased serotonin in the caudal region compared with the sham operated animals (green triangles). (*B*) Serotonin fibres in the rostral part of the lesion site were significantly increased at 1 week (red square) and 3 weeks (blue circle) compared with the sham operated group after lateral cervical hemisection. However, in the caudal region, 1 and 3 weeks after injury were similar to the sham operated group. 1 week after hemisection, there was a loss of serotonin but by 3 weeks levels had returned to values similar to sham operated animals. *N* = 5 or 6 per group. #$p < 0.05$, 1 week hemisection versus sham group. *$p < 0.05$, 3 week hemisection versus sham group. (*C, D*) The images were captured 1750 μm caudal to the lesion site. Double labelling shows serotonin fibres (green) in contact with ChAT immunoreactive motor neurons (red) in the ventral horn of vehicle- and DHA-treated rats. Insets, dashed boxes at higher magnification. (*E*) Quantitative analysis reveals that there is a significant increase in the density of serotonin fibres contacting motor neurons in the DHA-treated group compared with the control group. N = 5 or 6 per group. *$p < 0.05$, DHA versus vehicle group. †$p < 0.05$, sham versus vehicle group. #$p < 0.05$, DHA versus sham group. Scale bar, 100 μm. Reproduced from [42] with permission.

2.3. Pyramidotomy

The CST axons in rodents run in the medullary pyramids, before decussating and descending at the base of the dorsal columns. Unilateral pyramidotomy transects these CST axons and

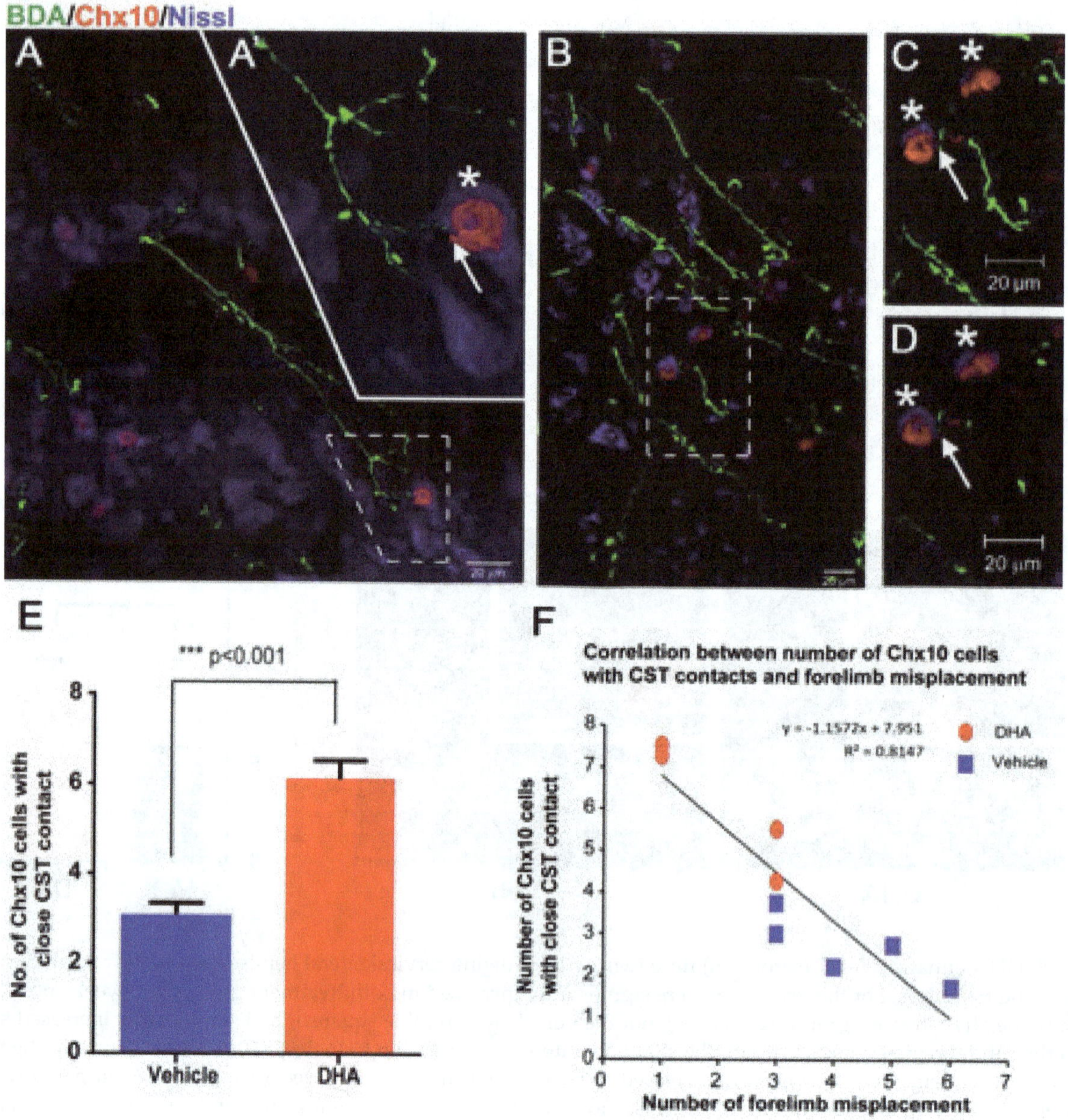

Figure 6. DHA enhances functional recovery via connection with Chx10 interneurons in pyramidotomy mice. (*A–D*), Confocal images of mouse cervical spinal cord transverse sections at the intermediate laminae of the CST-denervated side, showing examples of BDA-labelled CST collaterals (green) in the vicinity of blue fluorescent Nissl-stained cells (Neurotrace 435/455), some of which are V2a interneurons identified by immunostaining for Chx10 (red). (*A, B*) Dashed boxes represent high magnification in *A'*, and in *C, D,* which reveal contacts (arrows) between BDA-labelled collaterals and Chx10 interneurons (asterisks). (*A'*) *A* Z-stack comprising 10 × 0.66 μm optical images. (*C*), A stack comprising 25 × 0.72 μm optical images. (*D*, A) Single 0.72 μm optical image. Examination of the single optical image confirms that the BDA-labelled CST fibre contacts (arrow) one of the Chx10 interneurons. (*E*) Quantitative analysis revealed a significant increase in the number of Chx10 interneurons contacted by BDA-labelled CST collaterals following DHA treatment (red bar) compared with vehicle treatment (blue bar). (*F*) A strong negative correlation was observed between the numbers of Chx10 interneurons with BDA-labelled CST contacts and the numbers of forelimb misplacements. Data were taken from DHA-treated (red circle) and vehicle-treated (blue square) animals. ***$p<0.001$, DHA versus vehicle group. Scale bar, 20 μm. Reproduced from [42] with permission.

results in the loss of CST axons in the spinal cord on the contralateral side. Using BDA to label the CST axons on the non-lesioned side, we observed that a small number of CST axons respond to the pyramidotomy by sprouting across the midline to innervate the lesioned side (**Figure 6A**). The number of sprouting CST axons is doubled following DHA treatment [42]. Furthermore, we have shown that the sprouting axons contact a particular class of interneuron, namely the V2a propriospinal neurons described above. V2a neurons were identified by their expression of the Chx10 transcription factor (**Figure 6A–D**). V2a interneurons have been shown to play an important role in skilled reaching [22]. Following DHA treatment and pyramidotomy, an increased number of V2a interneurons receive contacts from CST axons (**Figure 6E**), and the recovery of forelimb movement shows a tight correlation with the number of V2a neurons that receive contacts (**Figure 6F**). It therefore appears that DHA treatment after pyramidotomy results in the formation of a novel circuit (CST to contralateral V2a interneurons) that promotes recovery of skilled reaching. This is in addition to the effects of DHA on sprouting 5-HT axons, and neuroprotective effects on neuronal cell bodies and axons.

3. Discussion

Motor pathways are so complex that it is difficult to establish a direct causal relationship between the effects of a therapeutic agent on spinal circuitry and an improvement in a particular motor task. However, the data reviewed above indicates that there is a strong correlation between the neuroprotective and neuroplasticity effects of DHA and the recovery of motor function. This dual effect of DHA, together with its established safety profile and the recent demonstration of the efficacy in SCI of a multinutrient combination containing DHA and EPA [44], makes DHA a particularly promising candidate for development as a therapeutic agent in SCI. There is a substantial literature on the neuroprotective effects of DHA (reviewed above) but the effects on neuroplasticity are more novel and less studied. We have shown that DHA treatment following SCI upregulates the microRNA miR-21 and suppresses phosphatase and tensin homolog (PTEN), a central negative regulator of the phosphatidylinositol 3-kinase (PI3K) signalling pathway [42]. However, these effects are quite widespread and it is not known how they result in beneficial axon sprouting. Bareyre and colleagues [45] have shown that new connections form after SCI, but inappropriate connections are lost because they are not used. A similar mechanism may mould the sprouting and connections promoted by DHA, in which case, there may be great benefit in combining DHA treatment with rehabilitation and task specific training.

3.1. Therapeutic implications

The magnitude of the effects induced by the acute administration of DHA and reported in various models of SCI is comparable with that described with various other therapeutic approaches which are already being explored in clinical trials in neurotrauma, such as progesterone, erythropoietin, riluzole and minocycline [46]. DHA has clear potential for clinical translation in SCI; therefore, it is appropriate to consider the issues which remain to be clarified in order to improve the chances of translational success.

It is important to note that in the studies published so far with DHA and reporting beneficial effects of this fatty acid in a variety of conditions, there are two types of administration: DHA administered using a chronic oral supplementation route and DHA administered as an acute bolus, using an injectable route. Are the cellular targets and mechanisms activated by DHA the same in the two types of treatment? When DHA is administered chronically, one of the consequences of this regime is the structural enrichment in DHA in membranes, and because DHA has unique molecular structural characteristics, this influences the dynamics of membrane components, and may change the activity of ion channels and G-protein-coupled receptors (GPCR). DHA incorporation in membranes changes the properties of specialized domains such as the lipid rafts and caveolae, and this can modify signalling [47]. When DHA is administered acutely as a bolus, its half-life in plasma is very short (approximately 2 min), as shown in PET imaging studies carried out in healthy volunteers [48]; therefore, efficacy may be due to the activation of different mechanisms. Long-chain omega-3 PUFA such as DHA and EPA have various specific molecular targets, including ion channels, GPCR and nuclear receptors [17, 47]. They include voltage-sensitive Na^+ and Ca^{2+} channels and two-pore domain background K^+ channels, such as TREK-1 (which is also a target for riluzole), the GPCRs GPR40 and GPR120, and transcription factors such as the retinoid X receptors (RXR) and peroxisome proliferator-activated receptors (PPAR). RXR can heterodimerize with PPAR or with retinoic acid receptors (RAR), and changes in the expression of these receptors have been reported after SCI [49]. Several studies indicate that the activation of retinoid signalling supports axonal regeneration [50].

The spontaneous partial recovery of function which occurs after SCI may be due to neuroplasticity, compensation and repair [51]. Rehabilitation through training is at present the most successful treatment for patients with SCI, to enhance the recovery of some neurological function. Rehabilitation enhances the spontaneous plasticity changes that occur after injury and enhances the activity of sensorimotor pathways, as documented in experimental SCI [52]. Exercise leads to a reconfiguration of cortical representation maps, it modifies the biophysical properties of motoneuron membranes, changes the activity of spinal inhibitory circuits and also increases the levels of neurotrophic factors, such as brain-derived neurotrophic factor (BDNF) and neurotrophin-3 (NT-3) [53]. Liu and collaborators [54] have shown that exercise increases the expression of miR21 and decreases PTEN mRNA levels, a profile of effects similar to our observations with DHA. Considering this similarity of action, a goal of future studies should be the exploration of a combination of DHA and exercise, to establish whether what could be achieved is true synergism or only additivity. The concept of combining treatment with exercise is supported by examples such as the successful combination of exercise with strategies such as the reduction in the glial scar components using chondroitinase ABC [55]. However, not all combinations achieve an optimum effect, as shown by the negative results obtained by combining exercise with antibodies against the myelin-derived inhibitor Nogo A [56]. Therefore, it will be essential to continue to characterize the targets and mode of action of DHA, so that it becomes clear what mechanisms could be harnessed and amplified by combining DHA (acute administration and chronic exposure) and rehabilitation training, to optimize outcome in SCI patients.

Acknowledgements

We acknowledge the generous support of Spinal Research, Corporate Action Trust, Barts Charity and Chang Gung Memorial Hospital (Taiwan) for the DHA studies in the various models of SCI discussed here.

Author details

John V. Priestley* and Adina T. Michael-Titus

*Address all correspondence to: j.v.priestley@qmul.ac.uk

Centre for Neuroscience and Trauma, Blizard Institute, Barts and The London School of Medicine and Dentistry, Queen Mary University of London, London, UK

References

[1] BrennaJT, SalemNJr., SinclairAJ, CunnaneSC. alpha-Linolenic acid supplementation and conversion to n-3 long-chain polyunsaturated fatty acids in humans. Prostaglandins Leukot Essent Fatty Acids. 2009; 80: 85–91.

[2] BrennaJT. Efficiency of conversion of alpha-linolenic acid to long chain n-3 fatty acids in man. Curr Opin Clin Nutr Metab Care. 2002; 5: 127–132.

[3] SimopoulosAP. Evolutionary aspects of omega-3 fatty acids in the food supply. Prostaglandins Leukot Essent Fatty Acids. 1999; 60: 421–429.

[4] SimopoulosAP. The importance of the omega-6/omega-3 fatty acid ratio in cardiovascular disease and other chronic diseases. Exp Biol Med (Maywood). 2008; 233: 674–688.

[5] FuruhashiM, HotamisligilGS. Fatty acid-binding proteins: role in metabolic diseases and potential as drug targets. Nat Rev Drug Discov. 2008; 7: 489–503.

[6] PelsersMM, GlatzJF. Detection of brain injury by fatty acid-binding proteins. Clin Chem Lab Med. 2005; 43: 802–809.

[7] FigueroaJD, IllanMS, LiceroJ, CorderoK, MirandaJD, DeLM. Fatty acid binding protein 5 (FABP5) modulates docosahexaenoic acid (DHA)-induced recovery in rats undergoing spinal cord injury. J Neurotrauma. March 2016, ahead of print.

[8] HorrocksLA, FarooquiAA. Docosahexaenoic acid in the diet: its importance in maintenance and restoration of neural membrane function. Prostaglandins Leukot Essent Fatty Acids. 2004; 70: 361–372.

[9] GawrischK, EldhoNV, HolteLL. The structure of DHA in phospholipid membranes. Lipids. 2003; 38: 445–452.

[10] SerhanCN, KrishnamoorthyS, RecchiutiA, ChiangN. Novel anti-inflammatory—pro-resolving mediators and their receptors. Curr Top Med Chem. 2011; 11: 629–647.

[11] SerhanCN, DalliJ, ColasRA, WinklerJW, ChiangN. Protectins and maresins: new pro-resolving families of mediators in acute inflammation and resolution bioactive metabolome. Biochim Biophys Acta. 2015; 1851: 397–413.

[12] BazanNG, MolinaMF, GordonWC. Docosahexaenoic acid signalolipidomics in nutrition: significance in aging, neuroinflammation, macular degeneration, Alzheimer's, and other neurodegenerative diseases. Annu Rev Nutr. 2011; 31: 321–351.

[13] McNamaraRK, CarlsonSE. Role of omega-3 fatty acids in brain development and function: potential implications for the pathogenesis and prevention of psychopathology. Prostaglandins Leukot Essent Fatty Acids. 2006; 75: 329–349.

[14] KuratkoCN, BarrettEC, NelsonEB, SalemNJr. The relationship of docosahexaenoic acid (DHA) with learning and behavior in healthy children: a review. Nutrients. 2013; 5: 2777–2810.

[15] MartinezM, VazquezE. MRI evidence that docosahexaenoic acid ethyl ester improves myelination in generalized peroxisomal disorders. Neurology. 1998; 51: 26–32.

[16] LauritzenI, BlondeauN, HeurteauxC, WidmannC, RomeyG, LazdunskiM. Polyunsaturated fatty acids are potent neuroprotectors. EMBO J. 2000; 19: 1784–1793.

[17] DyallSC, Michael-TitusAT. Neurological benefits of omega-3 fatty acids. Neuromolecular Med. 2008; 10: 219–235.

[18] DyallSC. Long-chain omega-3 fatty acids and the brain: a review of the independent and shared effects of EPA, DPA and DHA. Front Aging Neurosci. 2015; 7: 52.

[19] RossBM, SeguinJ, SieswerdaLE. Omega-3 fatty acids as treatments for mental illness: which disorder and which fatty acid? Lipids Health Dis. 2007; 6: 21.

[20] Harris-WarrickRM. Locomotor pattern generation in the rodent spinal cord. In: JaegerD, JungR, editors. Encyclopedia of Computational Neuroscience. New York; Springer; 2013. pp. 1–15.

[21] RybakIA, DoughertyKJ, ShevtsovaNA. Organization of the mammalian locomotor CPG: review of computational model and circuit architectures based on genetically identified spinal interneurons. eNeuro. 2015; 2(5) e0069-15.2015 1–21.

[22] AzimE, JiangJ, AlstermarkB, JessellTM. Skilled reaching relies on a V2a propriospinal internal copy circuit. Nature. 2014; 508: 357–363.

[23] CroneSA, QuinlanKA, ZagoraiouL, DrohoS, RestrepoCE, LundfaldL, EndoT, SetlakJ, JessellTM, KiehnO, SharmaK. Genetic ablation of V2a ipsilateral interneurons disrupts left-right locomotor coordination in mammalian spinal cord. Neuron. 2008; 60: 70–83.

[24] ZhangY, JiSR, WuCY, FanXH, ZhouHJ, LiuGL. Observation of locomotor functional recovery in adult complete spinal rats with BWSTT using semiquantitative and qualitative methods. Spinal Cord. 2007; 45: 496–501.

[25] FernandezE, PalliniR, LaurettiL, MercantiD, SerraA, CalissanoP, PiepmeierJM, TatorCH. Spinal cord transection in adult rats—effects of local infusion of nerve growth factor on the corticospinal tract axons. Neurosurgery. 1993; 33: 889–893.

[26] BoyceVS, ParkJ, GageFH, MendellLM. Differential effects of brain-derived neurotrophic factor and neurotrophin-3 on hindlimb function in paraplegic rats. Eur J Neurosci. 2012; 35: 221–232.

[27] KubasakMD, JindrichDL, ZhongH, TakeokaA, McFarlandKC, Munoz-QuilesC, RoyRR, EdgertonVR, Ramon-CuetoA, PhelpsPE. OEG implantation and step training enhance hindlimb-stepping ability in adult spinal transected rats. Brain. 2008; 131: 264–276.

[28] RapalinoO, LazarovSpieglerO, AgranovE, VelanGJ, YolesE, FraidakisM, SolomonA, GepsteinR, KatzA, BelkinM, HadaniM, SchwartzM. Implantation of stimulated homologous macrophages results in partial recovery of paraplegic rats. Nat Med. 1998; 4: 814–821.

[29] SlawinskaU, MajczynskiH, DjavadianR. Recovery of hindlimb motor functions after spinal cord transection is enhanced by grafts of the embryonic raphe nuclei. Exp Brain Res. 2000; 132: 27–38.

[30] FouadK, SchnellL, BungeMB, SchwabME, LiebscherT, PearseDD. Combining Schwann cell bridges and olfactory-ensheathing glia grafts with chondroitinase promotes locomotor recovery after complete transection of the spinal cord. J Neurosci. 2005; 25: 1169–1178.

[31] Lopez-ValesR, ForesJ, NavarroX, VerduE. Chronic transplantation of olfactory ensheathing cells promotes partial recovery after complete spinal cord transection in the rat. Glia. 2007; 55: 303–311.

[32] HadiB, ZhangYP, BurkeDA, ShieldsCB, MagnusonDS. Lasting paraplegia caused by loss of lumbar spinal cord interneurons in rats: no direct correlation with motor neuron loss. J Neurosurg. 2000; 93: 266–275.

[33] KingVR, HuangWL, DyallSC, CurranOE, PriestleyJV, Michael-TitusAT. Omega-3 fatty acids improve recovery, whereas omega-6 fatty acids worsen outcome, after spinal cord injury in the adult rat. J Neurosci. 2006; 26: 4672–4680.

[34] HuangWL, KingVR, CurranOE, DyallSC, WardRE, LalN, PriestleyJV, Michael-TitusAT. A combination of intravenous and dietary docosahexaenoic acid significantly improves outcome after spinal cord injury. Brain. 2007; 130: 3004–3019.

[35] LimSN, HuangW, HallJC, Michael-TitusAT, PriestleyJV. Improved outcome after spinal cord compression injury in mice treated with docosahexaenoic acid. Exp Neurol. 2013; 239: 13–27.

[36] PaternitiI, ImpellizzeriD, DiPR, EspositoE, GladmanS, YipP, PriestleyJV, Michael-TitusAT, CuzzocreaS. Docosahexaenoic acid attenuates the early inflammatory response following spinal cord injury in mice: in-vivo and in-vitro studies. J Neuroinflamm. 2014; 11: 6.

[37] BaskervilleTA, PriestleyJV, Michael-TitusAT. The effect of docosahexaenoic acid in a rat model of spinal cord injury by contusion. Soc Neurosci Abstr. 2012; 658.26/P15.

[38] HallJC, PriestleyJV, PerryVH, Michael-TitusAT. Effect of docosahexaenoic acid and eicosapentaenoic acid on the early inflammatory response following compression spinal cord injury in the rat. J Neurochem. 2012; 121: 738–750.

[39] WardRE, HuangW, CurranOE, PriestleyJV, Michael-TitusAT. Docosahexaenoic acid prevents white matter damage after spinal cord injury. J Neurotrauma. 2010; 27: 1769–1780.

[40] LiX, MurrayK, HarveyPJ, BallouEW, BennettDJ. Serotonin facilitates a persistent calcium current in motoneurons of rats with and without chronic spinal cord injury. J Neurophysiol. 2007; 97: 1236–1246.

[41] SaruhashiY, YoungW, PerkinsR. The recovery of 5-HT immunoreactivity in lumbosacral spinal cord and locomotor function after thoracic hemisection. Exp Neurol. 1996; 139: 203–213.

[42] LiuZH, YipPK, AdamsL, DaviesM, LeeJW, MichaelGJ, PriestleyJV, Michael-TitusAT. A single bolus of docosahexaenoic acid promotes neuroplastic changes in the innervation of spinal cord interneurons and motor neurons and improves functional recovery after spinal cord injury. J Neurosci. 2015; 35: 12733–12752.

[43] MontoyaCP, Campbell-HopeLJ, PembertonKD, DunnettSB. The "staircase test": a measure of independent forelimb reaching and grasping abilities in rats. J Neurosci Methods. 1991; 36: 219–228.

[44] PallierPN, PoddigheL, ZbarskyV, KostusiakM, ChoudhuryR, HartT, BurguillosMA, MusbahiO, GroenendijkM, SijbenJW, deWildeMC, QuartuM, PriestleyJV, Michael-TitusAT. A nutrient combination designed to enhance synapse formation and function improves outcome in experimental spinal cord injury. Neurobiol Dis. 2015; 82: 504–515.

[45] BareyreFM, KerschensteinerM, RaineteauO, MettenleiterTC, WeinmannO, SchwabME. The injured spinal cord spontaneously forms a new intraspinal circuit in adult rats. Nat Neurosci. 2004; 7: 269–277.

[46] PriestleyJV, Michael-TitusAT, TetzlaffW. Limiting spinal cord injury by pharmacological intervention. Handb Clin Neurol. 2012; 109: 463–484.

[47] CalderPC. Mechanisms of action of (n-3) fatty acids. J Nutr. 2012; 142: 592S–599S.

[48] UmhauJC, ZhouW, CarsonRE, RapoportSI, PolozovaA, DemarJ, HusseinN, BhattacharjeeAK, MaK, EspositoG, MajchrzakS, HerscovitchP, EckelmanWC, KurdzielKA,

SalemNJr. Imaging incorporation of circulating docosahexaenoic acid into the human brain using positron emission tomography. J Lipid Res. 2009; 50: 1259–1268.

[49] Van NeervenS, MeyJ. RAR/RXR and PPAR/RXR signaling in spinal cord injury. PPAR Res. 2007; 2007: 29275.

[50] PuttaguntaR & DiGS. Retinoic acid signaling in axonal regeneration. Front Mol Neurosci. 2011; 4: 59.

[51] CurtA, van HedelHJ, KlausD, DietzV. Recovery from a spinal cord injury: significance of compensation, neural plasticity, and repair. J Neurotrauma. 2008; 25: 677–685.

[52] IchiyamaRM, CourtineG, GerasimenkoYP, YangGJ, van den BrandR, LavrovIA, ZhongH, RoyRR, EdgertonVR. Step training reinforces specific spinal locomotor circuitry in adult spinal rats. J Neurosci. 2008; 28: 7370–7375.

[53] FouadK & TetzlaffW. Rehabilitative training and plasticity following spinal cord injury. Exp Neurol. 2012; 235: 91–99.

[54] LiuG, DetloffMR, MillerKN, SantiL, HouleJD. Exercise modulates microRNAs that affect the PTEN/mTOR pathway in rats after spinal cord injury. Exp Neurol. 2012; 233: 447–456.

[55] Garcia-AliasG, FawcettJW. Training and anti-CSPG combination therapy for spinal cord injury. Exp Neurol. 2012; 235: 26–32.

[56] MaierIC, IchiyamaRM, CourtineG, SchnellL, LavrovI, EdgertonVR, SchwabME. Differential effects of anti-Nogo-A antibody treatment and treadmill training in rats with incomplete spinal cord injury. Brain. 2009; 132: 1426–1440.

9

Music and Brain Plasticity: How Sounds Trigger Neurogenerative Adaptations

Mark Reybrouck, Peter Vuust and Elvira Brattico

Abstract

This contribution describes how music can trigger plastic changes in the brain. We elaborate on the concept of neuroplasticity by focussing on three major topics: the ontogenetic scale of musical development, the phenomenon of neuroplasticity as the outcome of interactions with the sounds and a short survey of clinical and therapeutic applications. First, a distinction is made between two scales of description: the larger evolutionary scale (phylogeny) and the scale of individual development (ontogeny). In this sense, listeners are not constrained by a static dispositional machinery, but they can be considered as dynamical systems that are able to adapt themselves in answer to the solicitations of a challenging environment. Second, the neuroplastic changes are considered both from a structural and functional level of adaptation, with a special focus on the recent findings from network science. The neural activity of the medial regions of the brain seems to become more synchronised when listening to music as compared to rest, and these changes become permanent in individuals such as musicians with year-long musical practice. As such, the question is raised as to the clinical and therapeutic applications of music as a trigger for enhancing the functionality of the brain, both in normal and impaired people.

Keywords: music, neuroplasticity, ontogenetic development, adaptation, connectivity, neurorehabilitation

1. Introduction

Going to concerts, listening to music in your living room, singing together or even playing an instrument is part of most people's everyday life. Recent research indicates that apart from just changing the current mood this may have long-lasting influences on the brain. This contribution, therefore, describes how music shapes the brain as the outcome of interactions with the sounds. These interactions can be multifarious, as in the case of performing, listening or mentally imaging music, but they all show complex and widespread activity in many areas of the brain. This activity, moreover, is related to training, previous exposure, personal preference, emotional involvement and many other modulating factors related to the cultural background and biological repertoire of each individual [1–7]. Musical training, moreover, is related to structural changes within auditory and motor areas of the brain and reinforces functional coupling of these regions during musical tasks as evidenced by many neuroimaging studies [8–10]. These changes have been observed also in white-matter tracts, such as the corpus callosum, the corticospinal tract and the arcuate fasciculus [11–13]. Studies (particularly those with a longitudinal design) showing the causal relation between the brain changes and the duration of musical training have convinced some researchers to consider musical training as a model for investigating practice-related brain plasticity in humans [14].

Music is a powerful stimulator of the brain. Acoustically, it consists of time-varying sound events that are characterised by a large number of features—more than hundred features can be computationally extracted that are tracked by several regions of the brain [15]. Many low-level features, such as timbre and pitch, are partly processed in Heschl's gyrus and the right anterior part of the superior temporal gyrus, in which the primary and non-primary auditory cortices are located [16, 17]. Besides auditory cortices, also motor regions, such as the supplementary motor area and the cerebellum, are involved during musical activities, including both playing and listening. Due to audio-motor coupling that is necessary for playing an instrument, listening is influenced by the motor demands intrinsic to musical practice, even to the extent that this would become manifest also in the brain responses to music listening alone [18, 19]. Moreover, practising and performing music is a complex, multimodal behaviour that requires extensive motor and cognitive abilities. It relies on immediate and accurate associations between motor sequences and auditory events leading to multimodal predictions [10, 20, 21], which engage broad networks of the brain [16, 22, 23]. Music training has thus been associated with changes in the brain, and some of these changes have been causally linked to the duration of the training, which makes the musician's brain a most interesting model for the study of neuroplasticity [9, 24]. This holds in particular for performing musicians, who provide a unique pool of subjects for investigating both the features of the expert brain and, when considering the length of the training, also the neural correlates of skill acquisition. Musicians' training and practice require the simultaneous integration of multimodal sensory and motor information in sensory and cognitive domains, combining skills in auditory perception, kinaesthetic control, visual perception and pattern recognition [25, 26]. In addition, musicians have the ability to memorise long and complex bimanual finger sequences and to translate musical symbols into motor sequences (see **Figure 1**). Some musicians are even able to perceive and identify tones in the absence of a reference tone, a rare ability termed absolute pitch [27, 28].

The brain changes that musical training entails are numerous and well-documented [2, 3, 5, 9, 24, 26–34]: they involve brain regions important for auditory processing, coordination of fast movements and cognitive control, as well as sensory-to-motor coupling mechanisms (see [35],

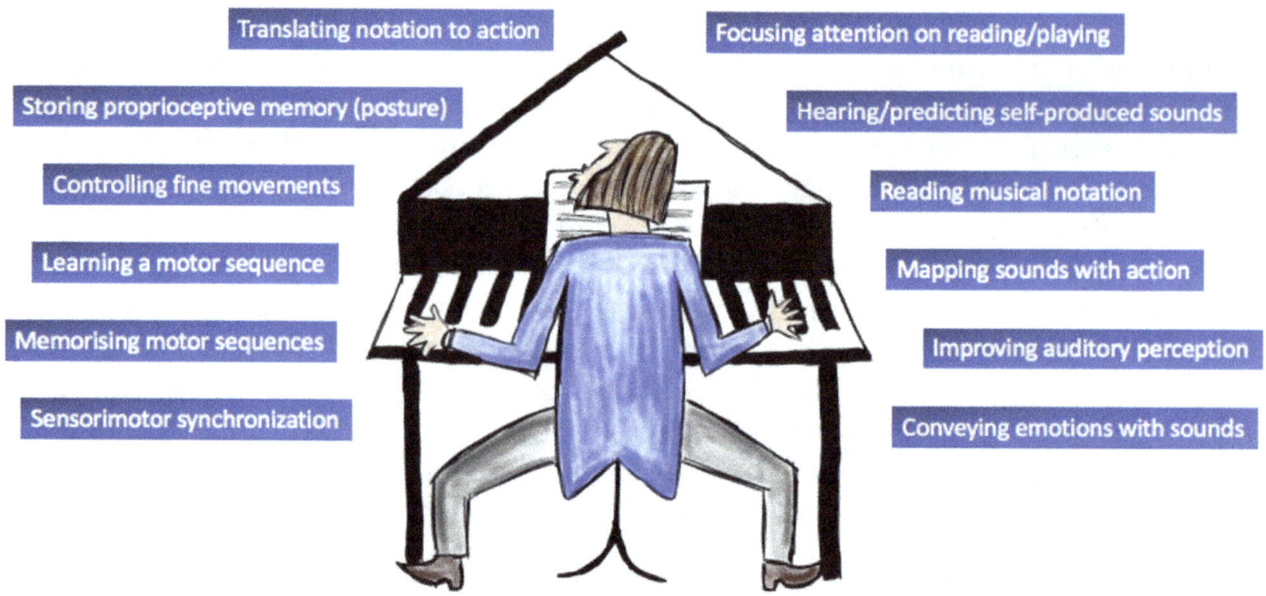

Figure 1. Illustration of several perceptual, motor, interoceptive and emotional skills that are acquired during musical training.

for an overview). While some of these changes might be what characterise individuals that decide to undertake a musical profession, and hence might exist at birth, others could be a direct result of training, as suggested by the significant relations between years of training and brain measures (e.g., [36]), as well as by longitudinal designs recording brain responses before and after music training (e.g., [29, 37]).

Here, we propose that the differences observed between the brains of musicians and non-musicians can be attributed to neuroplastic adaptations responding to the challenging demands of musical practice. Alternative explanations are also possible, such as that the differences exist even before training in those individuals that choose music as their profession, but accumulating evidence points at a causal relation between music training and brain changes. The behavioural correlates of these differences are multiple and can be seen especially in childhood (e.g., [38]). Besides, it has been shown that music may be beneficial in relation to a number of symptoms in several kinds of impairment, such as epilepsy, Alzheimer's disease, Parkinson's disease and senile dementia (see [39] for an overview). Hence, it is possible to conceive of dealing with music in educational, clinical and therapeutic terms.

In this contribution, we first expose the concept of adaptation, both from the phylogenetic and ontogenetic points of view. We then narrow down this concept by putting forward the hypothesis of music-induced neuroplasticity, with a first distinction between macrostructural and microstructural adaptations. Thereafter, we consider the reorganisation of the brain as the outcome of learning and skill acquisition, both at a structural and functional level of description with a major focus on the adult musician or listener as a model for the interaction between ontogeny and phylogeny. This latter, further, is considered from the point of view of network science with a major focus on the role of resting-state networks. Clinical and therapeutic applications, finally, are envisioned also.

2. Phylogenetic and ontogenetic claims: the role of adaptation

Brain plasticity is an adaptation to the environment with an evolutionary advantage. It allows an organism to be changed in order to survive in its environment by providing better tools for coping with the world [40]. This biological concept of adaptation can be approached from two different scales of description: the larger evolutionary scale of the human as a species (phylogeny) and the more limited scale of the human from newborn to old age (ontogeny). This phylogenetic/ontogenetic distinction is related to the "nature/nurture" and "culture/biology" dichotomy, which refers to the neurobiological claims of wired-in circuitry for perceptual information pickup as against the learned mechanisms for information processing and sense-making and immersion in a culture [41, 42].

These approaches may seem to be diverging at first glance, but they are complementary to some extent. This holds, in particular, for the here-hypothesised music-induced plasticity, which espouses a biocultural view that aims at a balance between genetic or biological constraints and historical/cultural contingencies. This places all human beings on equal ground (unity) by stating that diversity in culture is only an epiphenomenon of an underlying biological disposition that is shared by people all over the world [43]. The assumed unity is attributed to the neural constraints that underlie musical processing in general, but these constraints should not be considered as a static dispositional machinery. The picture that emerges from recent research is arguing, on the contrary, for a definition of the neural machinery as a dynamic system that is able to adapt in answer to the solicitations of a challenging environment [6]. The neurobiological approach to music, therefore, deals not only with the nature and evolution of the innate and wired-in neural mechanisms that are the hallmark of the hominid phylogenetic evolution but also with the ontogenetic development of these mechanisms [43]. As such, it makes sense to conflate neurobiological and developmental claims by taking the concept of adaptation as a working hypothesis.

The relation between adaptation and development, however, is asymmetrical in the sense that it is possible to conceive of development without adaptation, but no adaptation is conceivable without development. This development, further, can be natural, when it is the outcome of maturation, but it is possible also to intervene in its trajectory by combining development and learning. This is the case when an organism faces continued and long-term exposure to challenging environments, which triggers plastic changes in the structure and the functions of the brain. This brings us to the concept of brain plasticity, which refers to the fact that neuronal circuits are tuned in close interaction with the environment. It was introduced by William James, who defined plasticity as "the possession of a structure weak enough to yield to an influence, but strong enough not to yield all at once" [44] (p. 106). The idea was further developed by Ramón y Cajal, who claimed that to fully understand the phenomenon it is necessary to admit the formation of new pathways in the brain through ramification and progressive growth of the dendritic arborisation and the nervous terminals in addition to the reinforcement of pre-established organic pathways. The same idea was elaborated further by Donald Hebb, who proposed that neuronal cortical connections are strengthened and remodelled by experience. There is, however, another aspect of plasticity that goes beyond the level of synapses and that incorporates the level of cortical representation areas or cortical maps, which can be modified by sensory input and training [45]. It is suggested, in this regard, that additional neurons are recruited when they are needed and that rapid and transient alterations of cortical representations can be seen during learning tasks. Such short-term modulations are important in the acquisition of new skills, but they can lead also to structural changes in the intra-cortical and sub-cortical network once the skill has been established.

3. Neuroplasticity and music: macrostructural and microstructural adaptations

The evolutionary claims of adaptation—both at the phylogenetic and ontogenetic level—have received empirical evidence from neuroimaging and morphometric studies. In order to elucidate its underlying mechanisms, there is currently a whole body of research related to the psychobiological approach to the study of action, cognition and perception. A major claim in this research field is that the nervous system provides the immediate, necessary and sufficient mechanisms that underlie all mental processes, and that mental processes are reducible to the function, arrangement and interaction of neurons as the constituent building blocks of the nervous system [46]. This is the axiom of psychobiological equivalence, which claims an equivalence of maintained information from the neural to the psychological state [47]. The related research revolves around three major themes: (i) the localisation of functions in the brain, (ii) the representation or coding and (iii) the dynamic change or learning [46]. The first investigates which brain structures are responsive for particular processes. The second investigates how neural networks represent, encode or instantiate cognitive processes, both at macrostructural and microstructural level of description (see [48]). The third, finally, investigates how our brain adapts to experience and learning, what changes occur in its neural networks and how these changes correspond to externally observed behaviour.

The third theme—dynamic change or learning—concerns the neural correlates of skill acquisition and has been studied mainly at the level of perceptual processing and motor output. Yet, there is also the whole domain of creativity [49], musical aesthetics [6, 50–53] and human interaction [54, 55], which have been poorly investigated in relation to long-term music training. However, the topic is exemplary of a paradigm shift in current neuromusicological research, with a transition from a static conception of brain modules to a conception of reorganisational plasticity of the developing and adult brain [6]. Plasticity, in fact, is a fundamental organisational feature of the human brain, which can be modified throughout the life span in response to changes in environmental stimulation. This has been observed not only during a critical period in the developing brain but also even throughout the whole life span.

Skill learning, such as learning to play a musical instrument, can thus be used for the study of neuroplasticity. It typically starts early in life, while the brain is most sensitive to plastic changes, and continues often throughout life. It involves multiple sensory modalities and motor planning, preparation and execution systems [27, 56]. The role of environmental enrichment—being defined as a combination of complex inanimate and social stimulation [57]—on the other hand, should be stressed also as an emerging area of research. Music, in this view, can be considered as "sounding environment" [42], which is likely to drive brain plasticity. Even in the foetal phase of development, sounds can trigger ways of implicit learning [58]. Neonates and infants also learn to talk and sing quasi-effortless as the result of mere exposure, thus demonstrating implicit learning and developmental plasticity, which is even cross-modal to a large extent, in the sense that loss of one sensory modality may lead to neural organisation of the remaining modalities [2].

Neuroplasticity is also related to the field of sensory-motor learning, with a major role attributed to the challenges of a rich environment. It favours multiple interactions with the world—both at the sensory and at the motor level—stressing the interdependency of an organism and its environment through which it "enriches its repertory of genetic adaptations with acquired dispositions that are immediately at hand and mobilizable when confronted with a situation that can be foreseen or recognized as a familiar one" [59] (p. 925).

Musical training, accordingly, may be related to sensory and motor changes in the human brain of professional musicians. As a rule, music training involves years of sensory-motor training, often beginning in early childhood, with the aim to develop an expertise in a chosen instrument or mastery over the own voice, together with an improvement of the ability to attend to the fine-grained acoustics of musical sounds, including pitch, timing and timbre [3]. The brains of musicians might adapt to the demands of their instrumental practice at two levels: the gross anatomical differences between professional musicians and amateurs or laymen, and the subtle functional differences after enhanced musical practice and/or experience, which have to be sought in ever finer modifications of synaptic strength in distributed cortical networks. As such, it is possible to distinguish between macrostructural and microstructural adaptations. The macrostructural differences related to volume, morphology, density and connectivity of brain structures are measured with magnetic resonance imaging (MRI), whereas the microstructural differences in the functional activity of brain regions are measured with functional magnetic resonance imaging (fMRI), positron emission tomography (PET) and neurophysiology (electroencephalography, EEG and magnetoencephalography [MEG]) (see [5] for an overview). It is further hypothesised that functional reorganisation may cause structural adaptation. For instance, bimanual instrument training, such as for the piano, may cause an increase in cortical functionality for symmetric areas involved in motor, auditory and visuospatial processing, as well as in the white matter tracts of the corpus callosum [20] as compared with less bimanual training (such that for the violin) and especially as opposed to laypersons.

At the macrostructural level, studies show differences in the size of the primary motor cortex size, the cerebellum, the planum temporale, the corpus callosum, Heschl's gyrus and the arcuate fasciculus, all of which seem to correlate with the ability of musicians to identify and process acoustic variations [60]. The microstructural adaptations, on the other hand, happen at the level of individual neurons and synapses, with the aim to change the efficacy of neural connectivity. In general, the brain shows adaptation to extraordinary challenges by giving birth to new neurons (neurogenesis) and glial cells and by the formation and remodelling of new connections by the outgrowth of dendrites, axonal sprouting and increasing or strengthening of synaptic connections [61] (see **Box 1** for an overview). Such adaptations have been studied in the context of deafferentation studies—in the case of brain lesion—and in the case of motor skill learning [62]. In the former, some cortical remodelling has been found, including microstructural changes, such as the strengthening of existing synapses, the formation of new synapses (synaptogenesis), axonal sprouting and dendrite growth. In the latter, similar changes have been found, including an increased number of synapses per neuron and changes in the number of microglia and capillaries [63], which all lead to volumetric changes that are detectable also at the macrostructural level [27, 64].

The bulk of studies on neuroplasticity has been performed in the context of within-modality plasticity, particularly in the domain of sensory and motor modalities. They aim at demonstrating the adaptive capabilities of the human brain to shape the processing of sensory stimuli or to perform motor acts after repeated sensory exposure or action [9]. With regard to the sensory modality, animal studies have shown that environmental change critically affects brain development. Experience-driven neural activity, in fact, regulates the refinement of the neural circuitry by influencing various neural processes, such as synapse formation, pruning and synaptic plasticity (see **Box 1**) with modifications in synaptic connectivity as a result [65]. This enhanced connectivity, further, acts as a basis for learning and memory through alterations at the level of neural circuits [66], such as strengthening or weakening of the synaptic links or altering their number, changes in the number or properties of postsynaptic receptors in transmitter release and the formation of new synapses. The result is an increase in synaptic strength, which may be persistent and facilitate learning and memory so that experience-dependent plasticity could involve selective changes in pre-existing brain circuits [65].

As to the enhanced auditory skills, it has been argued that they may prime the brain for the processing of musical sounds and that these skills may percolate to other domains, such as speech, emotion and auditory processing in general [67, 68]. This has been observed already in the early stages of the auditory pathway, which are located mainly in the brainstem. Musicians have enhanced temporal and frequency coding in the auditory brainstem with

Myelinisation: the acquisition, development or formation of a myelin sheath around a nerve fibre. This fatty coating serves as insulation of individual fibres to enhance specificity of connections and increases markedly the quick and accurate transmission of electrical current from one nerve cell to another.

Pruning: a process that helps sculpt the adult brain and by which neurons and synaptic connections that are no longer used or useful are eliminated in order to increase the efficiency of neuronal transmissions.

Sprouting: a process by which a neuron generates additional branches or outgrowths to establish new links between existing neurons, as seen frequently in the case of growth of axons or dendrites from a damaged or intact neuron that projects to an area that is denervated.

Synaptic plasticity: strengthening or weakening of the synaptic links either by modulating the strength of synapses or by altering their numbers.

Synaptic efficacy: changes in the number or properties of postsynaptic receptors in transmitter release and the formation of new synapses (synaptogenesis).

Adult neurogenesis: birth of neurons from neural stem cells in the adult brain. In humans, adult neurogenesis has been shown to occur only in the hippocampus (particularly in the sub-granular zone of the dentate gyrus) and in the striatum. It differs from developmental neurogenesis.

Box 1. Overview of some basic mechanisms for refinement of the neural circuitry earlier (as early as 10 ms after acoustic onset) and larger responses than non-musicians to both speech and music stimuli. This has been shown for the onset response and the frequency-following response (FFR), i.e., a neuronal ensemble response that phase-locks to the incoming stimulus and that underlies perception of pitch as it relates to the sustained portion of a periodic sound with less or more stable frequencies [68, 69].

The role of auditory brainstem processing of behaviourally relevant sounds such as speech and music is important here. It can be measured by using the onset response and the FFR to see how the brainstem represents pitch, timing and timbre [68]. It has been shown that both temporal and spectral characteristics of sounds are preserved in this subcortical response (see [70] for an overview), reflecting the physical properties of sound with an unrivalled fidelity. As a rule, it occurs automatically at pre-attentive levels of auditory processing but is shaped by both long-term and short-term experience [71–73]. Subcortical function, moreover, is neither passive nor hardwired but interacts dynamically with higher-level cognitive processes refining the transcription of sounds into neural code. Hence, the responses do not originate merely in the brainstem but receive feedback from top-down cortical influences even at the earliest stages of auditory processing [3] via corticofugal feedback pathways [74, 75]. As such, it can be demonstrated that musical practice changes the early sensory encoding of auditory stimuli [68] relying on a top-down feedback system—consisting of efferent effects on cochlear biomechanics—that is continuously and automatically engaged to extract and represent regularities in the auditory system [3]. Musical training is thus not limited to the modification of cortical organisation but the modifications extend to subcortical sensory structures and generalise to early processing of speech and sounds in general.

Moreover, early auditory evoked responses and particularly the negative–positive complex (N19-P30) in the auditory evoked potential [76] localised in the primary auditory cortex (the anteromedial portion of Heschl's gyrus) have been found to be larger in musicians compared to amateurs and non-musicians. Moreover, it has been found that the generating neural tissue, namely the grey matter volume of the primary auditory cortex, was broader in volume for professional musicians [77] as compared to laypersons. It thus seems that music can trigger both macrostructural and microstructural or functional changes, not as separate and distinct levels of adaptations, but as phenomena that are dynamically and tightly interconnected.

4. Music facilitates neural connectivity

Music can trigger plastic changes in the brain, as evidenced by the rich history of structural and functional neuroimaging studies of the past decades. Recent advances in functional neuroimaging have furthermore provided new tools for measuring the functional interactions and communication between distinct regions in the brain and for examining their functional connectivity [78]. In an attempt to study the brain as a complex network of functionally and structurally interconnected regions, a fuller understanding of its organisation and function is proposed by relying on the contributions of network science [79], which investigates complex systems in terms of their elements and the relationships and interactions between these elements.

Functional connectivity can be defined as the temporal dependence of neuronal activity patterns of anatomically separated and removed regions in the brain, reflecting the level of communication between them [80]. It makes it possible to examine the brain as an integrative network of functionally interacting regions and to gain new insights into large-scale neuronal communication in the human brain. Such whole-brain connectivity patterns can be studied by measuring the synchronisation of spontaneous fMRI or MEEG time-series reflecting neural activity of anatomically separated brain regions, which are recorded during rest. These resting–state networks are believed to reflect the functional communication between brain regions [78, 81] and suggest an ongoing information processing and functional connectivity between them even at rest, which is related to neuronal firing. The pattern of correlations between distinct brain areas, moreover, points at the existence of organisational networks in the brain [81], which seems to be analogous to the networks that are engaged during the performance of sensory-motor and cognitive tasks, and which are dependent upon the brain's anatomical connectivity [10]. Such spontaneous neuronal interaction has been first investigated in motor cortices but were later extended to other cortical systems, such as the visual and auditory networks, the default mode network (DMN) and attention and memory related regions. It has been suggested that at least 10–12 resting-state networks (RSNs) can be detected in the cerebral cortex in resting state, which implicates that they represent some intrinsic form of brain connectivity with temporal correlations between spatially discrete regions [82].

DMN has been related to specific brain functions, such as self-referential thoughts, emotional perspectives and levels of self-awareness. DMN is believed to be a neural circuit that constantly monitors the sensory environment and displays high activity during lack of focused attention on external events [83]. It seems to function as a toggle switch between outwardly focused mind states and the internal or subjective sense of self [84] and can be used to explore the functional connections of the complex integrative network of functionally linked brain regions, which continuously share information with each other. As such, there are interconnected resting-state neuronal communities or functional brain networks with functional communication between them. Being organised according to an efficient topology, they combine efficient local information processing with efficient global information integration with the most pronounced functional connections found between those regions that share common functions.

Overall, resting-state fMRI oscillations reflect ongoing functional communication between distinct brain regions [78], which makes them indicative of the level of cognitive functioning in general. There seems to be, in fact, a link between an efficient organisation of the brain network and intellectual performance—this is the neural efficiency hypothesis—so that functional connectivity patterns may be used as a powerful predictor for cognitive performance [85]. This resting-state connectivity, further, is not to be considered as an established and fixed property, but as a state that can be modulated by recent experiences and learning episodes, both within and between the networks they recruit. Such modulation points in the direction of a learning consolidation function of resting-state brain activity, as evidenced by the findings that high learners manifest stronger pre-task resting-state functional connectivity between the involved regions than low learners [10]. It thus seems that, even in the absence of external stimuli or demands, the brain is constantly sharing information. It thus consolidates recent learning and maintains the association of activity of brain areas that are likely to be used together in future [86].

Initial research suggests that musical training might enhance this pattern of increased resting-state connectivity by triggering heightened connections at a functional level between those brain regions that are structurally and functionally altered as the result of training. This is manifested even during a task-free condition, pointing to the "silent" imprint of musical training on the human brain [35]. Research on the differences between musicians and non-musicians in their functional connectivity during rest, however, is still in its infancy [10, 82]. By selecting predefined seed regions for computing connectivity analysis, increased connectivity between contralateral homologue regions has been found in musicians between prefrontal, temporal, inferior-parietal and premotor areas [35]. It is to be questioned, however, whether the study of predefined regions or seed regions does not neglect residual whole-brain dynamics. However, for the seed regions for which plastic changes in musicians have been found already—as evidenced by increased grey matter volume—connectivity analyses have revealed brain areas whose resting-state time series activity was more closely synchronised with one of them. Four networks were found to supply integrative interpretations for the cognitive functions during musical practice: (i) autobiographical memory-related regions belonging to the default mode network, recruited by the encoding, storage and recall of melodies with an emotional and biographical quality; (ii) areas that belong to the salience network with access to semantic memory that is related to the storage of music in terms of verbal labels and auditory structure; (iii) regions that are implied in language processing and the resting-state auditory network and (iv) structures that belong to the executive control network, and which could subserve the motor modulation required for an emotionally expressive interpretation of music. The question whether this practice-related plasticity is triggered by local grey matter volume, however, is not yet satisfactorily resolved, in the sense that other variables may be implicated in the expertise-related resting-state functional reorganisation of musician's plastic brain [10].

5. Clinical and therapeutic applications

To stretch further our hypothesis about music-induced neuroplastic adaptation, music, as a cognitive-demanding activity stimulating neuroplasticity, may be able to slow down, arrest or even reverse the detrimental effects of ageing on learning and memory capacity of the elderly [33]. Recent studies have provided evidence that music-induced plasticity may help also to overcome neurological impairments, such as neurodevelopmental disorders and acquired brain injuries [56]. For instance, attentive music listening recruits multiple forms of working memory, attention, semantic processing, target detection and motor function, relying mainly on bilateral brain areas—superior temporal gyrus, intraparietal sulcus, precentral sulcus, inferior sulcus and gyrus, and frontal operculum—which all serve general functions rather than music-specific cortical regions [87, 88]. Complex musical tasks, moreover, engage the co-activation of many processes involving widely distributed and partly interchangeable substrates of the brain [89]. This may explain, to some extent, the sparing of some musical functions in cases of progressive destruction of some areas in degenerative diseases of the brain. This has been shown most typically in the case of Alzheimer's disease (AD), which is characterised by a general and progressive decline in cognitive function, with the first symptom as an impaired episodic memory. Music, in this case, has been reported as one of the domains in which general skill and memory are preserved in spite of otherwise severe impairment [90]. This preserved musical processing, moreover, is not limited to procedural memory but often includes also stories of music, which can be used as an effective mnemonic device [91].

Hence, music may shape the development of normal and healthy human beings over the lifespan, but its potential as a non-pharmacological interventional aid for caregivers to help the cognitive and emotional capacity of patients with neurological and psychiatric brain disorders is receiving growing interest [15]. The use of resting-state fMRI techniques, e.g., with a main focus on the default mode network, seems to be well-suited to examine possible functional disconnectivity effects in disorders such as Alzheimer's disease, depression, dementia and schizophrenia. Also, other neurogenerative diseases like multiple sclerosis and amyotrophic lateral sclerosis seem to show changed connectivity in the default network as well as in other resting-state networks [78]. This may suggest that neurodegenerative diseases would attack interconnected cortical networks rather than single regions in the brain [92] and can thus be targets of a music intervention aimed at stabilising abnormal patterns of functional connectivity between compromised brain areas.

Music has been used already as a treatment for some psychiatric and neurological pathologies, such as schizophrenic disorders, Alzheimer's disease, Parkinson's disease, cerebral ischemia, pain, autism, anxiety and depression [15]. Music, furthermore, has been reported to improve also the well-being and cognitive functions in healthy adults, such as autobiographical memory, semantic memory, language ability and cognitive functions, and to alleviate neuropsychiatric symptoms, such as agitation, apathy, depression and anxiety (see [39] for an overview). Effects of music on AD are exemplary of the mechanisms that might mediate the impact of music on human well-being. Latent benefits of musical mnemonics as an aid to standard mnemonic methods, which may seem to be insufficient for AD patients, have been reported (for a review, see [15]). The mechanisms behind these memory-enhancing effects, however, are still not fully understood, but there is strong evidence for a benefit of music as a mnemonic device in a variety of clinical settings [91]. A possible explanation is that the areas of the brain associated with music cognition are preferentially spared in the case of AD. It has been suggested that procedural memory and priming effects for musical stimuli remain intact, whereas short-term and long-term episodic memory for melodic excerpts is impaired [93].

This dissociation between memory and general performance in AD patients holds in particular for listening to their favourite songs, which seems to recruit previously encoded memories. These memories seem to support and sustain brain introspection via connectivity within the default mode network and also to effectively reprocess autobiographic and episodic memories [84]. An additional explanation for this dissociation is that in patients with general cortical and hippocampal atrophy, which impairs standard episodic learning, musically-associated stimuli allow for a more diversified encoding. Music processing, in that case, encompasses a neural network that is recruiting from multiple areas of the brain, including cortical as well as subcortical areas. Musical stimuli and stimuli accompanied by music seem to create a more robust association at the stage of encoding and support a more composite encoding and retrieval process by inducing oscillatory synchrony in those neural networks that are associated with learning and memory [91, 94].

6. Conclusion and perspectives

Neuroplasticity is now an established topic in music and brain studies. Revolving around the concept of adaptation, it has been found that the brain is able to adapt its structure and function to cope with the solicitations of a challenging environment. This concept can be studied in the context of music performance studies and long-term and continued musical practice. It has been shown that some short-term plastic changes can even occur in the case of merely listening to music—without actually performing—(e.g., [95]) and in the short-time perspective of both listening and performing (e.g., [96]). Attentive listening to music in a real-time situation, in fact, is very demanding: it recruits multiple forms of memory, attention, semantic processing, target detection and motor function [18, 97]. As such, we propose here that music represents a sort of enriched environment that invites the brain to raise its general level of conscious functioning.

Traditional research on musical listening and training, however, has focussed mainly on structural changes, both at the level of macro- and microstructural adaptations. This has been well-documented with morphometric studies, which aimed at showing volumetric changes of target areas in the brain as the outcome of intensive musical practice. Recent contributions, however, have shown that the brain can be studied also from the viewpoint of network science. The brain, in this view, is not to be considered as an aggregate of isolated regions, but as a dynamic system that is characterised by multiple functional interactions and communication between distinct regions of the brain. Whole-brain connectivity patterns can be studied by measuring the co-activation of separate regions. Much is to be expected from the study of resting-state networks with a special focus on the default mode network. These networks seem to be indicative of the level of cognitive functioning in general and are subject to the possibility of modulation by experience and learning, both in the developing and in the mature brain. We propose that music has the potential to alter the organisation of these brain networks and enhance the connectivity of the brain, both in normal people and in those with an impaired brain.

A major emerging topic, therefore, is the tension between neurogenerative and neurodegenerative forces with the critical question as to the possible role of music as an intervening force to develop, maintain or even restore the connectivity in brain tissue. The idea that age-related cognitive decline may be slowed, arrested or even reversed through appropriately designed training or activities, such as musical practice, is supported already by some research. Moreover, the finding that the adult brain can undergo continual modifications highlights the potential of music intervention for inducing the plastic changes that can ultimately attenuate the impairments due to brain injury. Much more research, however, is still needed towards an integration of findings from neuroscience, education, music therapy and development.

Author details

Mark Reybrouck[1,2]*, Peter Vuust[3] and Elvira Brattico[3]

*Address all correspondence to: mark.reybrouck@kuleuven.be

1 Musicology Research Group, KU Leuven – University of Leuven, Belgium

2 IPEM Institute for Systematic Musicology, Ghent University, Belgium

3 Department of Clinical Medicine, Center for Music in the Brain, Aarhus University and The Royal Academy of Music, Aarhus/Aalborg, Denmark

References

[1] Altenmüller E. Apollo's gift and curse: Brain plasticity in musicians. Karger's Gazette. 2009;**70**:8-10. DOI: http://www.karger.com/gazette/70/altenmueller/art_4.htm

[2] Johansson B. Music and brain plasticity. European Review. 2006;**14**:49-64. DOI: 10.1017/s1062798706000056

[3] Kraus N, Chandrasekaran B. Music training for the development of auditory skills. Nature Reviews Neuroscience. 2010;**11**:599-605. DOI: 10.1038/nrn2882

[4] Miendlarzewska EA, Trost WJ. How musical training affects cognitive development: Rhythm, reward and other modulating variables. Frontiers in Neuroscience. 2013;**7**:279. DOI: 10.3389/fnins.2013.00279

[5] Merrett DL, Peretz I, Wilson SJ. Moderating variables of music training-induced neuroplasticity: A review and discussion. Frontiers in Psychology. 2013;**4**:606. DOI: 10.3389/fpsyg.2013.00606

[6] Reybrouck M, Brattico E. Neuroplasticity beyond sounds: Neural adaptations following long-term musical aesthetic experiences. Brain Sciences. 2015;**5**:69-91. DOI: 10.3390/brainsci5010069

[7] Vuust P, Liikala L, Näätänen R, Brattico P, Brattico E. Comprehensive auditory discrimination profiles recorded with a fast parametric musical multi-feature mismatch negativity paradigm. Clinical Neurophysiology. 2016;**127**:2065-2077. DOI: http://dx.doi.org/10.1016/j.clinph.2015.11.009

[8] Bangert M, Peschel T, Schlaug G, Rotte M, Drescher D, Hinrichs H, Heinze H-J, Altenmüller E. Shared networks for auditory and motor processing in professional pianists: Evidence from fMRI conjunction. NeuroImage. 2006;**30**:917-926. DOI: 10.1016/j.neuroimage.2005.10.044

[9] Münte TF, Altenmüller E, Jancke L. The musician's brain as a model of neuroplasticity. Nature Reviews Neuroscience. 2002;**3**:473-477. DOI: 10.1038/nrn843

[10] Fauvel B, Groussard M, Chételat G, Fouquet M, Landeau B, Eustache F, Desgranges B, Platel H. Morphological brain plasticity induced by musical expertise is accompanied by modulation of functional connectivity at rest. NeuroImage. 2014;**90**:179-188. DOI: 10.1016/j.neuroimage.2013.12.065

[11] Bengtsson SL, Nagy Z, Skare S, Forsman L, Forssberg H, Ullén F. Extensive piano practicing has regionally specific effects on white matter development. Nature Neuroscience. 2005;**8**:1148-1150. DOI: 10.1038/nn1516

[12] Imfeld A, Oechslin M, Meyer M, Loenneker T, Jancke L. White matter plasticity in the corticospinal tract of musicians: A diffusion tensor imaging study. NeuroImage. 2009; **46**:600-607. DOI: 10.1016/j.neuroimage.2009.02.025

[13] Öztürk HA, Tascioglu B, Aktekin M, Kurtoglu Z, Erden I. Morphometric comparison of the human corpus callosum in professional musicians and nonmusicians by using in vivo magnetic resonance imaging. Journal of Neuroradiology. 2002;**29**:29-34

[14] Fauvel B, Groussard M, Eustache F, Desgranges B, Platel H. Neural implementation of musical expertise and cognitive transfers: Could they be promising in the framework of normal cognitive aging? Frontiers in Human Neuroscience. 2013;**7**:693. DOI: http://dx.doi.org/10.3389/ fnhum.2013.00693

[15] Matrone C, Brattico E. The power of music on Alzheimer's disease and the need to understand the underlying molecular mechanisms. Journal of Alzheimer's Disease & Parkinsonism. 2015;**5**:1-7. DOI: 10.4172/2161-0460.1000196

[16] Alluri V, Toivianen P, Jääskeläinen I, Glerean E, Sams M, Brattico E. Large-scale brain networks emerge from dynamic processing of musical timbre, key and rhythm. NeuroImage. 2012;**59**:3677-3689. DOI: S1053-8119(11)01300-0 [pii]

[17] Brattico E. Cortical Processing of Musical Pitch as Reflected by Behavioural and Electrophysiological Evidence. Yliopistopaino: Helsinki; 2006

[18] Alluri V, Toiviainen P, Burunat I, Kliuchko M, Vuust P, Brattico E. Connectivity patterns during music listening: Evidence for action-based processing in musicians. Human Brain Mapping. 2017;**38**:2955-2970. DOI: 10.1002/hbm.23565

[19] Burunat I, Tsatsishvili V, Brattico E, Toiviainen P. Coupling of action-perception brain networks during musical pulse processing: Evidence from region-of-interest-based independent component analysis. Frontiers in Human Neuroscience. 2017;**11**:230. DOI: 10.3389/fnhum.2017.00230

[20] Burunat I, Brattico E, Puoliväli T, Ristaniemi T, Sams M, Toiviainen P. Action in perception: Prominent Visuo-motor functional symmetry in musicians during music listening. PLoS One. 2015;**30**:1-18. DOI: https://doi.org/10.1371/journal.pone.0138238

[21] Pantev C, Herholz SC. Plasticity of the human auditory cortex related to musical training. Neuroscience & Biobehavioral Reviews. 2011;**35**:2140-2154. DOI: 10.1016/j.neubiorev.2011.06.010

[22] Pallesen KJ, Brattico E, Bailey CJ, Korvenoja A, Koivisto J, Gjedde A, Carlson S. Cognitive control in auditory working memory is enhanced in musicians. PLoS One. 2010;**5**:e11120. DOI: https://doi.org/10.1371/journal.pone.0011120

[23] Abrams DA, Ryali S, Chen T, Chordia P, Khouzam A, Levitin D, Menon V. Inter-subject synchronization of brain responses during natural music listening. European Journal of Neuroscience. 2013;**37**:1458-1469. DOI: 10.1111/ejn.12173

[24] Habib M, Besson M. What do music training and musical experience teach us about brain plasticity? Music Perception. 2009;**26**:279-285. DOI: 10.1525/mp.2009.26.3.279

[25] Barrett K, Ashley R, Strait D, Kraus N. Art and science: How musical training shapes the brain. Frontiers in Psychology. 2013;**4**(713). DOI: https://doi.org/10.3389/fpsyg.2013.00713

[26] Gaser C, Schlaug G. Brain Structures differ between musicians and non-musicians. The Journal of Neuroscience. 2003;**23**:9240-9245

[27] Schlaug G. The brain of musicians. A model for functional and structural adaptation. Annals of the New York Academy of Sciences. 2001;**930**:281-299

[28] Schlaug G, Marchina S, Norton A. Evidence for plasticity in white-matter tracts of patients with chronic Broca's aphasia undergoing intense intonation-based speech therapy. Annals of the New York Academy of Sciences. 2009;**1169**:385-394. DOI: 10.1111/j.1749-6632.2009.04587.x

[29] Hyde K, Lerch J, Norton A, Forgeard M, Winner E, Evans A, Schlaug G. Musical training shapes structural brain development. Journal of Neuroscience. 2009;**29**:3019-3025. DOI: https://doi.org/10.1523/JNEUROSCI.5118-08.2009

[30] Gärtner H, Minnerop M, Pieperhoff P, Zilles K, Altenmüller E, Amunts K. Brain morphometry shows effects of long-term musical practice in middle-aged keyboard players. Frontiers in Psychology. 2013;**4**. DOI: 10.3389/fpsyg.2013.00636

[31] Jäncke L. Music drives brain plasticity. F1000Reports Biology. 2009;**1**. DOI: 10.3410/B1-78

[32] Stewart L. Do musicians have different brains? Clinical Medicine. 2008;**8**:304-308

[33] Wan C, Schlaug G. Music making as a tool for promoting brain plasticity across the life span. The Neuroscientist. 2010;**16**:566-577. DOI: 10.1177/1073858410377805

[34] Pascual-Leone A. The brain that makes music and is changed by it. In: Peretz I, Zatorre R, editors. The Cognitive Neuroscience of Music. Oxford – New York: Oxford University Press; 2003. pp. 396-409

[35] Klein C, Liem F, Hänggi J, Elmer S, Jäncke L. The "silent" imprint of musical training. Human Brain Mapping. 2016;**37**:536-546. DOI: 10.1002/hbm.23045

[36] Brattico E, Pallesen KJ, Varyagina O, Bailey C, Anourova I, Jarvenpaa M, Eerola T, Tervaniemi M. Neural discrimination of nonprototypical chords in music experts and laymen: An MEG study. Journal of Cognitive Neuroscience. 2009;**21**:2230-2244. DOI: 10.1162/jocn.2008.21144

[37] Lahav A, Saltzman E, Schlaug G. Action representation of sound: Audiomotor recognition network while listening to newly acquired actions. Journal of Neuroscience. 2007; **27**:308-314. DOI: 10.1523/JNEUROSCI.4822-06.2007

[38] Schellenberg EG, Peretz I. Music, language and cognition: Unresolved issues. Trends in Cognitive Sciences. 2008;**12**:45-46

[39] Ueda T, Suzukamo Y, Sato M, Izumi S. Effects of music therapy on behavioral and psychological symptoms of dementia: A systematic review and meta-analysis. Aging Research Reviews. 2013;**12**:628-641. DOI: 10.1016/j.arr.2013.02.003

[40] Fleagle J. Primate Adaptation and Evolution. San Diego: Academic Press; 1999

[41] Reybrouck M. From sound to music: An evolutionary approach to musical semantics. Biosemiotics. 2013;**6**:585-606. DOI: https://doi.org/10.1007/s12304-013-9192-6

[42] Reybrouck M. Music as environment: An ecological and biosemiotic approach. Behavioral Sciences. 2015;**5**:1-26. DOI: 10.3390/bs5010001

[43] Brown S, Merker B, Wallin N. An introduction to evolutionary musicology. In: Wallin N, Merker B, Brown S, editors. The Origins of Music. Cambridge, MA – London: The MIT Press; 2000. pp. 3-24

[44] James W. The Principles of Psychology. Vol. 1. New York: Holt; 1890

[45] Kaas J. Plasticity of sensory and motor maps in adult mammals. Annuals Reviews of Neurosciences. 1991;**114**:137-167. DOI: 10.1146/annurev.ne.14.030191.001033

[46] Uttal W. The Psychobiology of Mind. Hillsdale, NJ: Lawrence Erlbaum; 1978

[47] Reybrouck M. Musical universals and the axiom of psychobiological equivalence. In: Leroy J-J, editor. Topicality of Musical Universals/Actualité des Universaux musicaux Paris. France: Editions des Archives Contemporaines; 2013. pp. 31-44

[48] Deco G, Kringelbach M. Great expectations: Using whole-brain computational connectomics for understanding neuropsychiatric disorders. Neuron. 2014;**84**:892-905. DOI: 10.1016/j.neuron.2014.08.034

[49] Sachs ME, Ellis RE, Schlaug G, Loui P. Brain connectivity reflects human aesthetic responses. Social Cognitive and Affective Neuroscience. 2016;**11**:1-8. DOI: 10.1093/scan/nsw009

[50] Brattico E. From pleasure to liking and back: Bottom-up and top-down neural routes to the aesthetic enjoyment of music. In: Nadal M, Houston JP, Agnati L, Mora F, Cela Conde CJ, editors. Art, Aesthetics, and the Brain. Oxford – New York: Oxford University Press; 2015. pp. 303-318

[51] Brattico E, Bogert B, Jacobsen T. Toward a neural chronometry for the aesthetic experience of music. Frontiers in Psychology. 2013;**4**:1-21. DOI: doi.org/10.3389/fpsyg.2013.00206

[52] Brattico P, Brattico E, Vuust P. Global sensory qualities and aesthetic experience in music. Frontiers in Neuroscience. 2017;**11**:59. DOI: 10.3389/fnins.2017.00159

[53] Brattico E, Pearce M. The neuroaesthetics of music. Psychology of Aesthetics, Creativity, and the Arts. 2013;**7**:48-61 http://dx.doi.org/10.1037/a0031624

[54] Brattico E, Vuust P. Brain-to-brain coupling and culture as prerequisites for musical interaction. In: Lesaffre M, Leman M, Maes P-J, editors. The Routledge Companion to Embodied Music Interaction. Abingdon-on-Thames, UK: Routledge; 2016

[55] Konvalinka I, Roepstorff A. The two-brain approach: How can mutually interacting brains teach us something about social interaction? Frontiers in Neuroscience. 2012;**6**:215. DOI: 10.3389/fnhum.2012.00215

[56] Schlaug G. Musicians and music making as a model for the study of the brain. Progress in Brain Research. 2015;**217**:37-54. DOI: 10.1016/bs.pbr.2014.11.020

[57] van Praag H, Kempermann G, Gage F. Neural consequences of environmental enrichment. Nature Reviews Neuroscience. 2000;**1**:191-198. DOI: 10.1038/35044558

[58] Gerhardt K, Abrams R. Fetal exposures to sound and vibroacoustic stimulation. Journal of Perinatology. 2000;**20**:20-S29

[59] Paillard J. La conscience. In: Richelle M. Requin J, Robert M, editors. Traité de psychologie expérimentale. Vol. 2. Paris: Presses Universitaires de France; 1994. pp. 639-684

[60] Schneider P, Sluming V, Roberts N, Bleeck S, Rupp A. Structural, functional, and perceptual differences in Heschl's gyrus and musical instrument preference. Annals of the New York Academy of Sciences. 2005;**1060**:387-394. DOI: 10.1196/annals.1360.033

[61] Chen JL, Nedivi E. Neuronal structural remodeling; is it all about access? Current Opinion in Neurobioly. 2010;**20**:557-562. DOI: 10.1016/j.conb.2010.06.002

[62] Ziemann U, Hallet M, Cohen LG. Mechanisms of deafferentation-induced plasticity in human motor cortex. Journal of Neuroscience. 1998;**18**:7000-7007

[63] Segal M. Dendritic spines: Morphological building blocks of memory. Neurobiology of Learning and Memory. 2017;**138**:3-9. DOI: 10.1016/j.nlm.2016.06.007

[64] Hutchinson S, Hui-Lin Lee L, Gaab N, Schlaug G. Cerebellar volume in musicians. Cerebral Cortex. 2003;**13**:943-949. DOI: https://doi.org/10.1093/cercor/13.9.943

[65] Chaudhury S, Chandra Nag T, Wadhwa S. Effect of prenatal auditory stimulation on numerical synaptic density and mean synaptic height in the posthatch day 1 chick hippocampus. Synapse. 2008;**63**:152-159. DOI: 10.1002/syn.20585

[66] Martin SJ, Morris RG. New life in an old idea: The synaptic plasticity and memory hypothesis revisited. Hippocampus. 2002;**12**:609-636. DOI: 10.1002/hipo.10107

[67] Hannon EE, Trainor LJ. Music acquisition: Effects of enculturation and formal training on development. Trends in Cognitive Science. 2007;**11**:466-472. DOI: 10.1016/j.tics.2007.08.008

[68] Musacchia G, Sams M, Skoe E, Kraus N. Musicians have enhanced subcortical auditory and audiovisual processing of speech and music. Proceedings of the National Academy of Sciences of the USA. 2007;**104**:15894-15898. DOI: 10.1073/pnas.0701498104

[69] Chandrasekaran B, Kraus N. The scalp-recorded brainstem response to speech: Neural origins and plasticity. Psychophysiology. 2010;**47**:236-246. DOI: 10.1111/j.1469-8986.2009.00928.x

[70] Skoe E, Kraus N. Auditory brain stem response to complex sounds: A tutorial. Ear and Hearing. 2007;**31**:302-324. DOI: 10.1097/AUD.0b013e3181cdb272

[71] Song JH, Skoe E, Wong PC, Kraus N. Plasticity in the adult human auditory brainstem following short-term linguistic training. Journal of Cognitive Neuroscience. 2008;**20**:1892-1902. DOI: 10.1162/jocn.2008.20131

[72] Strait DL, Kraus N, Skoe E, Ashley R. Musical experience and neural efficiency: Effects of training on subcortical processing of vocal expressions of emotion. European Journal of Neuroscience. 2009;**29**:661-668. [PubMed: 19222564] DOI: 10.1111/j.1460-9568.2009.06617.x

[73] Tzounopoulos T, Kraus N. Learning to encode timing: Mechanisms of plasticity in the auditory brainstem. Neuron. 2009;**62**:463-469. DOI: 10.1016/j.neuron.2009.05.002

[74] Suga N. Role of corticofugal feedback in hearing. Journal of Comparative Physiology. 2008;**194**:169-183. DOI: 10.1007/s00359-007-0274-2

[75] Suga N, Ma X. Multiparametric corticofugal modulation and plasticity in the auditory system. Nature Reviews Neuroscience. 2003;**4**:783-794. DOI: 10.1038/nrn1222

[76] Rupp A, Hack S, Gutschalk A, Schneider P, Picton T, Stippic C, Scherg M. Fast temporal interactions in human auditory cortex. Neuroreport. 2000;**11**:3731-3736

[77] Schneider P, Scherg M, Dosch HG, Specht HJ, Gutschalk A, Rupp A. Morphology of Heschl's gyrus reflects enhanced activation in the auditory cortex of musicians. Nature Neuroscience. 2002;**5**:688-694

[78] van den Heuvel M, Hulshoff Pol H. Exploring the brain network: A review on resting-state fMRI functional connectivity. European Neuropsychopharmacology. 2010;**20**:519-534. DOI: 10.1016/j.euroneuro.2010.03.008

[79] Bassett DS, Gazzaniga MS. Understanding complexity in the human brain. Trends in Cognitive Science. 2011;**15**:200-209. DOI: http://dx.doi.org/10.1016/j.tics.2011.03.006

[80] Friston KJ, Frith CD, Liddle PF, Frackowiak RS. Functional connectivity: The principal-component analysis ofl arge (PET) data sets. Journal of Cerebral Blood Flow & Metabolism. 1993;**13**:5-14. DOI: 10.1038/jcbfm.1993.4

[81] Damoiseaux JS, Rombouts SA, Barkhof F, Scheltens P, Stam CJ, Smith SM, Beckmann CF. Consistent resting-state networks across healthy subjects. Proceedings of the National Academy of Science of USA. 2006;**103**13:848-853

[82] Luo C, Qiu C, Guo Z, Fang J, Li Q, Lei X, Xia Y, Lai Y, Gong Q, Zhou D, Yao D. Disrupted functional brain connectivity in partial epilepsy: A resting-state fMRI study. PLoS One. 2012;**7**:e28196. DOI: 10.1371/journal.pone.0028196

[83] Raichle M. The brain's default network. Annual Review of Neuroscience. 2015;**8**:433-447. DOI: 10.1196/annals.1440.011

[84] Wilkins RW, Hodges DA, Laurienti PJ, Steen M, Burdette JH. Network science and the effects of music preference on functional brain connectivity: From beethoven to eminem. Scientific Reports. 2014;**4**. Article number: 6130. DOI: 10.1038/srep0613

[85] van den Heuvel MP, Stam CJ, Kahn RS, Hulshoff Pol HE. Efficiency of functional brain networks and intellectual performance. Journal of Neuroscience. 2009;**29**:7619-7624

[86] Fox MD, Raichle ME. Spontaneous fluctuations in brain activity observed with functional magnetic resonance imaging. Nature Reviews Neuroscience. 2007;**8**:700-711. DOI: 10.1038/nrn2201

[87] Janata PB, Tillmann B, Bharucha JJ. Listening to polyphonic music recruits domain-general attention and working memory circuits. Cognitive, Affective and Behavioral Neuroscience. 2002;**2**:121-140

[88] Karmonik C, Brandt A, Anderson J, Brooks F, Lytle J, Silverman E. Music listening modulates functional connectivity and information flow in the human brain. Brain Connectivity. 2016;**6**:632-641. DOI: 10.1089/brain.2016.0428

[89] Cuddy L, Duffin J. Music, memory, and Alzheimer's disease: Is music recognition spared in dementia, and how can it be assessed? Medical Hypotheses. 2005;**64**:229-235. DOI: 10.1016/j.mehy.2004.09.005

[90] Jacobsen JH, Stelzer J, Fritz TH, Chetelat G, La Joie R, Turner R. Why musical memory can be preserved in advanced Alzheimer's disease. Brain. 2015;**138**(Pt 8):2438-2450. DOI: 10.1093/brain/awv135

[91] Simmons-Stern N, Budson A, Ally B. Music as a memory enhancer in patients with Alzheimer's disease. Neuropsychologia. 2010;**48**:3164-3167. DOI: 10.1016/j.neuropsy chologia.2010.04.033

[92] Seeley W, Crawford RK, Zhou J, Miller BL, Greicius MD. Neurodegenerative diseases target large-scale human brain networks. Neuron. 2009;**62**:42-52. DOI: 10.1016/j.neuron. 2009.03.024

[93] Baird A, Samson S. Memory for music in Alzheimer's disease: Unforgettable? Neuropsycholigal Review. 2009;**19**:85-101. [PubMed: 19214750]

[94] Thaut MH, Peterson DA, McIntosh GC. Temporal entrainment of cognitive functions: Musical mnemonics induce brain plasticity and oscillatory synchrony in neural networks underlying memory. Annals of the New York Academy of Sciences. 2005;**1060**:243-254. [PubMed: 16597771] DOI: 10.1196/annals.1360.017

[95] Brattico E, Tervaniemi M, Picton TW. Effects of brief discrimination-training on the auditory N1 wave. Neuroreport. 2003;**14**:2489-2492. DOI: 10.1097/01.wnr.0000098748.87269.a1

[96] Lappe C, Herholz SC, Trainor L, Pantev C. Cortical plasticity induced by short-term unimodal and multimodal musical training. Journal of Neuroscience. 2008;**28**:9632-9639. DOI: 0.1523/JNEUROSCI.2254-08.2008

[97] Burunat I, Alluri V, Toiviainen P, Numminen J, Brattico E. Dynamics of brain activity underlying working memory for music in a naturalistic condition. Cortex. 2014;**57**: 254-269. DOI: 10.1016/j.cortex.2014.04.012

10

Dendritic Spine Modifications in Brain Physiology

Jun Ju and Qiang Zhou

Abstract

An essential feature for an organism to survive is to adapt and learn. Studies in the past decades have revealed that synaptic plasticity is a key cellular mechanism underlying learning and memory functions in the adult, and the refinement of neural connections during development. Memory and refinement of connections can last for a long period of time, and hence requires the corresponding structural changes to take place. Alterations in dendritic spine morphology (enlargement or shrinkage) and/or spine density (increase or decrease) have been shown to occur with synaptic modifications, and have been proposed to enable persistent, long-term modifications of synapses. In this chapter, we will review the basics of spine plasticity and its functional contributions to synaptic modification, with focus on modifications of spine morphology (enlargement and shrinkage).

Keywords: spine formation, synaptic plasticity, AMPA receptor trafficking, cytoskeleton, long-term potentiation, long-term depression

1. Introduction

Dendritic spines are small protruding structures from the dendrites, around 1 μm in diameter. Spines are the primary site of excitatory inputs onto neurons and about 90% of excitatory synapses occur on spines of the excitatory neurons in the adult cortex [1].

Based on the size, spine head size and spine neck length, they can be roughly divided into three distinct types: mushroom, thin and stubby spine. Mushroom type spines have large spine heads and narrow spine necks, thin spines have small spine heads and thin spine necks, while stubby spines bear no distinction between spine heads and necks [2, 3]. In reality, the distribution of spines is not in these distinct sets but in a continuous distribution.

A major component of dendritic spines is cytoskeleton, which is critical to the structure and function of spines. Cytoskeletons consist of actin filaments and microtubules. Actin filaments are highly enriched in spine heads, while microtubules are found mostly in the dendritic shafts [4, 5]. Actin filaments inside spines are of two pools, G-actin and F-actin. G-actin is a monomer form of actin and F-actin is the polymer form, while they are found in the tip and base of spines, respectively [6]. Actin filaments bind to the scaffold proteins such as PSD-95 and Shanks, which anchor receptors and signaling molecules at the synapses [7]. Actin filaments are dynamic since actin monomer dissociates from the pointed end while new actin monomers are recruited into the barbed end. Certain actin-binding proteins regulate this dynamic process [8].

Spines are dynamic features in that they are in a constant motion (termed morphing), and their sizes fluctuate around a mean value [9, 10]. Dendritic filopodia are highly motile and flexible, and their lifetime is on the order of minutes to hours [11, 12]. This high motility may allow filopodia to explore the space around them in search for potential presynaptic inputs to form connections [13]. To understand this dynamic nature and to monitor these changes accurately, two-photon imaging has become an invaluable tool. With two-photon imaging, spine morphology and dynamics can be studied in much more details using time-lapse and repetitive imaging. This approach has revealed spine modifications under physiological or pathological conditions or events [14–16] and has greatly advanced our understanding of spine function and allowed in-depth study on the underlying structure–function relationship. During brain development dendritic spines are dynamic in their genesis and elimination, while in adolescence spines show much higher elimination than formation which results in a net spine loss or pruning. In contrast, the rate of spine genesis and elimination in adult is much lower and about equal, and this balance maintains the stability of spine density [17, 18].

Spine is considered as a unique calcium compartment, because the transfer of electrical charge is limited by the spine neck. The length of spine neck controls the degree of interaction between spines and their parent dendrite. In general, short spines and parent dendrites show similar responses to glutamate, while long spines exhibit faster and larger responses [19]. Spine plasticity is evidenced by their rapid (on the order of seconds) and persistent (for months to years) changes in response to physiological or pathological stimuli. Large spines has been suggested to be the site of stable long-term memory storage [1] while filopodia are considered by most to be an immature form of spine. Filopodia may transform into mature spines or are eliminated [20]. Hence, we define spine plasticity in two forms: alterations in their morphology/size and alterations in their density. We note that both forms of plasticity reflect modification of synaptic connections. In neurodegenerative and psychiatric diseases, spine density and spine morphology are altered, and changes in spine density and morphology may at least partially account for altered brain functions in these diseases [1, 21–24]. Therefore, better understanding of spine pathology may provide better therapeutic intervention.

In this chapter, we will discuss signaling mechanisms underlying the formation and maintenance of spines, plasticity of spine morphology and its relationship to modification of synaptic strength.

2. Development of dendritic spines during brain development

The relative sequence of synapse and spine genesis during brain development is still in debate. Some evidences suggest that spine genesis lags behind synapse genesis. Fiala et al.

showed that axonal fibers made synaptic contacts with long filopodia, which subsequently were transformed into mature spines [25]. Durand et al. reported during the first postnatal week in rats, synapses on the excitatory neurons are functional and plastic in the absence of dendritic spines [26]. Hence synaptic function and plasticity can take place without spines. After induction of long-term enhancement of synaptic connections in area CA1, new spines appeared on the postsynaptic dendrite [27]. Maletic-Savatic found that with axonal inputs activation, these small filopodia-like protrusions enlarged and became dendritic spines [28]. For those filopodia that do not connect with axonal inputs, they did not turn into mature spines and were absorbed back into dendrites [12]. Interestingly, increase of spine synapse might inhibit the mobility of nearby filopodia on the same dendrite and diminish the formation of synapses [29]. These results indicate that synapse formation or strengthening promotes the formation or maturation of spines, and lend support for the notion that synapse genesis occurs prior to spine genesis.

Do spines form from filopodia, or from existing synapses on the dendritic shafts? In mature cultures, some stable spines could emerge without going through the dynamic filopodia stage [12]. The series sample analysis in young hippocampal area CA1 also revealed that most of synapses are on dendritic shafts, with rare synapses on stubby and mushroom spines [3]. Despite all this, the transformation from dendritic shaft synapses to spines has not been supported by direct observations [30]. On the other hand, several *in vitro* studies revealed that during the initial 1–2 weeks in culture, the long and headless filopodia bear no synaptic contacts associated with the presynaptic axons. Over the subsequent 4 weeks, these dynamic filopodia turned into stable, mushroom-like spines [29, 31, 32]. Fiala et al. also found that in the hippocampal CA1, synapses were present on both filopodia and dendrites. From PN1 to PN12, the number of shaft synapses and filopodia synapses was decreased, while the number of stubby and spine synapses was significantly increased [25]. Thus, it is likely that during early development, shaft synapses are the dominant form of synaptic contact. With development, and likely the need for increasing contact area, spine synapse replace shaft synapses to become the major form of synapses, at least in the adult cortex. Recently, shaft synapses are shown to define the locations where dendritic spines are formed [30] (**Figure 1**), providing more evidence for the transition from shaft synapse to spine synapse as a major process in synapse formation and maturation.

The initial surge of spine genesis leads the generation of more spines than what eventually is retained in the adult brain, and pruning of excessive spines after spine genesis allows a better adaptation to the environment [33]. This pruning process could be evoked by low-frequency glutamatergic stimulation and requires activation of NMDA receptors [34–36].

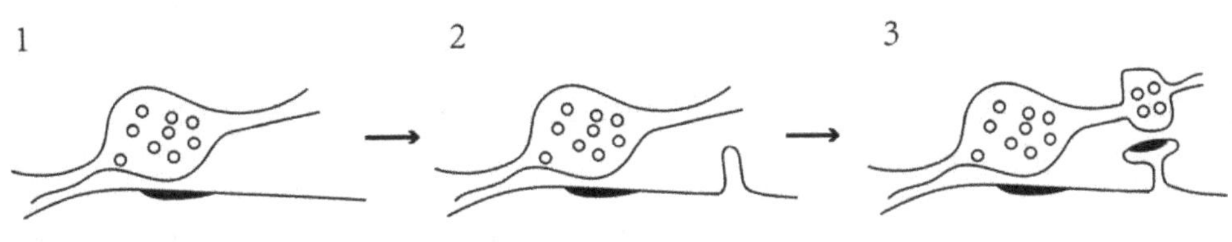

Figure 1. Dendritic spines are derived from filopodia with the assistance of shaft synapses. (1) presynaptic axon forms synapses with dendritic shaft. (2) a dendritic protrusion occurs adjacent to the dendritic shaft synapse. (3) the dendritic protrusion contacts with the presynaptic axon and eventually a mushroom dendritic spine is generated. Modified from [30].

In young adolescent mice (1-month old), within a 2 week period of time, 13–20% of total spines were eliminated with 5–8% formed in the barrel, motor and frontal cortices, and this imbalance led to a significant spine loss in many brain regions. However, in the adult mice (4–6 months old), 3–5% of spines were eliminated and formed in 2 weeks [18]. Most evidences support that dendritic spines are stable in the adulthood [37, 38]. Grutzendler et al. reported that spines in the primary visual cortex of young adolescence have a turnover rate of 27% per month but this rate dropped to only 4% in the adult [15]. In contrast, Trachtenberg et al. found that adult spines are highly dynamic with about 20% turnover per day in the mouse barrel cortex [16]. This discrepancy is likely due to differences in the methodology in that the use of cranial window in the latter study triggered inflammatory responses in the brain which resulted in elevated turnover rates. It should be pointed out that spine turnover rate differs in various brain regions. For example, Holtmaat et al. reported that spines turn over more slowly (both generation and elimination) in the visual cortex than in the somatosensory cortex, with the fraction of transient spines (lifetime ≤ 4 days) also lower in visual cortex [17].

3. Signaling events during spine formation and maintenance

Motility of dendritic spines is regulated by the dynamic balance between G-actin and F-actin [39]. F-actin consists of two pools, a large dynamic pool in the tip of the spine head and a small stable pool in the base of spine [6] [40]. With LTP induction, the stable F-actin is severed into short segments and reorganized to expand the spine [41]. Thus, the dynamics of actin cytoskeleton controls dendritic spine morphological remodeling and plenty of signaling molecules participate in this process [42–44].

Spine morphology is regulated by actin binding and cytoskeleton proteins. Drebrin was the first identified to modify dendritic spines since overexpression of drebrin in cultured neurons increased the length of spines [45]. Spines in the drebrin knockout mice exhibited normal morphology but altered plasticity [46]. Takahashi et al. reported that drebrin entered filopodia and formed an actin filament cluster to recruit postsynaptic components (including scaffolding protein PSD95), and this process enables the transition from filopodia to mature spines. Based on this observation, filopodia are classified into two types, an immature diffuse-type and a mature cluster-type. A filopodium with a drebrin cluster, whose maximum intensity was higher than twice the average intensity of the filopodium, was classified as a cluster-type filopodium. Otherwise, it was classified as a diffuse-type filopodium. The cluster-type filopodia were likely to be converted to mature spines [47]. In addition, overexpression of drebrin in neurons caused F-actin to accumulate in the growth cone, whereas knockdown of drebrin reduced F-actin level [48]. Drebrin binds to F-actin to generate thick bundles of F-actin [49], and drebrin also competes with other actin binding proteins such as ADF/cofilin which depolymerizes F-actin [50, 51].

Besides drebrin, other actin-binding proteins including myosin II, Abi-1 and spinophilin regulate actin polymerization in the dendritic spines. Myosin II belongs to the family of molecular motors which is highly expressed in dendritic spines, and regulates dendritic spine morphology and synaptic plasticity [52]. Blockade of myosin II with shRNA suppressed the formation of mushroom-like spines and increased the presence of filopodia [53]. Abi-1 is a member of the c-Abl tyrosine interactor (Abi) protein family, which interacts with scaffolding proteins and F-actin in the spines [54]. Knocking down of Abi-1 by RNAi shifted spines to an immature form [55]. Spinophilin has an actin-binding domain at its N terminus and can bundle F-actin filaments [56]. Knockout of spinophilin in mice increased the presence of filopodia [57].

Actin polymerization is regulated by actin binding proteins, whose active and inactive states are regulated by small GTPases. Of the Rho family of small GTPases, three are most actively involved in spine morphogenesis, RhoA, Rac1 and Cdc42. These three GTPases are distinguished by two opposite activities: RhoA inhibits whereas Rac1 and Cdc42 promote spine growth. Tashiro et al. reported that in hippocampal neurons, Rac1 increased spine density but reduced spine length, while RhoA decreased both spine density and spine length [58]. Interestingly, RhoA and Cdc42 play opposite roles in stress fiber formation by controlling the phosphorylation of myosin light chain. RhoA inhibits myosin phosphatase via the Rho kinase while Rac1 and Cdc42 activate it via the serine/threonine kinase PAK [59, 60]. Thus, Rac1 and RhoA might have opposite effects on the same target proteins and hence opposite effects in regulating spine density. Similarly, Nakayama et al. found that Rac1 is essential for the maintenance of dendritic spines while enhanced RhoA activity led to significant simplification of dendrites [61].

Receptor tyrosine kinases also regulate spine morphology. Among them, the erythropoietin-producing hepatocellular carcinoma (Eph) receptors have unique activity on synapse. They consist of type A and type B receptor subclasses based on their binding capability to Ephrin A and Ephrin B ligands. Moeller et al. reported that activation of EphB2 in the cultured hippocampal neurons led to shortening of filopodia [62]. Furthermore, activation of EphB likely phosphorylates guanine exchange factors (GEFs) such as kalirin7, which further stimulates Rho family GTPases Rac1 and Cdc42 [63]. Opposite to EphB2, activation of EphA4 by its ligand, ephrin-A3, located in the perisynaptic processes of astrocytes, decreased spine length and density. Loss of EphA4 led to spine elongation and disorganization [64]. Similarly, in the hippocampus of ephrin-A3-null mice, EphA4 phosphorylation was decreased and abnormal spine elongation was observed [65]. Thus, either loss of EphA4 or ephrin-A3 induces identical dendritic spine deficits.

In summary, we have reviewed three types of important and representative signaling molecules in spine function. The first signaling pathway is mediated by actin binding proteins, the second is the family of small GTPases (including Rac1, RhoA and Cdc42, which determine the activity states of actin binding proteins), and the third is receptor tyrosine kinases. The absence or malfunctioning of the above three signaling pathways leads to altered spine morphogenesis and function.

4. Spine plasticity

Spine plasticity may be exhibited in two forms—changes in spine density and spine dimension. Change in spine density reflects modification of connection density between the presynaptic and postsynaptic neurons, which happens most commonly during brain development (increase, decrease/pruning) and aging/degeneration (decrease). Changes in spine morphology/dimension, especially the size of spine head, have been widely reported, and are believed to be associated with changes in the strength of synapses that reside on these altered spines. In this chapter, we will focus on alterations of spine dimension.

4.1. Changes in spine morphology

Due to the heterogeneity of spine size/morphology, the most convincing way to demonstrate that spine morphology is altered is to compare the same set of spines before and after a manipulation, such as synaptic plasticity-inducing stimuli in brain slices or learning *in vivo*. By using time-lapse two-photon imaging on the same set of spines, Yang et al. found new spines were formed after *in vivo* experience in the form of sensory or motor, and a fraction of these newly appeared spines persisted for months after the experience. More importantly, of the appearance of these new spines is specifically related to the *in vivo* experience or training [66]. In addition, Hayashi-Takagi et al. showed that motor learning on rotarod led to an enhanced *Arc* signaling, together with an expansion of a subset of spines in the motor cortex. By expressing a photoactivatable GTPase Rac1 in spines, they further showed that prolonged photo-activation of Rac1 resulted in reversal of spine expansion and loss of motor memory. This is a striking demonstration that potentiated synapses and enlarged spines are likely the underlying biological substrates of stored memory and formed memory can be erased by reversing these changes [67].

Many studies have examined spine modifications with the induction of long-term potentiation (LTP) and long-term depression (LTD), since this procedure allows the examination of the same set spines associated with fast, large and long-lasting changes in synaptic strength. These two forms of synaptic plasticity refer to the increase and decrease in synaptic strength respectively, and are generally regarded as the cellular basis of synaptic modifications underlying developmental remodeling of neuronal connections, and learning and memory function in the adult brain [68]. When studied in brain slices (acute or organotypic culture), LTP or LTD is induced by stimulation of the presynaptic inputs with distinct patterns. In some studies, changes in the synaptic strength were also monitored, and thus changes in synaptic function and spine morphology can be related to each other in the same set of spines/synapse, or even a single synapse/spine [34, 69–71]. In general, spines exhibit the capacity of bi-directional changes in that spine enlargement is observed with LTP while spine shrinkage with LTD [72–74] (**Figure 2**). Either uncaging of caged glutamate onto a single spine [75] or electrical stimulation of a population of synapses [70, 71] had confirmed the above observations. Uncaging of glutamate directly enhances postsynaptic AMPAR function, and since it bypasses presynaptic release, and thus has provided the unambiguous evidence that postsynaptic changes can underlie the expression of LTP [69, 75]. These observations further indicate that morphological and functional changes are likely driven by the same stimuli or process (see below).

In general, there is a good correlation between the strength of a given synapse (measured by electrophysiological responses) and the size of spine. Electrophysiological responses are further determined by the number/density of AMPA receptors at a given synapse. Takumi et al. found a linear relationship between AMPAR density and the diameter of PSD [76]. Matsuzaki et al.

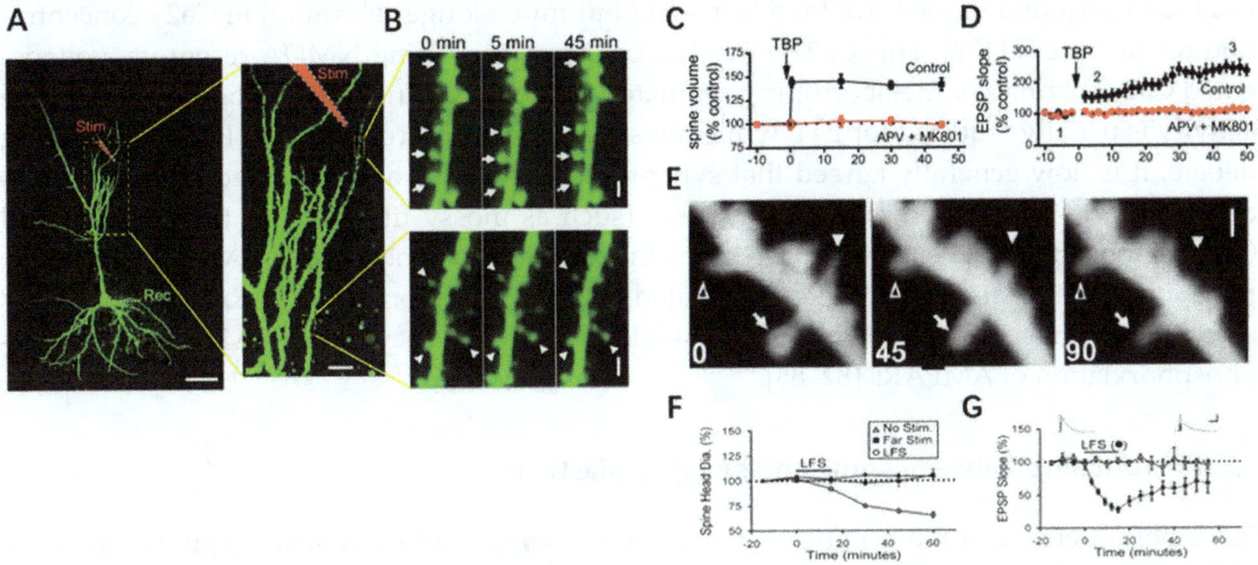

Figure 2. Bi-directional modification of spine size by synaptic plasticity. (A) Recording, synaptic stimulation and fluorescence imaging of the same set of synapses and spines in acute hippocampal slices. (B) Spine enlargement associated with LTP induction by theta burst stimulation, this enlargement is persistent and long-lasting. In addition, enlargement was restricted to spines close (upper) but not far away from the stimulation site (lower). (C) Change in spine volume before and after LTP induction and its requirement of activation of NMDARs since it was prevented by bath application of NMDAR antagonists APV and MK-801. (D) Increase in synaptic strength (EPSPs) as a result of LTP induction. LTP occurred in two phases, an initial rapid increase (indicated by 2 on the plot) and a slower gradual increase (indicated by 3). LTP was also sensitive to NMDAR blockade. (E) Spine shrinkage associated with LTD, it is persistent and long-lasting. (F) Shrinkage of spines occurred to those spines close to, but not to those far away from the stimulating electrode, or those had not received any stimulation. Compared to the almost instantaneous enlargement of spine heads after LTP, spine shrinkage develops slowly and takes much longer to reach a plateau. (G) Low frequency stimulation led to depression of EPSPs. Taken from [34, 71].

reported that the number of AMPAR in spines is of a large range. In addition, mushroom spines are enriched with AMPARs, compared to the low distribution of them in the thin spines and filopodia. These observations support a strong relationship between number of AMPAR and volume of spines [77]. In addition, it provides direct evidence that mushroom spines are functionally mature while thin spines and filopodia are not.

4.2. Synaptic plasticity

Synapses can change their strength by the activity patterns that they receive, and this modification allows synaptic strength to be adjusted to better suit the need for adaptation. Originally put forwarded by Donald Hebb and later adopted as "fire together, wire together" model, the current model of synaptic modification states that neurons sharing spike activity have increased connections between these two partners [78]. After the discovery of LTP in 1973, this activity-driven increase in synaptic strength has been extensively studied, both in acute brain slices and *in vivo* [68]; and has been used widely as a tool to induce synaptic modification in order to study the associated processes. Various molecules have been identified to be required for the induction and expression of LTP [68]. In general, Ca2+ entry or elevated intracellular Ca2+ concentration is required to convert electrical activity into intracellular signaling that determines the direction of synaptic changes. Usually a large but transient elevation in

Ca2+ concentration induces LTP while a small but much longer elevation in Ca2+ concentration results in LTD [79]. This Ca2+ entry can be through opening NMDA receptors, voltage-gated Ca2+ channels or metabotropic glutamate receptors [68]. Increase in postsynaptic kinase activity is usually required for LTP while phosphatase activity required for LTD. After a long debate, it is now generally agreed that synaptic modifications are expressed in the postsynaptic neurons, except in a few specific cases (such as mossy fiber LTP in the hippocampal CA3 region) [80, 81]. Postsynaptic changes involve the translocation of AMPARs and their phosphorylation state, in that LTP is associated with translocation of AMPARs to synapse and/or increased phosphorylation of AMPARs while LTD with endocytosis of AMPARs and/or dephosphorylation of AMPARs [82–85].

4.3. Relationship between spine and synapse plasticity

Since both increase in the synaptic strength and enlargement of dendritic spine occur with LTP, an obvious question is whether changes in synaptic physiology/function are casually related to changes in spine morphology/structure. More specifically, are these two processes driven by the same initial process? Does the occurrence or persistence of one process require the occurrence/presence of the other? It is now well established that influx of Ca2+ through synaptic NMDARs during LTP induction drives AMPAR phosphorylation and/or insertion [68], and polymerization of action filaments inside spines which drives enlargement of spine heads [74] (**Figure 3**). Thus, the initial changes in function and structure are driven by the same signaling process. This initial increase in synaptic response and spine volume occurs very rapidly (less than 1 min) [71].

Dendritic spine heads accumulate F-actin during the rapid expansion phase of synaptic modification. Potentiation of single synapse/spine with uncaging of glutamate led to a significant expansion of the spine head and a shortening and widening of the spine neck [86, 87]. Spine expansion takes place rapidly after LTP, as fast as it can be measured (~ 20 sec after LTP induction) [71]. F-actin concentration inside the spine head rises, together with the entry of actin-severing, actin-depolymerizing/–polymerizing, actin-capping proteins, while actin-stabilizing proteins leave the spines [6, 39, 86, 88–90]. Actin-depolymerizing agent, cofilin, is highly elevated in spines during this initial process [89]. Interestingly, unlike the expression of LTP, this initial spine expansion did not require postsynaptic exocytosis or PKA signaling [71], suggesting the involvement of different signaling pathways in spine enlargement than that supports LTP. After this initial rapid expansion, the next phase of events lasts up to 1 h, with spine head volume decreased from the initial increase, but still larger than the pre-LTP baseline. In addition, the total actin concentration in the spine may drop to the baseline level [89].

LTD is associated with the shrinkage of spines and removal of synaptic AMPARs via internalization [34, 36, 39]. During the induction of LTD with low frequency synaptic stimulation, Ca2+ influx through the activated NMDARs is required for both LTD and spine shrinkage [34, 70]. Ca2+ entry through synaptic NMDARs leads to the activation of calcineurin which is also required for both LTD and spine shrinkage, while activation of protein phosphatase 2A is required for LTD expression but not spine shrinkage, while elevated cofilin activity is required for spine shrinkage but not LTD [34, 39, 70, 91]. Consistent with the above conclusion, Sdrulla

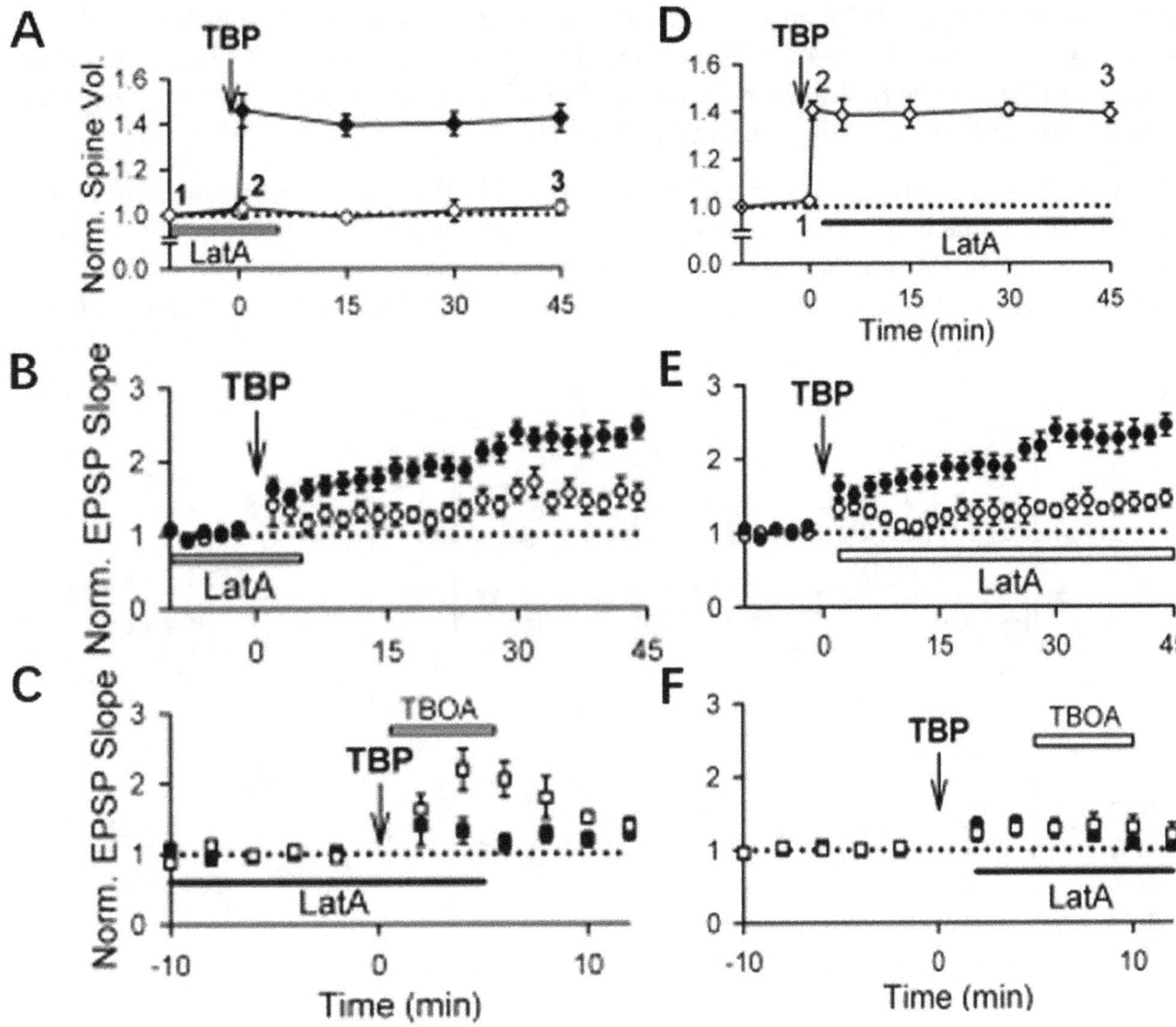

Figure 3. Time-dependent reversal of synaptic and spine modification. (A) Spine shrinkage induced by low frequency stimulation (LFS) can be readily reversed by subsequent high frequency stimulation (HFS). (B) Spine enlargement induced by HFS is also readily reversed by subsequent LFS. (C) Spine enlargement induced by TBP can be reversed by LFS only if LFS is given within a time window of about 15 min after TBP. (D) this critical reversal window also holds for reversing TBP-induced LTP. (E) LFS given outside this reversal window does not affect spine size. (F) LFS given outside the reversal window does not reverse LTP either. Taken from [34, 71].

and Linden demonstrated that LTD expression and spine changes in cerebellar Purkinje cells could be induced independently of each other, and induction of one did not affect the other [92]. Wang et al. reported that trafficking of AMPARs to and away from PSDs was activity-independent and not associated with alterations in spine size. The significance of this finding requires further investigation [70].

One interesting and important feature of synaptic modification is its reversibility. This reversibility is defined by reversal of synaptic modification after its induction [34, 93]. There are a few aspects to this reversal: (1) reversal applies to both LTP and LTD, and spine enlargement and spine shrinkage [34, 71] (**Figure 4**). More specifically, low frequency stimulation reverses LTP and spine enlargement, while high frequency stimulation reverses LTD and spine shrinkage. (2) There is a critical time window only during which reversal can occur [34, 71, 93, 94] (**Figure 4**). In hippocampal slices, the window for LTP reversal is about 15–30 min [71]. (3) The typical stimuli that can induce reversal are not capable altering basal synaptic strength or spine dimension [71, 93, 95, 96].

Although it is generally believed that expression of LTP requires the addition of synaptic AMPARs, some evidences suggest that these newly added AMPARs are not delivered directly into the PSDs inside spines, but rather they are either delivered to regions outside synapses (i.e., the perisynaptic regions; [82] or onto dendritic shaft [83]. These AMPARs

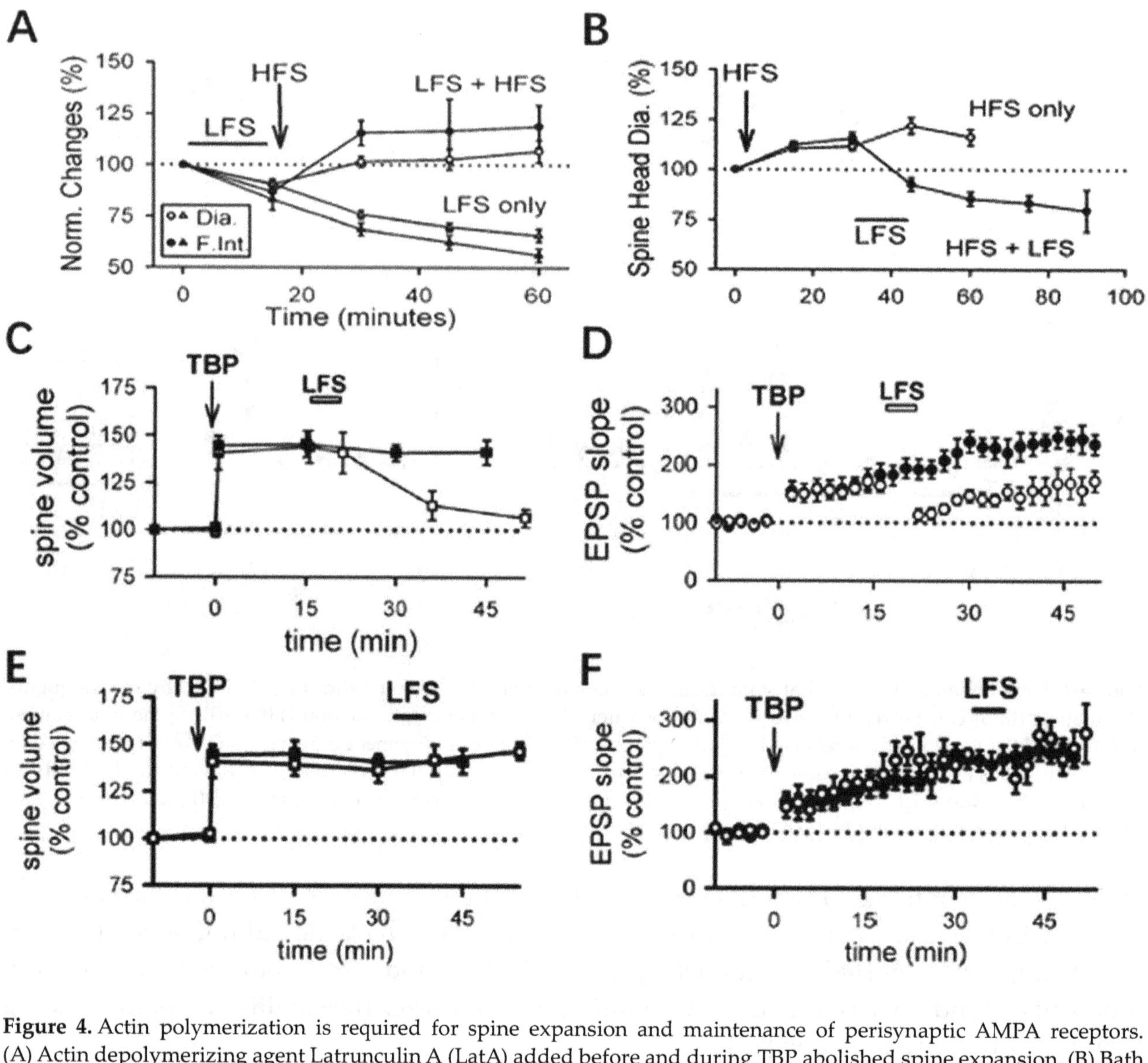

Figure 4. Actin polymerization is required for spine expansion and maintenance of perisynaptic AMPA receptors. (A) Actin depolymerizing agent Latrunculin A (LatA) added before and during TBP abolished spine expansion. (B) Bath perfusion of LatA before and during TBP impaired enhancement of synaptic response (EPSPs). (C) Bath perfusion of LatA 2 min after TBP did not disrupt the delivery of AMPARs to perisynaptic site, as revealed by the increased in responses to application of glutamate transporter blocker TBOA (open symbols). (D) Bath perfusion of LatA 2 min after TBP did not affect spine enlargement, indicating that persistent spine enlargement does not require persistent actin polymerization. (E) Bath perfusion of LatA 2 min after TBP prevented the occurrence of gradual increase in EPSP enhancement which requires the synaptic addition of new AMPARs. (F) Addition of LatA 2 min after TBP removed the newly delivered perisynaptic AMPARs as revealed by the absence of increase in response to TBOA. Taken from [83].

then move laterally into spines/PSDs. Thus, with LTP induction, two rapid processes (within 30 sec) occurs independent of each other: spine expansion which requires actin polymerization and activation of NMDARs but not postsynaptic PKA activation, and delivery of AMPARs to the perisynaptic regions which requires activation of NMDARs and postsynaptic PKA signaling but not actin polymerization. The next 15 min or so (reversal time window) determines whether LTP and spine expansion can be stabilized into a long-term change. During this period, translocation of the newly delivered perisynaptic AMPARs stabilized spine expansion, while removal of these receptors led to collapse of enlarged spines [71]. On the other hand, reversal of spine enlargement also removed these perisynaptic AMPARs. Hence, there is a mutual interaction between perisynaptic AMPARs and spine enlargement in that the presence of one is required to sustain the other (**Figure 3**). Yang et al. found that postsynaptic PKC activity is required for the translocation of perisynaptic AMPARs to synapse, and in the absence of PKC activity, these AMPARs remain perisynaptic. Importantly, as long as the perisynaptic AMPARs are present, both LTP and spine expansion exist in a labile state in that they can either be reverted to the baseline state (no plasticity), or they can enter a stabilized state of persistent increase in synaptic strength and spine size (persistent plasticity). Low frequency synaptic stimulation given within a 15 min "grace period" post-LTP induction reversed spine expansion and removed AMPARs from the perisynaptic regions and hence blocked the conversion of short-term plasticity to a long-term one (**Figure 5**) [71, 82].

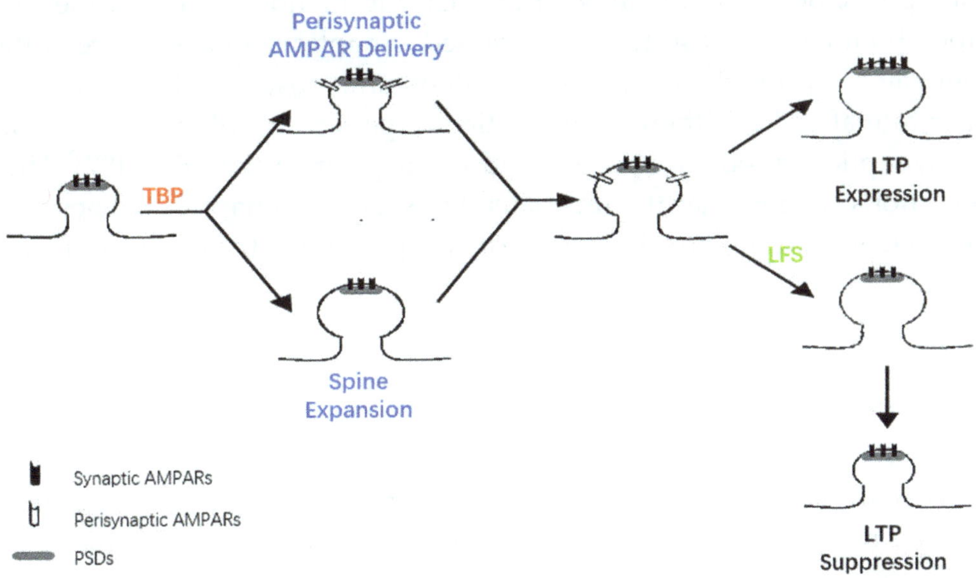

Figure 5. Two-step model for coordinated expression of synaptic potentiation and spine enlargement. TBP triggers two initial processes, spine enlargement and perisynaptic delivery of AMPARs. These two processes occur simultaneously and mostly independent of each other. In the absence of any disturbance, perisynaptic AMPARs translocate into synapse, which stabilizes both AMPARs and spine enlargement, and this leads to persistent potentiation of synaptic responses and spine enlargement. On the other hand, when low frequency synaptic stimulation (LFS) is given within this "grace period" when both processes are in a liable state, it readily removes perisynaptic AMPARs. As a result, synaptic potentiation is aborted and spine enlargement collapses, and no LTP and spine enlargement. This model shows the interaction between functional and structural aspects of synapse modification is critical to the persistency and long-lasting occurrence of synaptic modification.

The above results are consist with a model (**Figure 5**) in which (1) the expression of functional plasticity (LTP) and structural plasticity (spine enlargement) are initially two independent processes only share the activation of NMDARs; (2) these two processes then enter an interactive state that the continuous presence of one is required for the persistence of the other; (3) the above state is liable in that interference (such as low frequency stimulation) can revert both changes back to the baseline; (4) once both processes are stabilized, synapse modification has entered a state resistant to reversal. We like to note that during the "grace period" coordinated changes in synaptic plasticity (function and structure) are cross-checked to ensure that they do occur together, and in the situation only one such process occurs (perhaps can be viewed as a mistake), the other process will be aborted albeit in process. This double-proof mechanism is essential to ensure that only appropriate changes are allowed to be sustained, and may thus be especially important in face of the highly dynamic nature of synaptic modifications, such as those occurring during early neural development [94].

Sustained reduction in synaptic strength may eventually lead to the loss of synaptic connections, and this loss is manifested as a reduction in spine density. Spine loss appears to be a protracted process and hence it is difficult to study. Even if monitoring changes in the same set of synapses/spines, it is usually more difficult to exclude the possibility that the reduced synaptic function and spine number is caused by deterioration of the health of the preparation, or by some other unknown or uncontrolled processes that occur randomly during the long period (>hours) between LTD induction and spine loss. Nonetheless, a few studies have examined this process. By using organotypical slices and monitoring both presynaptic boutons and spines, Becker et al. showed that LTD induction increased the turnover rate of presynaptic boutons and resulted in decreased synaptic contacts between the pre- and post-synaptic sites. Although presynaptic boutons and postsynaptic spines disappear at much greater rate after LTD, there is no particular pattern to follow, since disappearance of either presynaptic boutons or spines could occur prior to the other [97]. Therefore, the above observations suggest that the mismatch between presynaptic and postsynaptic sites is more likely a key factor in the elimination of synapse, while the exact sequence might not play much role.

5. Conclusions

Dendritic spines are small protrusions on the dendritic shaft as major excitatory inputs site on the excitatory neurons in the adult cortex. Spines play critical roles in the excitatory synaptic transmission and plasticity. Genesis of spines occurs during brain development, and is subjected to activity-dependent modulation to determine their fates, either to transit to mature spines or be eliminated. Spines are the site where physiological/functional and morphological/structural modifications meet and integrate, during both physiological (such as memory formation) and pathological (such as neurodegeneration) processes. Interestingly, early changes in functional and structural aspects of synapse modification occur independently, but they subsequently interact with each other to sustain changes in both. This highly interactive nature ensures that the end result is a coherent modification of synapse function and structure. Extensive progress has been made on our understanding of the structure and function of spine which vastly has advanced our understanding of neuronal and synaptic communication and plasticity. In addition, changes in spine density and dimension may serve as a marker of pathological processes and hence have potential therapeutic/diagnostic values.

Acknowledgements

This work was supported by grants from Peking University Shenzhen Graduate School and grants from Shenzhen government (ZDSYS201504301539161 and KQTD2015032709315529).

Competing interests

The authors declare that they have no competing interests.

Author details

Jun Ju and Qiang Zhou*

*Address all correspondence to: zhouqiang@pkusz.edu.cn

School of Chemical Biology and Biotechnology, Peking University Shenzhen Graduate School, Shenzhen, China

References

[1] Tackenberg C, Ghori A, Brandt R. Thin, stubby or mushroom: Spine pathology in Alzheimer's disease. Current Alzheimer Research. 2009;**6**(3):261-268

[2] Peters A, Kaiserman-Abramof IR. The small pyramidal neuron of the rat cerebral cortex. The perikaryon, dendrites and spines. The American Journal of Anatomy. 1970;**127**(4):321-355

[3] Harris KM, Jensen FE, Tsao B. Three-dimensional structure of dendritic spines and synapses in rat hippocampus (CA1) at postnatal day 15 and adult ages: Implications for the maturation of synaptic physiology and long-term potentiation. The Journal of Neuroscience. 1992;**12**(7):2685-2705

[4] Cohen RS, Chung SK, Pfaff DW. Immunocytochemical localization of actin in dendritic spines of the cerebral cortex using colloidal gold as a probe. Cellular and Molecular Neurobiology. 1985;**5**(3):271-284

[5] Caceres A et al. Immunocytochemical localization of actin and microtubule-associated protein MAP2 in dendritic spines. Proceedings of the National Academy of Sciences of the United States of America. 1983;**80**(6):1738-1742

[6] Honkura N et al. The subspine organization of actin fibers regulates the structure and plasticity of dendritic spines. Neuron. 2008;**57**(5):719-729

[7] Verpelli C et al. Scaffold proteins at the postsynaptic density. Advances in Experimental Medicine and Biology. 2012;**970**:29-61

[8] Lee SH, Dominguez R. Regulation of actin cytoskeleton dynamics in cells. Molecules and Cells. 2010;**29**(4):311-325

[9] Verkuyl JM, Matus A. Time-lapse imaging of dendritic spines in vitro. Nature Protocols. 2006;**1**(5):2399-2405

[10] Matus A. Actin-based plasticity in dendritic spines. Science. 2000;**290**(5492):754-758

[11] De Roo M et al. Activity-dependent PSD formation and stabilization of newly formed spines in hippocampal slice cultures. Cerebral Cortex. 2008;**18**(1):151-161

[12] Dailey ME, Smith SJ. The dynamics of dendritic structure in developing hippocampal slices. The Journal of Neuroscience. 1996;**16**(9):2983-2994

[13] Yoshihara Y, De Roo M, Muller D. Dendritic spine formation and stabilization. Current Opinion in Neurobiology. 2009;**19**(2):146-153

[14] Mizrahi A et al. High-resolution in vivo imaging of hippocampal dendrites and spines. The Journal of Neuroscience. 2004;**24**(13):3147-3151

[15] Grutzendler J, Kasthuri N, Gan WB. Long-term dendritic spine stability in the adult cortex. Nature. 2002;**420**(6917):812-816

[16] Trachtenberg JT et al. Long-term in vivo imaging of experience-dependent synaptic plasticity in adult cortex. Nature. 2002;**420**(6917):788-794

[17] Holtmaat AJ et al. Transient and persistent dendritic spines in the neocortex in vivo. Neuron. 2005;**45**(2):279-291

[18] Zuo Y et al. Development of long-term dendritic spine stability in diverse regions of cerebral cortex. Neuron. 2005;**46**(2):181-189

[19] Korkotian E, Segal M. Structure-function relations in dendritic spines: Is size important? Hippocampus. 2000;**10**(5):587-595

[20] Marrs GS, Green SH, Dailey ME. Rapid formation and remodeling of postsynaptic densities in developing dendrites. Nature Neuroscience. 2001;**4**(10):1006-1013

[21] Glantz LA, Lewis DA. Decreased dendritic spine density on prefrontal cortical pyramidal neurons in schizophrenia. Archives of General Psychiatry. 2000;**57**(1):65-73

[22] Kalus P et al. The dendritic architecture of prefrontal pyramidal neurons in schizophrenic patients. Neuroreport. 2000;**11**(16):3621-3625

[23] Scheff SW et al. Synaptic loss in the inferior temporal gyrus in mild cognitive impairment and Alzheimer's disease. Journal of Alzheimer's Disease. 2011;**24**(3):547-557

[24] Zou C et al. Neuroinflammation impairs adaptive structural plasticity of dendritic spines in a preclinical model of Alzheimer's disease. Acta Neuropathologica. 2016;**131**(2):235-246

[25] Fiala JC et al. Synaptogenesis via dendritic filopodia in developing hippocampal area CA1. The Journal of Neuroscience. 1998;**18**(21):8900-8911

[26] Durand GM, Kovalchuk Y, Konnerth A. Long-term potentiation and functional synapse induction in developing hippocampus. Nature. 1996;**381**(6577):71-75

[27] Engert F, Bonhoeffer T. Dendritic spine changes associated with hippocampal long-term synaptic plasticity. Nature. 1999;**399**(6731):66-70

[28] Maletic-Savatic M, Malinow R, Svoboda K. Rapid dendritic morphogenesis in CA1 hippocampal dendrites induced by synaptic activity. Science. 1999;**283**(5409):1923-1927

[29] Ziv NE, Smith SJ. Evidence for a role of dendritic filopodia in synaptogenesis and spine formation. Neuron. 1996;**17**(1):91-102

[30] Reilly JE, Hanson HH, Phillips GR. Persistence of excitatory shaft synapses adjacent to newly emerged dendritic protrusions. Molecular and Cellular Neurosciences. 2011;**48** (2):129-136

[31] Collin C, Miyaguchi K, Segal M. Dendritic spine density and LTP induction in cultured hippocampal slices. Journal of Neurophysiology. 1997;**77**(3):1614-1623

[32] Papa M et al. Morphological analysis of dendritic spine development in primary cultures of hippocampal neurons. The Journal of Neuroscience. 1995;**15**(1 Pt 1):1-11

[33] Rakic P et al. Concurrent overproduction of synapses in diverse regions of the primate cerebral cortex. Science. 1986;**232**(4747):232-235

[34] Zhou Q, Homma KJ, Poo MM. Shrinkage of dendritic spines associated with long-term depression of hippocampal synapses. Neuron. 2004;**44**(5):749-757

[35] Wiegert JS, Oertner TG. Long-term depression triggers the selective elimination of weakly integrated synapses. Proceedings of the National Academy of Sciences of the United States of America. 2013;**110**(47):E4510-E4519

[36] Nagerl UV et al. Bidirectional activity-dependent morphological plasticity in hippocampal neurons. Neuron. 2004;**44**(5):759-767

[37] Peters A, Sethares C, Moss MB. The effects of aging on layer 1 in area 46 of prefrontal cortex in the rhesus monkey. Cerebral Cortex. 1998;**8**(8):671-684

[38] Masliah E et al. Quantitative synaptic alterations in the human neocortex during normal aging. Neurology. 1993;**43**(1):192-197

[39] Okamoto K et al. Rapid and persistent modulation of actin dynamics regulates postsynaptic reorganization underlying bidirectional plasticity. Nature Neuroscience. 2004; **7**(10):1104-1112

[40] Frost NA et al. Single-molecule discrimination of discrete perisynaptic and distributed sites of actin filament assembly within dendritic spines. Neuron. 2010;**67**(1):86-99

[41] Chen JH et al. Two-photon correlation spectroscopy in single dendritic spines reveals fast actin filament reorganization during activity-dependent growth. PLoS One. 2015;**10**(5) e0128241

[42] Chazeau A, Giannone G. Organization and dynamics of the actin cytoskeleton during dendritic spine morphological remodeling. Cellular and Molecular Life Sciences. 2016;**73**(16):3053-3073

[43] Penzes P, Rafalovich I. Regulation of the actin cytoskeleton in dendritic spines. Advances in Experimental Medicine and Biology. 2012;**970**:81-95

[44] Chazeau A et al. Nanoscale segregation of actin nucleation and elongation factors determines dendritic spine protrusion. The EMBO Journal. 2014;**33**(23):2745-2764

[45] Hayashi K, Shirao T. Change in the shape of dendritic spines caused by overexpression of drebrin in cultured cortical neurons. The Journal of Neuroscience. 1999;**19**(10):3918-3925

[46] Aoki C et al. Drebrin a knockout eliminates the rapid form of homeostatic synaptic plasticity at excitatory synapses of intact adult cerebral cortex. The Journal of Comparative Neurology. 2009;**517**(1):105-121

[47] Takahashi H et al. Drebrin-dependent actin clustering in dendritic filopodia governs synaptic targeting of postsynaptic density-95 and dendritic spine morphogenesis. The Journal of Neuroscience. 2003;**23**(16):6586-6595

[48] Mizui T et al. Drebrin E is involved in the regulation of axonal growth through actin-myosin interactions. Journal of Neurochemistry. 2009;**109**(2):611-622

[49] Mikati MA, Grintsevich EE, Reisler E. Drebrin-induced stabilization of actin filaments. The Journal of Biological Chemistry. 2013;**288**(27):19926-19938

[50] Sharma S et al. Atomic force microscopy reveals drebrin induced remodeling of f-actin with subnanometer resolution. Nano Letters. 2011;**11**(2):825-827

[51] Grintsevich EE, Reisler E. Drebrin inhibits cofilin-induced severing of F-actin. Cytoskeleton (Hoboken). 2014;**71**(8):472-483

[52] Zhang H et al. A GIT1/PIX/Rac/PAK signaling module regulates spine morphogenesis and synapse formation through MLC. The Journal of Neuroscience. 2005;**25**(13):3379-3388

[53] Ryu J et al. A critical role for myosin IIb in dendritic spine morphology and synaptic function. Neuron. 2006;**49**(2):175-182

[54] Park E, Chi S, Park D. Activity-dependent modulation of the interaction between CaMKIIalpha and Abi1 and its involvement in spine maturation. The Journal of Neuroscience. 2012;**32**(38):13177-13188

[55] Proepper C et al. Abelson interacting protein 1 (Abi-1) is essential for dendrite morphogenesis and synapse formation. The EMBO Journal. 2007;**26**(5):1397-1409

[56] Satoh A et al. Neurabin-II/spinophilin An actin filament-binding protein with one pdz domain localized at cadherin-based cell-cell adhesion sites. Journal of Biological Chemistry. 1998;**273**(6):3470-3475

[57] Feng J et al. Spinophilin regulates the formation and function of dendritic spines. Proceedings of the National Academy of Sciences of the United States of America. 2000; **97**(16):9287-9292

[58] Tashiro A, Minden A, Yuste R. Regulation of dendritic spine morphology by the rho family of small GTPases: Antagonistic roles of Rac and rho. Cerebral Cortex. 2000;**10** (10):927-938

[59] Manser E et al. Expression of constitutively active alpha-PAK reveals effects of the kinase on actin and focal complexes. Molecular and Cellular Biology. 1997;**17**(3):1129-1143

[60] Dutartre H et al. Cytokinesis arrest and redistribution of actin-cytoskeleton regulatory components in cells expressing the rho GTPase CDC42Hs. Journal of Cell Science. 1996;**109**(Pt 2):367-377

[61] Nakayama AY, Harms MB, Luo L. Small GTPases Rac and rho in the maintenance of dendritic spines and branches in hippocampal pyramidal neurons. The Journal of Neuroscience. 2000;**20**(14):5329-5338

[62] Moeller ML et al. EphB receptors regulate dendritic spine morphogenesis through the recruitment/phosphorylation of focal adhesion kinase and RhoA activation. The Journal of Biological Chemistry. 2006;**281**(3):1587-1598

[63] Irie F, Yamaguchi Y. EphB receptors regulate dendritic spine development via intersectin, Cdc42 and N-WASP. Nature Neuroscience. 2002;**5**(11):1117-1118

[64] Murai KK et al. Control of hippocampal dendritic spine morphology through ephrin-A3/EphA4 signaling. Nature Neuroscience. 2003;**6**(2):153-160

[65] Carmona MA et al. Glial ephrin-A3 regulates hippocampal dendritic spine morphology and glutamate transport. Proceedings of the National Academy of Sciences of the United States of America. 2009;**106**(30):12524-12529

[66] Yang G, Pan F, Gan WB. Stably maintained dendritic spines are associated with lifelong memories. Nature. 2009;**462**(7275):920-924

[67] Hayashi-Takagi A et al. Labelling and optical erasure of synaptic memory traces in the motor cortex. Nature. 2015;**525**(7569):333-338

[68] Malenka RC, Nicoll RA. Long-term potentiation--a decade of progress? Science. 1999;**285**(5435):1870-1874

[69] Kasai H et al. Structure-stability-function relationships of dendritic spines. Trends in Neurosciences. 2003;**26**(7):360-368

[70] Wang XB, Yang Y, Zhou Q. Independent expression of synaptic and morphological plasticity associated with long-term depression. The Journal of Neuroscience. 2007; **27**(45):12419-12429

[71] Yang Y et al. Spine expansion and stabilization associated with long-term potentiation. The Journal of Neuroscience. 2008;**28**(22):5740-5751

[72] Wang XB, Zhou Q. Spine remodeling and synaptic modification. Molecular Neurobiology. 2010;**41**(1):29-41

[73] Yang Y, Zhou Q. Spine modifications associated with long-term potentiation. The Neuroscientist. 2009;**15**(5):464-476

[74] Yuste R, Bonhoeffer T. Morphological changes in dendritic spines associated with long-term synaptic plasticity. Annual Review of Neuroscience. 2001;**24**:1071-1089

[75] Harvey CD et al. The spread of Ras activity triggered by activation of a single dendritic spine. Science. 2008;**321**(5885):136-140

[76] Takumi Y et al. Different modes of expression of AMPA and NMDA receptors in hippocampal synapses. Nature Neuroscience. 1999;**2**(7):618-624

[77] Matsuzaki M et al. Dendritic spine geometry is critical for AMPA receptor expression in hippocampal CA1 pyramidal neurons. Nature Neuroscience. 2001;**4**(11):1086-1092

[78] Hebb DO. The Organization of Behavior: A Neuropsychological Theory. New York: Wiley and Sons; 1949

[79] Lisman J. A mechanism for the Hebb and the anti-Hebb processes underlying learning and memory. Proceedings of the National Academy of Sciences of the United States of America. 1989;**86**(23):9574-9578

[80] Schmitz D et al. Presynaptic kainate receptors impart an associative property to hippocampal mossy fiber long-term potentiation. Nature Neuroscience. 2003;**6**(10):1058-1063

[81] Mellor J, Nicoll RA. Hippocampal mossy fiber LTP is independent of postsynaptic calcium. Nature Neuroscience. 2001;**4**(2):125-126

[82] Yang Y et al. Delivery of AMPA receptors to perisynaptic sites precedes the full expression of long-term potentiation. Proceedings of the National Academy of Sciences of the United States of America. 2008;**105**(32):11388-11393

[83] Makino H, Malinow R. AMPA receptor incorporation into synapses during LTP: The role of lateral movement and exocytosis. Neuron. 2009;**64**(3):381-390

[84] Malinow R, Malenka RC. AMPA receptor trafficking and synaptic plasticity. Annual Review of Neuroscience. 2002;**25**:103-126

[85] Malenka RC. Synaptic plasticity and AMPA receptor trafficking. Annals of the New York Academy of Sciences. 2003;**1003**:1-11

[86] Matsuzaki M et al. Structural basis of long-term potentiation in single dendritic spines. Nature. 2004;**429**(6993):761-766

[87] Tonnesen J et al. Spine neck plasticity regulates compartmentalization of synapses. Nature Neuroscience. 2014;**17**(5):678-685

[88] Mizui T et al. Myosin II ATPase activity mediates the long-term potentiation-induced exodus of stable F-actin bound by drebrin A from dendritic spines. PLoS One. 2014;**9**(1) e85367

[89] Bosch M et al. Structural and molecular remodeling of dendritic spine substructures during long-term potentiation. Neuron. 2014;**82**(2):444-459

[90] Meyer D, Bonhoeffer T, Scheuss V. Balance and stability of synaptic structures during synaptic plasticity. Neuron. 2014;**82**(2):430-443

[91] Halpain S, Hipolito A, Saffer L. Regulation of F-actin stability in dendritic spines by glutamate receptors and calcineurin. The Journal of Neuroscience. 1998;**18**(23):9835-9844

[92] Sdrulla AD, Linden DJ. Double dissociation between long-term depression and dendritic spine morphology in cerebellar Purkinje cells. Nature Neuroscience. 2007;**10**(5):546-548

[93] Zhou Q, Poo MM. Reversal and consolidation of activity-induced synaptic modifications. Trends in Neurosciences. 2004;**27**(7):378-383

[94] Zhou Q, Tao HW, Poo MM. Reversal and stabilization of synaptic modifications in a developing visual system. Science. 2003;**300**(5627):1953-1957

[95] Abel T, Nguyen PV. Regulation of hippocampus-dependent memory by cyclic AMP-dependent protein kinase. Progress in Brain Research. 2008;**169**:97-115

[96] Nguyen PV, Woo NH. Regulation of hippocampal synaptic plasticity by cyclic AMP-dependent protein kinases. Progress in Neurobiology. 2003;**71**(6):401-437

[97] Becker N et al. LTD induction causes morphological changes of presynaptic boutons and reduces their contacts with spines. Neuron. 2008;**60**(4):590-597

11

Neuroplasticity of Primary Sensory Neurons in Visceral Nociception

Victor V. Chaban

Abstract

Chronic visceral pain is the most common complication of many functional disorders that do not have a defined pathophysiological cause. Functional pain syndromes include common disorders, such as irritable bowel syndrome (gastroenterology), chronic pelvic pain (gynecology), interstitial cystitis/painful bladder syndrome (urology), fibromyalgia (rheumatology), across multiple medical disciplines. Patients suffering from functional diseases may progress to cognitive decline and depression through neuroplastic changes not only at the level of the central nervous system but also in the periphery. Moreover, most functional diseases are much more prevalent in women than men suggesting estrogen modulation of nociceptive pathways. Defining the etiology of functional diseases for possible therapeutic interventions will have a significant impact on our understanding of observed gender differences and on improving patient's quality of life.

Keywords: neuroplasticity, functional diseases, visceral pain, sensory neurons

1. Introduction

Despite considerable efforts made by the medical research community and pharmaceutical industry to develop effective therapeutical treatments aimed to treat chronic visceral pain resulted from functional disease, there is little progress to date. Functional syndromes are estimated to affect up to 15–20% of the population worldwide. Symptom description of interstitial cystitis/painful bladder syndrome (IC/PBS, urgency, frequency, and bladder pain generally relieved by voiding) is parallel to the description of irritable bowel syndrome-diarrhea (IBS-D) predominance (urgency, frequency and abdominal pain) relieved by defecation. IBS stands in contrast to a bowel's structural disorder: unlike ulcerative colitis and Crohn's disease, which are forms of inflammatory bowel disease (IBD), it does not cause changes in bowel tissue. The cause of functional disorders is unknown. Chronic abdominal complaints are without a structural or biochemical cause. Bloating, mucous in stools, diarrhea, constipation or alternating diarrhea and constipation, depression, anxiety or stress are also common symptoms of IBS. Hypersensitivity of visceral primary afferent neurons could result from excessive production of different modulatory neurotransmitters in response to changes in their signal transduction pathways [1]. Nociceptors are small-to-medium size dorsal root ganglia (DRG) neurons, whose peripheral processes detect nociceptive physical and chemical stimuli. There is often no clear relationship between the severity of the chronic pelvic pain and pathology in the pelvic viscera, and there are also noticeable gender differences in the prevalence of functional diseases that affect more women than men. Most of studies in this area were focused on the central nervous system (CNS); however, our recent data that estrogen can gate primary afferent response to modulate nociception support the idea about the involvement of the peripheral nervous system (PNS) in the etiology of a wide range of the functional and inflammatory diseases [2]. This potentially could involve neuroplastic changes in primary sensory neurons and can be a novel target for therapeutic interventions for patients suffering from chronic visceral pain associated with functional diseases. Despite a successful reduction of pain using available analgesics, visceral pain relapses in most patients. Currently, it is a time for paradigm shift what we consider as visceral nociception, and in this report, author looks for possible new mechanisms of peripheral modulation of primary afferent sensory neurons in development of chronic pelvic pain.

2. Neuroplasticity in peripheral nervous system

Traditionally, the main mechanism involved in development of chronic visceral pain is thought to be neuroinflammation. This pathway effects peripheral and central nerve sensitization and/or dysfunction of inhibitory descending pathways [3]. However, in clinical studies, visceral nociception strongly affects negative sensations that difficult to correlate with visceral traumata. Most nociceptive systems involved in peripheral sensitization originate in free sensory nerve endings of target organs that send their signals toward primary afferent sensory neurons within the lumbar-sacral regions of dorsal root ganglia (L_1-S_3 DRG).

Visceral sensitization may develop as a result of interaction between the nervous and immune systems. All visceral afferents can be sensitized by proinflammatory mediators, such as serotonin, histamine, nitric oxide and ATP, leading to neuropathic hyperalgesia. During inflammation, mast cells and leukocytes secrete inflammatory mediators such as cytokines and prostaglandins that activate polymodal nociceptors triggering the response of normally silent mechano-insensitive receptors. Mast cell mediators can also activate vanilloid receptors (TRPV1), purinergic ($P2X_3$) and bradykinin (BK2) at PNS, causing hyperalgesia.

The serotonergic pathway, one of the main inhibitory mechanisms in the CNS, may also be functionally important in facilitating peripherally mediated visceral pain [4]. Most antidepressants gradually increase serotonin level in the brain. Indeed, depression has been reported to be associated with immunosuppression. Serotonin plays a major role in the gut-brain axis by modulating intestinal movement and the perception of visceral pain. An imbalance of serotonin in the gut, an improper reaction of the digestive system to serotonin, or a faulty serotoninergic network between the gut and the brain may be a cause of depression associated with functional diseases. Enteric nervous systems that innervate gastrointestinal tract include differentiated (visceral) primary afferent neurons that innervate intrinsic and extrinsic pathways implicated in the pathology of many inflammatory as well as functional diseases. There is a noticeable correlation between inflammation induced by gut infection and symptom occurrence of functional disorders such as IBS [5]. New data changed the previous paradigm that each primary afferent neuron innervates only one viscus. The concept of viscero-visceral cross-sensitization is well accepted and has been documented clinically [6]. Inflammation in one organ can induce peripheral (in addition to central) sensitization affecting another viscera. Therefore, nociceptive mechanisms involved in the progression of functional diseases are complicated by comorbid disorders. Both components of pain—discriminative and affective—concomitantly affect motor and cognitive systems. These systems can be gated by estrogen to modulate perception of pain, pain threshold and tolerance.

3. Gender differences in visceral pain

The chronic pelvic pain (CPP) from pelvic structures is more prevalent in female subjects compared to males. In clinical studies, this sexual dimorphism is well recognized: the incidence of functional disorders is 2–3 times higher in women with IBS and even greater with IC/PBS. A large body of literature supports that concept indicating estrogen modulation of different nociceptive pathways [2]. In our previous studies, we found that estrogen receptors (ERα and ERβ) are present in small-to-medium size DRG neurons (presumably nociceptors) and ATP-sensitive DRG neurons respond to 17β-estradiol (E_2) [7], which correlated well with the idea that visceral afferents are E_2 sensitive. Our data clearly suggest that in addition to CNS actions, E_2 can act in the periphery to modulate nociception [1]. Specifically, E_2 acts in DRG neurons to modulate L-type VGCC and through group II metabotropic glutamate receptors [8]. One prominent way E_2 modulates neuronal excitability is through the interaction with antinociceptive opioids such as enkephalins, β-endorphin and pronociceptive nociceptin/orphanin. Furthermore, our hypothesis is that increased nociceptive input from an inflamed organ (i.e. uterus) sensitizes neurons that receive convergent input from an unaffected organ (i.e. colon). In summary, our data suggest that potential site of visceral cross-sensitivity is the dorsal root ganglion [9]. DRG neurons could be responsible for changes observed in the perception of pain during the etiology of different functional syndromes associated with pain.

Several lines of evidence indicate that E_2 directly influences the functions of primary afferent neurons. Both estrogen receptors (ERα and ERβ) are present in DRG and visceral pain is affected by hormonal level in cycling females [1, 2]. Even a large body of literature supports the idea that E_2 modulates nociceptive responses in pelvic pain syndromes, the exact mechanism remains unresolved. Within the context of our hypothesis, E2 modulation of nociceptive response depends on the type of pain, its durations and the involvement of other nociceptive-mediated mechanisms.

4. Primary afferent nociceptors as target in modulation of nociception

Visceral nociceptive signal transduction depends on type of pain (type of sensory fiber), severity, duration and effects of other endogenous nociceptive-mediated molecules. Extrinsic primary afferent fibers can be directly modulated by activation of different chemosensitive or mechanosensitive receptors in target organs. There are 31 pairs of polymodal nerves carrying sensory motor and autonomic signal transduction in human spinal cord. This information is further transferred to the CNS by the spinothalamic ascending pathways to the primary sensory motor cortex for integration and analysis. In DRG neurons, afferent and efferent processes function as a single axon-proximal and distal part connected to somata as an offshoot. DRG first synapses with a dorsal horn neuron through the contralateral spinothalamic tract. These primary sensory neurons have been studied intensively in pain sensory physiology. Small-to-medium size DRG neurons express a variety of receptors involved in pain perception such as ATP-sensitive P2X3, capsaicin-sensitive TRPV1 or acid-sensitive ASIC channels. Since DRG neurons are responsive to estrogen [10] through ERα type [11] and show sensitization, it makes them a suitable model to study gender differences in nociception. Interestingly, TRPV1 and P2X3 transduction is significantly altered during inflammatory response. DRG is also an important site for primary afferent fiber convergence and visceral organ cross-sensitization. Even the role of DRG in neuromodulation of nociception is a novel topic in visceral and chronic pain, we hope to convince the scientific community that the DRG is an active structure rather than passive. The future studies may reveal more neuroplastic changes at the level of first-order sensory neurons. New hypotheses will drive translational research that should improve the outcomes of clinical interventions to relive patients from suffering.

5. Discussion

Pain is a complex and personal experience. Chronic visceral pain affects mood, and social and professional life. A delicate balance between biochemical and physiological changes and cognitive approaches is the most appropriate strategy to study clinical aspects of nociception. Pain in women can originate due to inflammation of a pelvic organ (gut, uterus and bladder) that can heighten the sensitivity of noninflamed organ that are innervated by the same afferent neuronal pathway [12]. Commonly, the overlapping of pelvic pain occurs between the lower gut, uterus and urinary bladder. Common convergence of different visceral primary afferents onto one spinal secondary neuron transmitting signals to the supraspinal nuclei can either synthesize or attenuate intrinsic cellular functions via activation of $P2X_3$ receptors by ATP and TRPV1 receptors by capsaicin within the L_1-S_3 DRG neurons. Furthermore, in addition to ATP, prostaglandin E2 (PGE2) is synthesized and realized during distention and contributes to hyperalgesia. We showed that PGE2 enhanced calcium responses induced by pronociceptive molecules such as ATP and capsaicin [2]. Together, our studies opened up a new paradigm of neuroplasticity: modulation of primary sensory neurons by sex steroids that may lead to structural changes within DRG. Estrogen can gate primary afferent nociceptors to enhance or decrease nociception.

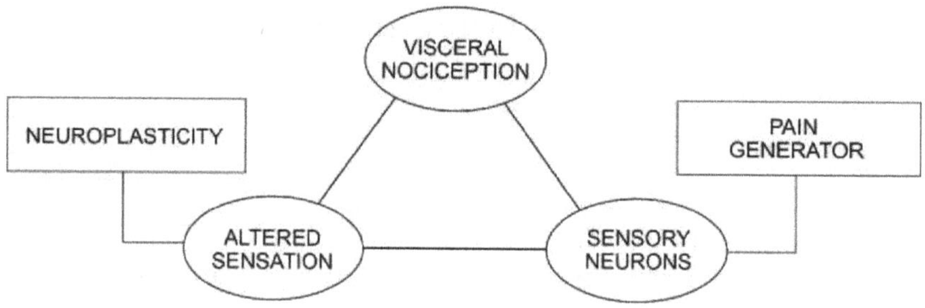

Figure 1. Conceptual model of regulatory mechanisms mediating neuroplasticity of visceral nociception at the level of primary afferent sensory neurons.

Pelvic pain is very subjective and thus difficult to standardize for any scientific modeling since its etiology affects different systems. In addition to nervous, urinary, gastrointestinal, reproductive and psychological systems are involved. Nociceptive behavior is highly complex: the affective experience leads to avoidance and often protective escape. New data will hopefully lead to the development of effective gender-specific therapies. Involvement of peripheral nervous system in mediating and/or regulating chronic visceral pain associated with nociception through structural and physiological changes at the level of DRG is confirmed. The new principle of neuroplasticity at the level of peripheral nervous system is important to understand the etiology of many chronic diseases associated with visceral pain (**Figure 1**). Peripheral sensitization at the level of primary afferent neurons (pain generator) leads to neuroplastic changes with major structural alterations. The observation that 17β-estradiol increased survival of DRG neurons [13] put this sex steroid hormone as potential neuroplastic modulator of sensory afferent neurons. Estradiol may act as transmitter molecule by changing excitability of DRG [14]. DRG neuroplasticity also contributes to hyperalgesia [15]. Noteworthy, treating pain can restore normal nervous system function. As with all new stories, the unusual concept gets most attention of medical and clinical communities. We convey the message by driving translational science into the new horizon and propose a multicomponent conceptual model of neuroplasticity associated with functional disorders.

Acknowledgements

This work is supported by National Institute of Health grant: SC1 NS 063939 (PI—Victor Chaban).

Author details

Victor V. Chaban[1,2*]

*Address all correspondence to: victorchaban@cdrewu.edu

1 Department of Internal Medicine, Charles R. Drew University of Medicine and Science, USA

2 Department of Medicine, University of California, Los Angeles, USA

References

[1] Chaban V, editor. Irritable Bowel Syndrome-Novel Concepts for Research and Treatment. Rijeka: InTech; 2017. 85 p. ISBN 978-953-51-2827-4

[2] Chaban V. Unraveling the Enigma of Visceral Pain. New York: Nova Publishers; 2016. 77 p. ISBN: 978-63489-430-8. Library of U.S. Congress Control Number: 2015951299

[3] Schaible HS. Peripheral and central mechanisms of pain generation. In: Stein C, editor. Analgesia. Heidelberg: Springer; 2007. pp. 435-463

[4] Sommer C. Serotonin in pain and pain control. Handbook of Behavioral Neuroscience. 2010;**21**:457-471

[5] Brierley S, Linden D. Neuroplasticity and dysfunction after gastrointestinal inflammation. Nature Review: Gastroenterology and Hepatology. 2014;**11**(10):611-627

[6] Brumovsky P, Gebhart G. Visceral organ cross-sensitization—An integrated perspective. Autonomic Neuroscience. 2010;**153**(1-2):106

[7] Chaban V. Visceral pain modulation in female primary afferent sensory neurons. Current Trends in Neurology. 2015;**9**:111-114

[8] Chaban V, Li J, McDonald J, Rapkin A, Micevych P. Estradiol attenuates ATP-induced increase of intracellular calcium through group II metabotropic glutamate B receptors in rat DRG neurons. Journal of Neuroscience Research. 2011;**89**(11):1707-1710

[9] Li J, McDonald J, Rapkin A, Micevych P, Chaban V. Inflammation in the uterus induces pERK and substance P activation in DRG neurons innervating both uterus and colon in rats. Journal of Neuroscience Research. 2008;**86**:2746-2752

[10] Chaban V, Mayer E, Ennes H, Micevych P. Estradiol inhibits ATP-induced $[Ca^{2+}]i$ increase in DRG neurons. Neuroscience. 2003;**118**(6):941-948

[11] Chaban V, Micevych P. Estrogen receptor-α mediates estradiol attenuation of ATP-induced Ca^{2+} signaling in dorsal root ganglion neurons. Journal of Neuroscience Research. 2005;**81**(1):31-37

[12] Chaban V. Estrogen modulation of visceral nociception. In: Ritzner, Weizman, editors. Neuroactive Steroids in Brain Function, and Mental Health: New Perspectives for Research and Treatment. Berlin: Springer; 2008. pp. 89-102

[13] Patrone C, Anderson S, Korhonen L, Lindholm D. Estrogen receptor-dependent regulation of sensory neuron survival in developing dorsal root ganglion. Proceeding National Academy of Sciences USA. 1999;**96**:10905-10910

[14] Micevych P, Christensen A. Membrane-initiated estradiol actions mediate structural plasticity and reproduction. Frontiers in Neuroendocrinology. 2012;**33**(4):331-341

[15] Kim Y, Anderson M, Park K, Zheng Q, Agarwal A, Gong C, Young L, Shaoqiu, LaVinka P, Zhou F, Bergles D, Hanani M, Guan Y, Spray D, Dong X. Coupled activation of primary sensory neurons contributes to chronic pain. Neuron. 2016;**91**(5):1085-1096

Permissions

All chapters in this book were first published in NINR, by InTech Open; hereby published with permission under the Creative Commons Attribution License or equivalent. Every chapter published in this book has been scrutinized by our experts. Their significance has been extensively debated. The topics covered herein carry significant findings which will fuel the growth of the discipline. They may even be implemented as practical applications or may be referred to as a beginning point for another development.

The contributors of this book come from diverse backgrounds, making this book a truly international effort. This book will bring forth new frontiers with its revolutionizing research information and detailed analysis of the nascent developments around the world.

We would like to thank all the contributing authors for lending their expertise to make the book truly unique. They have played a crucial role in the development of this book. Without their invaluable contributions this book wouldn't have been possible. They have made vital efforts to compile up to date information on the varied aspects of this subject to make this book a valuable addition to the collection of many professionals and students.

This book was conceptualized with the vision of imparting up-to-date information and advanced data in this field. To ensure the same, a matchless editorial board was set up. Every individual on the board went through rigorous rounds of assessment to prove their worth. After which they invested a large part of their time researching and compiling the most relevant data for our readers.

The editorial board has been involved in producing this book since its inception. They have spent rigorous hours researching and exploring the diverse topics which have resulted in the successful publishing of this book. They have passed on their knowledge of decades through this book. To expedite this challenging task, the publisher supported the team at every step. A small team of assistant editors was also appointed to further simplify the editing procedure and attain best results for the readers.

Apart from the editorial board, the designing team has also invested a significant amount of their time in understanding the subject and creating the most relevant covers. They scrutinized every image to scout for the most suitable representation of the subject and create an appropriate cover for the book.

The publishing team has been an ardent support to the editorial, designing and production team. Their endless efforts to recruit the best for this project, has resulted in the accomplishment of this book. They are a veteran in the field of academics and their pool of knowledge is as vast as their experience in printing. Their expertise and guidance has proved useful at every step. Their uncompromising quality standards have made this book an exceptional effort. Their encouragement from time to time has been an inspiration for everyone.

The publisher and the editorial board hope that this book will prove to be a valuable piece of knowledge for researchers, students, practitioners and scholars across the globe.

List of Contributors

Denis Larrivee
Loyola University Chicago, USA

Max F.K. Happel
Department Systems Physiology of Learning, Leibniz-Institute for Neurobiology, Magdeburg, Germany
Institute for Biology, Otto-von-Guericke University Magdeburg, Magdeburg, Germany

Renato Frischknecht
AG Perisynaptic Extrazellular Matrix, Department Neurochemistry and Molecular Biology, Leibniz-Institute for Neurobiology, Magdeburg, Germany

Alexandra E. Proshchina, Yuliya S. Krivova, Valeriy M. Barabanov and Sergey V. Saveliev
Research Institute of Human Morphology, Moscow, Russia

Olga G. Leonova
Engelhardt Institute of Molecular Biology, Russian Academy of Sciences, Moscow, Russia

Michael I. Sandstrom, Kevin A. Anderson and Parnit K. Bhupal
Neuroscience and Experimental Psychology Programs, Central Michigan University, Mount Pleasant, MI, USA

Gary L. Dunbar
Neuroscience and Experimental Psychology Programs, Central Michigan University, Mount Pleasant, MI, USA
Field Neurosciences Institute, Saginaw, MI, USA

Naveen Jayaprakash
Biomedical Science, Marquette University, Milwaukee, WI, USA

Montserrat González Platas and María Yaiza Pérez Martin
Neurology Service, Hospital Universitario de Canarias, La Laguna, Santa Cruz de Tenerife, Spain

Lora T. Likova
Smith-Kettlewell Eye Research Institute, San Francisco, CA, USA

Robert H. Miller, Molly Karl, Ahdeah Pajoohesh-Ganji and Mohammad Abu-Rub
School of Medicine and Health Sciences, George Washington University, Washington, DC, USA

Reshmi Tognatta
Gladstone Institute, San Francisco, CA, USA

John V. Priestley and Adina T. Michael-Titus
Centre for Neuroscience and Trauma, Blizard Institute, Barts and The London School of Medicine and Dentistry, Queen Mary University of London, London, UK

Mark Reybrouck
Musicology Research Group, KU Leuven – University of Leuven, Belgium
IPEM Institute for Systematic Musicology, Ghent University, Belgium

Peter Vuust and Elvira Brattico
Department of Clinical Medicine, Center for Music in the Brain, Aarhus University and The Royal Academy of Music, Aarhus/Aalborg, Denmark

Jun Ju and Qiang Zhou
School of Chemical Biology and Biotechnology, Peking University Shenzhen Graduate School, Shenzhen, China

Victor V. Chaban
Department of Internal Medicine, Charles R. Drew University of Medicine and Science, USA
Department of Medicine, University of California, Los Angeles, USA

Index

www.ingramcontent.com/pod-product-compliance
Lightning Source LLC
LaVergne TN
LVHW060557210926
848485LV00005B/1329
* 9 7 8 1 6 3 9 8 9 3 7 3 7 *